# The Lure of the South

# The Lure of the South

## *Health, the Victorians and the Continent*

Richard Aspin

BLOOMSBURY ACADEMIC
LONDON • NEW YORK • OXFORD • NEW DELHI • SYDNEY

BLOOMSBURY ACADEMIC
Bloomsbury Publishing Plc
50 Bedford Square, London, WC1B 3DP, UK
1385 Broadway, New York, NY 10018, USA
29 Earlsfort Terrace, Dublin 2, Ireland

BLOOMSBURY, BLOOMSBURY ACADEMIC and the Diana logo are trademarks of Bloomsbury Publishing Plc

First published in Great Britain 2025



Cover image: Edward Lear, a View of Menton
© Artepics via Alamy Stock Photo



A catalogue record for this book is available from the British Library.

A catalog record for this book is available from the Library of Congress.

ISBN: HB: 978-1-3504-4472-0
ePDF: 978-1-3504-4473-7
eBook: 978-1-3504-4474-4

Typeset by Newgen KnowledgeWorks Pvt. Ltd., Chennai, India

# Contents

# Maps

# Preface

In his contribution to a special issue of *Anthropology & Medicine* dedicated to medical travel, historian George Weisz distinguished between 'medical' and 'health' tourism by adducing the importance of place. The former, he noticed, involves travelling to access medical expertise or services, whether personal or institutional, in a location that is normally incidental to the quality of the product or service sought; the latter is almost always place-dependent[1]. Medical tourism is a very recent phenomenon, for the most part; health tourism by contrast is as old as the hills. Its deep roots are exemplified by the practice of visiting healing springs in antiquity.[2] Medieval pilgrimage has been viewed as a form of health tourism, and tellingly the word was sometimes invoked by early Victorian invalid travellers to describe their peregrinations. In contrast to medieval pilgrims, these travellers were peripatetic, without a fixed destination, the word 'pilgrimage' serving to characterize their wandering quest for what might today be construed as 'wellness'. The Victorian pilgrims were not however oblivious of place. Their travels were almost invariably centred on the Mediterranean, the heart of classical civilization, for this region above all held the promise of restoring their sagging spirits and zest for life. These health pilgrims, or invalid grand tourists, were followed by others with more modest if perhaps sometimes more urgent ambitions, searching for a 'change of air' to arrest a dread disease or merely a refuge from the northern winter. They strove to leave places that were cold, foggy and depressing – often all three; they dreamt of reaching places that were balmy, sun-filled and life-giving – the lure of the south.

This book explores the motivations, hopes, fears and experiences of British health-seekers in Europe of every invalid status. These people have not always received a favourable press from either contemporaries or historians. For medical commentators at the time, they were frequently upbraided for ignorance and carelessness, condemned as slavish followers of the herd as far as selecting a destination was concerned and oblivious of sensible medical directions about behaviour, diet and the like. Historians have been tempted to dismiss them as credulous, bullied by their medical advisers and ultimately deluded. Rarely have they been allowed to speak for themselves, except in their occasional capacity as published writers and novelists. This work attempts to remedy that deficiency by privileging first-hand testimony from invalids and their companions in exile. Sourcing such unpublished material has never been easy because of the way archival collections are organized and described. There is no such thing as an archive of invalidity. No university library specializes in collecting the papers of patients. No entrant in the *Oxford Dictionary of National Biography* is given the occupational title 'invalid' or 'consumptive patient'. It is however practicable now to identify enough potential sources, owing to the widespread adoption of searchable databases by archive repositories, enabling vastly improved access to the often rich catalogue descriptions of family and other papers that archivists have been producing for many years. Such sources have been profitably exploited by other students of Victorian continental tourism, such as Marjorie Morgan,[3] but without a particular focus on invalid travellers.

Victorian health-seekers travelled the world. The justification for restricting coverage of their activities to a particular region rests partly on practicality – the number of potential invalid destinations would simply be too large to document in any detail without some artificial limitation. Furthermore, this study takes a few liberties in defining the 'continent of Europe'. Some popular health destinations, such as Egypt, have been excluded for sound geographical reasons; others such as Algiers and Madeira have been included as, although interlopers in strict geographical terms, they were an integral part of the European cultural zone at the time and indeed ruled from their respective continental metropole. Besides, it would have been perverse to exclude Madeira from consideration since it was the foremost destination for British consumptive patients in the first half of the nineteenth century. Inclusion of Madeira points to a broader principle adopted in determining the boundaries of coverage. As well as being 'European', destinations had to be southern (bordering the Mediterranean), foreign – in other words not part of the British Empire, like Malta – and popular, if only briefly, like Algiers and Malaga. This means that many destinations in northern France and the Low Countries that attracted British health-seekers have been excluded.

Conversely, Pau, in south-west France, is a long way – geographically, culturally and climatically – from the Mediterranean world, but its importance as an invalid destination demanded inclusion.[4] Since the Pyrenean spas were closely associated with Pau, providing both a summer refuge and therapeutic resources for British invalids wintering there, they are included in the story, as well as any other continental spa that was popular with British visitors, on the basis that they often served a similar function for patients travelling to and from the Mediterranean.

A focus on Europe addresses a secondary aim of the book, which is to explore aspects of the relationship between Britain and her nearest neighbours at a time when the political, economic and societal distance between them had perhaps never been greater. The rupture of the French wars had been merely the final coping stone to an edifice of difference that Britain – or perhaps more especially England – had been constructing for centuries. The British return to the Continent after 1815 involved not so much a reacquaintance as a process of discovery by a generation with little first-hand experience of continental travel, let alone extended residence, burdened by the baggage of centuries of accumulated expectation, received opinion and prejudice. Moreover, the horrors of the French Revolution and its aftermath could not be entirely forgotten, even by the most well-disposed tourist. British visitors headed south with the grisly knowledge that some unspeakable horror might have occurred within living memory in the very place through which they passed. Those who travelled for health shared these preoccupations, as well as the special hopes and fears attending their own personal medical journey. Their extra vulnerability as patients may even have amplified their sensibility to difference, lending their testimony an added piquancy.

The book concentrates on the half-century or so from about 1830 to 1880. The former date signals the approximate start of the phenomenon of wintering in the south by significant numbers of British invalids and the beginnings of a genre of specialist literature directed at the intending expatriate patient and his medical advisers. The latter date marks very roughly the point from which 'genuine' invalids began to disappear from the health resorts of the south, increasingly favouring the sanatoria of central Europe. This coincided with and was to a large extent caused by a change in the medical consensus regarding the treatment of pulmonary consumption, still the biggest cause of death in Britain in 1880, as in 1830, and the disease which sent the majority of 'genuine' invalids to the south. This development marked the end of the era of 'change of air' as a prescription for consumption and of trusting, albeit without much confidence, in the southern climate to help the patient when medicine had failed. It goes without saying that this transition was far from uniform – it impacted different resorts at different stages and was gradual rather than sudden – but it seems nonetheless an important caesura in the trajectory of health tourism in Europe. Indeed, in so far as some of the new sanatoria were run by specialist consultants in locations which, although usually scenic, had not been chosen chiefly for their climatic qualities, the transition might be seen as a turn from 'health' to 'medical' tourism, in Weisz's definition.

A few words on the nomenclature of nationality are in order. Students of the Victorian period will be familiar with the routine conflation of the terms 'English' and 'British' by contemporaries. I have endeavoured to use the latter term where it is clear that contemporary commentators have had all the inhabitants of Great Britain (and usually Ireland as well) in mind, as for instance in estimates of visitor numbers at resorts, or have been obviously referring to a condition or aspect of Britain rather than of England alone, such as the weather or the government. On rare occasions where there has been some ambivalence I have kept to the contemporary usage, sometimes with inverted commas. Original quotations remain unmodified of course. If any infelicities have slipped through I trust they will be forgiven.

# Acknowledgements

The idea for this book emerged from the fusion of two sources of interest, a personal one in travel in Europe and Britain's relations with her continental neighbours and a professional one in the history of health, as a member of staff at the Wellcome Library in London. The question of Britain's place in Europe, apparently settled by the Maastricht Treaty in 1992, seemed at first to have rendered the issue one of merely historical significance until, shortly before embarking on research for the book, the Brexit referendum result helpfully reminded me that nothing in history is settled. On the contrary everything is up for renegotiation, dependant on the uncertain churn of subterranean currents of sentiment. A project that might have appeared somewhat detached before 2016 suddenly seemed topical. As I studied the antics of our Victorian forebears stepping onto the European Continent as if into terra incognita, I thought perhaps we had not put so much distance between ourselves and our ancestors after all.

I would like to acknowledge the advice and support of former colleagues at Wellcome, who encouraged me to embark on the research for the book in retirement, including Julia Sheppard, Simon Chaplin and Jennifer Haynes, as well as fellow members of the library's research team, especially Elma Brenner and Ross Macfarlane, who have been generous with their suggestions and expertise. I thank the staff of the National Archives, Kew, the London Metropolitan Archives, and the county archive offices of Bedfordshire, Gloucestershire, Hampshire, Lancashire, Northamptonshire, Surrey and Wiltshire, for their assistance and professionalism, especially in view of the challenges posed by the Covid-19 lockdown. My thanks are also due to the librarians and archivists of the British Library, Lambeth Palace Library, the Royal College of Physicians of London Library and the Library of the Society of Friends. Meriel Lees, city archivist of Stoke-on-Trent, kindly supplied a digital copy of Louisa Campbell's journal describing her visit to Kissingen. I am indebted to Astrid Krüger, of the Stadtarchiv Bad Homburg, for help with the *Homburger Kur-und Bad-Listen* online resource, and to Cefyn Embling-Evans, archivist of Holy Trinity church Funchal, for assistance with the church's records deposited at the Archivo e Biblioteca da Madeira, now accessible online via the ABM's website. The restrictions on visiting physical collections during much of 2020 and 2021 brought home the immense boon to scholarship provided by the recent growth in online access to research materials and the debt owed by researchers to those many librarians, archivists, IT specialists, managers and funders, whose foresight and skill has transformed the research landscape for the humanities. I would single out in particular the Wellcome Library's online collections and the Medical Heritage Library, hosted by the Internet Archive.

I am indebted to the several reviewers of the text at various stages for their recommendations for improvement. I am grateful to my dear friend Susan Hamlyn for reading parts of the text in draft, making many helpful comments and saving me from multiple stylistic blunders and grammatical errors. Those that remain are of course my own. It is a pleasure to acknowledge the invaluable help of my son Thomas in creating the maps. My deepest thanks are due to my wife Janet, who has lived with this project for several years and has been unfailingly encouraging. The book is dedicated to her.

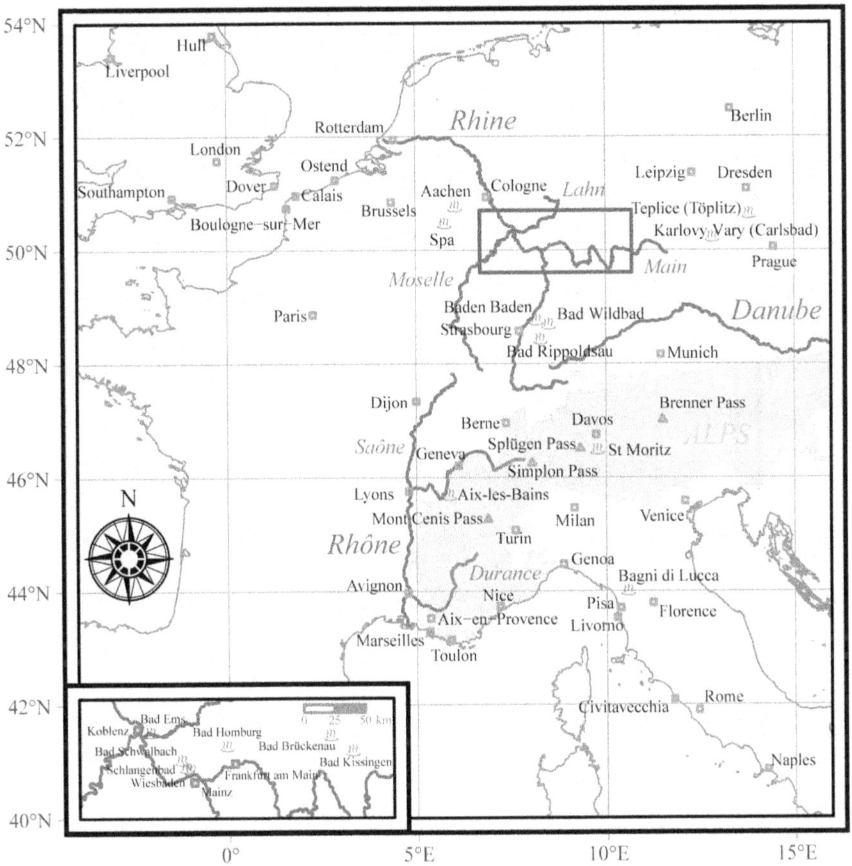


**Map 1** The German spas and the routes to Italy

Source: Author.

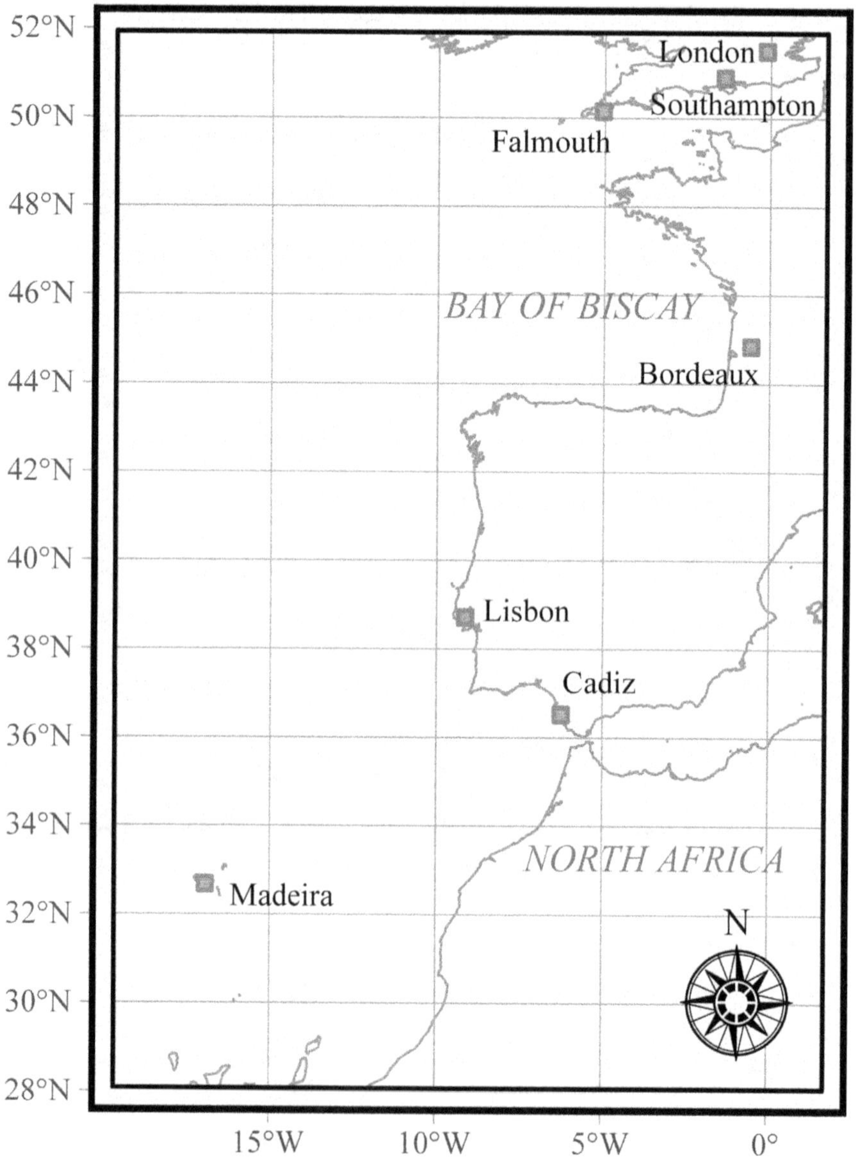


**Map 2** The sea lane to Madeira

Source: Author.

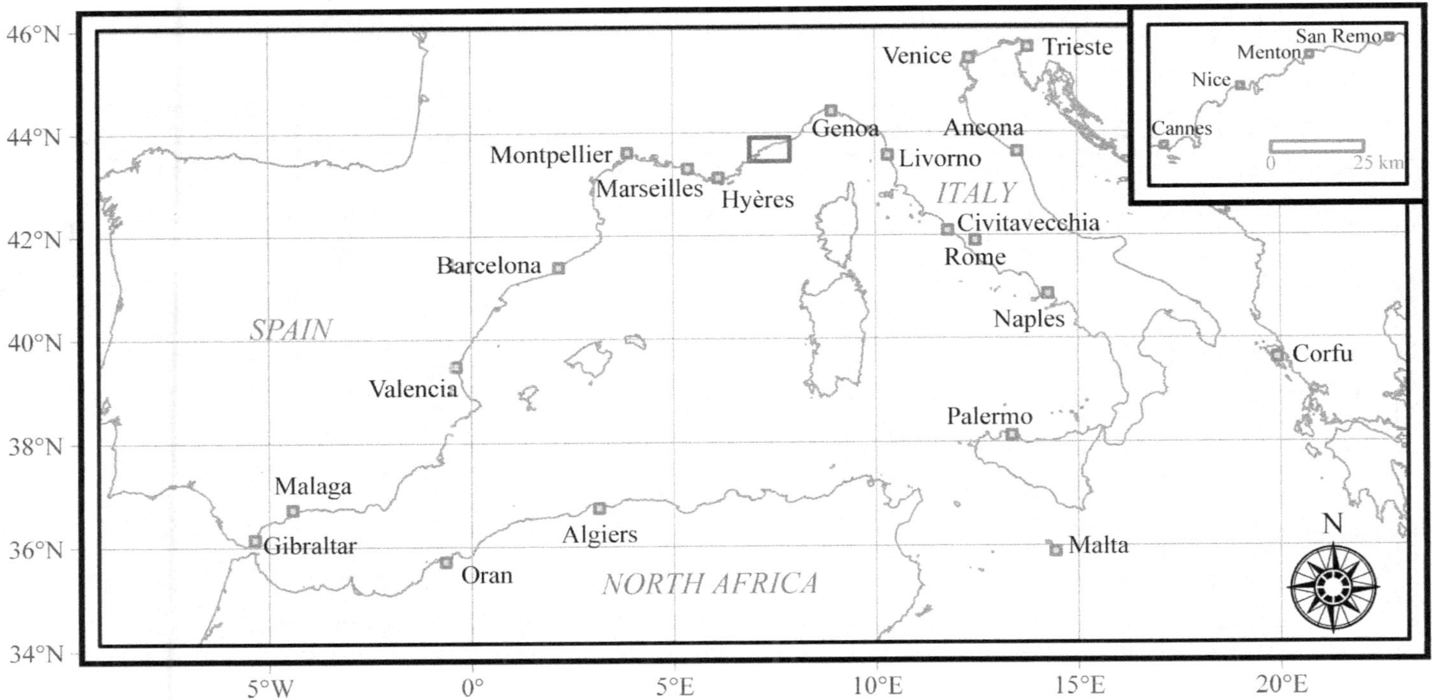


**Map 3** The Western Mediterranean

Source: Author.

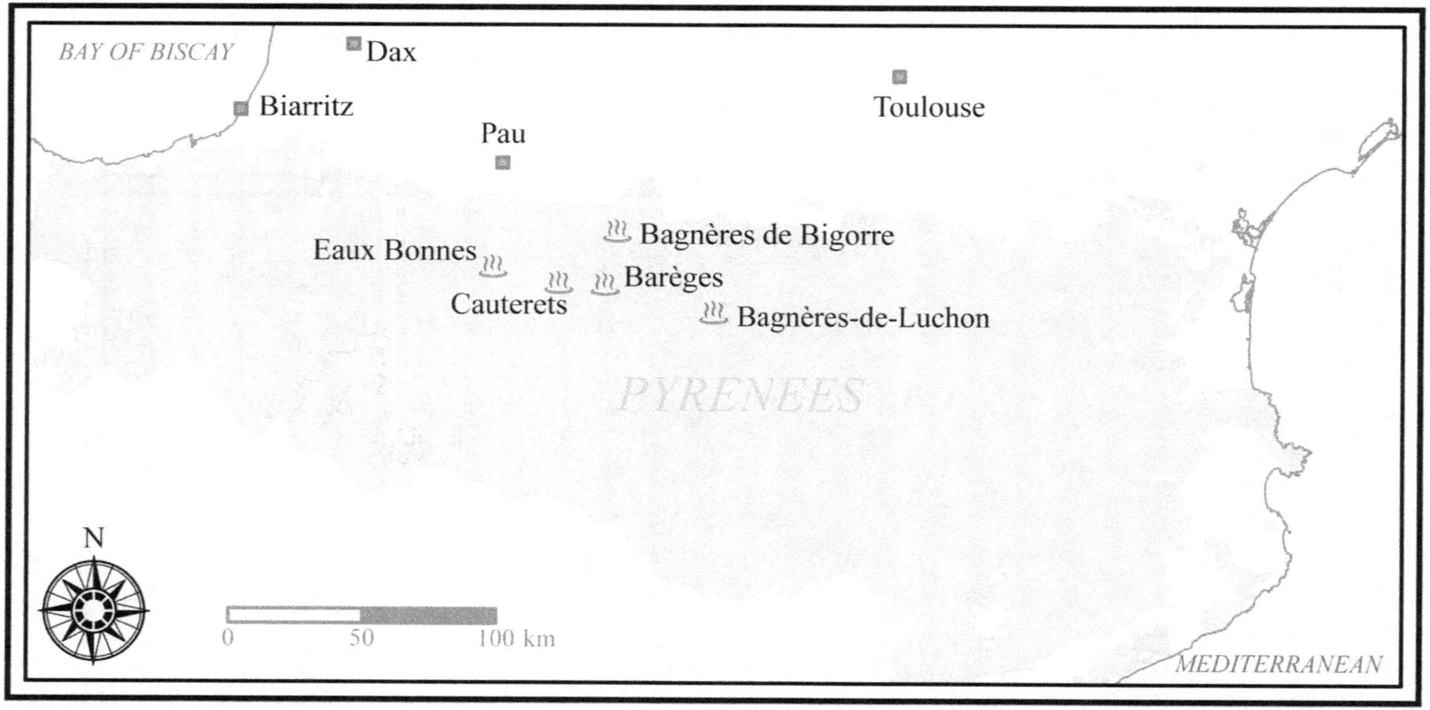


**Map 4** Spas of the French Pyrenees

Source: Author.

# Introduction

Health tourism was a Victorian growth industry. It is well known that as societies become richer, they spend proportionately more of their resources on healthcare. This was just as true in the nineteenth century as in the twenty-first. At the same time as it was becoming richer, Victorian Britain was becoming more populous, more urbanized, industrialized and polluted. Arguably it was also becoming more competitive and anxious. These developments impacted all levels of society, albeit differentially. The increase in national wealth may have been very unevenly distributed, but the consequences of urbanization and industrialization were widely shared. Even those with inherited wealth and ample acres in rural England tended to migrate to the capital for the London season. The life and fortune of the burgeoning professional and middle classes usually depended on the world of urban Britain, however much they might hanker for the suburbs. The human desire for improved physical or mental health, for relief from chronic illness or simply for a brief intermission of peace and quiet in stressful lives, was not new. But the Victorian middle classes, as well as suffering from some of the baleful effects of the advanced economy they had helped to create, also reaped differentially the largest material rewards from industrial development, making them, in the words of Peter Bailey, 'the most substantial beneficiaries of the new bounty (of leisure)'.[1] Once released from the burden of unremitting toil to make a living, those without inherited means could join their upper-class compatriots in contemplating a vacation from work in order to privilege their health.

The Victorians were heirs to the medical landscape of their Georgian forebears. Among its salient features was a framework of orthodox doctrine that emphasized the importance of regulation of lifestyle to maintain good health – attention to diet, exercise, sleep, bodily evacuations, environment and mental equilibrium – as well as a prodigious reliance on drugs that to a considerable extent conflicted with orthodox principles. In both cases, however, much of the burden of treatment rested with the patient rather than the doctor.[2] Patients were obviously best acquainted with their own body and lifestyle and consequently best equipped to manage both, with suitable advice. Meanwhile drugs, including powerful metallic preparations such as arsenicals and mercurials, were routinely available, both by prescription and over the counter, as well as a growing range of patent medicines of dubious provenance. Such a background might have been purpose-built to encourage those in search of better health to seek out new sites for self-cure and find an alternative to a regime of unsatisfactory self-dosing.

Although an eighteenth-century medic might advise a visit to a spa to take the waters to improve digestion or a trip to the seaside for a change of air, neither course implied therapeutic value in travel per se, however essential a journey might be to complying with the advice. The putative health benefits of travel itself, especially for mental well-being, remained on the margins of Georgian medicine. It was the aesthetic and sensual appeal of travel, as exemplified by the attractions of the Grand Tour, that propelled travelling for health into the mainstream in the nineteenth century, based not on any well-developed theory of therapeutics but on post-hoc rationalization of an activity that in the words of Vladimir Janković 'exuded a prophylactic appeal unmatched by even the best home treatment'.[3]

At the same time, there were a large number of patients for whom a journey for health could never be more than a means to an end. They suffered from organic disease, or some other debilitating condition, that all logic demanded be treated at home, in the comfort of familiar surroundings, supported by family and friends, with access to regular professional advice. Many such patients were consumptive – sufferers from pulmonary tuberculosis – a disease that seems to have enjoyed a resurgence in the early nineteenth century. However, consumption was a slippery disease, difficult to diagnose definitively, sometimes propelling its victims to an early death, sometimes lingering for years, with unexplained intermissions and returns. Those threatened with consumption, or in an early stage of the disease, or enjoying some respite from its symptoms, might be encouraged to travel for better air, a better climate or better opportunities to throw off the burden of disease by vigorous outdoor activity, just as American consumptives were urged to head west, where 'pioneers, explorers and health seekers were practically interchangeable'.[4]

But if a continental grand tour for health might have made sense for a patient with early but as yet undiagnosed signs of the disease, something more was required to encourage confirmed cases to leave home, especially once they were seriously ill. The medical rationale was 'change of air', or moving to a healthier environment, a prescription that aligned with the principles of orthodox medicine, provided the patient could bear the journey and the living conditions in their intended destination were tolerable, but did not necessarily indicate a foreign site for cure. The overseas dimension of 'change of air' was a function of fashion rather than medicine. Increased availability of surplus wealth and leisure time among the upper-middle and professional classes in Victorian Britain encouraged a search for new experiences and sensations, which naturally followed the contours that had been established in an earlier period by social superiors – grand touring in Italy, spa-visiting in the Rhineland and wintering at Nice. The sick, who might in an earlier age have remained at home, were swept up by the tourist tide, as more or less willing participants in a phenomenon that owed relatively little, at least initially, to the prescriptions of medicine. 'Medicine and travel co-constructed each other',[5] as travellers sought out new sites for winter expatriation in the south, which medicine retrospectively colonized and validated.

Victorian health tourism at home, from the growth of spa visiting to the development of the British seaside, has been the subject of considerable study by historians of health.[6] Study of Victorian health-seekers on the Continent has likewise tended to focus on spa visiting or on the British presence in individual resorts.[7] The history of Victorian health tourism in the south of Europe as a generalized phenomenon has received less attention. Exceptions to the rule include Vladimir Janković's important treatment of British climatotherapy, *Confronting the Climate* (2010), which among other things investigates the rise and decline of Madeira as a site of invalid expatriation. This work however addresses the issue of travelling abroad for better air as part of the development of environmental medicine and consequently concentrates on the debates and disputes among medical theorists and practitioners. The patient's voice has been largely mediated by literary and cultural historians. Foremost among these is John Pemble, whose *The Victorian Passion* (1987) remains the most comprehensive coverage of the British engagement with the Mediterranean world in the period, including its importance as an invalid destination.[8] The danger of a cultural focus for our purposes is of course that it privileges the professional writer's lens, thus risking lending undue weight to creative construction of the evidence. Writers, artists and even doctors were often patients themselves, but their witness, even if embodied in unpublished records or in posthumous editions of private correspondence, is unlikely to be representative of the generality of invalids. Doctors of course – at least those whose evidence can now be readily accessed – were usually published writers as well. Any one of a range of personal and professional considerations might have been to the fore when they put pen to paper – altruistic, reputational and pecuniary. Their evidence is indispensable but insufficient.

A more rounded view requires finding additional witnesses who are not writing for publication or posterity but for family and friends, occasionally for themselves. The benchmark for putting the patient's voice centre stage is Sheila Rothmans's *Living in the Shadow of Death* (1994), which uses a vast range of archival sources to tell the story of the American tuberculous patient in the nineteenth and early twentieth centuries. As Rothman remarks, 'to move the patient to the center of a history requires breaking out of the language and constructs of medicine'.[9] Integral to this is to try to liberate the patient from being defined by medicine, or even health, alone. As well as health-seekers, patients in the south were also travellers, tourists, employers, shoppers, excursionists, church-goers, readers, gossips and meddlers, and even if too ill themselves to partake fully in these activities, they usually depended on accompanying family for whom these were almost daily concerns. The central chapters of this book address the full range of issues that impinged on expatriate life abroad. They are organized thematically, following a putative patient as he or she selects a destination, prepares to leave the British Isles, travels south, finds lodgings, negotiates the local cuisine, hires servants, consults doctors, muses on the miseries of illness and pain of exile and meets and mixes with compatriots and strangers. The final chapter attempts an evaluation of the health outcomes of expatriation in the south, including the likelihood of death. The book cannot claim to rely so comprehensively on unpublished sources as Rothman's, but it is the first work to attempt a broad survey of the British patient experience in the warm south during the period of its greatest appeal as a sanatorium.

Arguably, reliance primarily on medical witnesses has led historians to overestimate the role of professional medicine in driving and sustaining the phenomenon of winter expatriation. The notion of being 'ordered' or 'directed' south by one's medical consultant appealed to the vanity of doctors and probably also served the patient's interests as well, enabling him to justify an extended period of 'leisure' to himself or his friends and family. It may also have served the purposes of family members concerned to persuade a reluctant patient to travel.[10] When however we burrow below the layer of published literature, whether by doctors or patients, and look at private sources, there is little evidence of medical direction. As with Rothman's patients, 'physicians appeared more as companions than authorities', only moving into a significant directorial role in the 1880s.[11] If patients were dupes, as John Pemble seems to suggest, they were not so much victims of doctors who had either run out of ideas about how to help their patient progress at home or, more self-servingly, had a vested interest in luring invalids to their lucrative practice in the sun, as dupes of fashion. Later in the century, doctors did indeed increasingly impose their will and cure regimes on tuberculous patients, aided by their increased confidence in managing the disease and doubtless declining expectations among patients themselves that the Mediterranean winter climate was their best hope for recovery. For the period covered by this book, however, patients and their families – however hesitant, unconvinced and confused they often were – were not merely the fuel of the phenomenon of winter expatriation in the south but the engine.

# 1

# Travel, climate and health

## The invalid grand tourist

To the early Victorian observer the European Continent seemed to be awash with British travellers and tourists. From the custom house at Calais or the deck of a Rhine steamer to the strand at Nice or the streets of Rome, there appeared to be no escape from the sound of English voices or the sight of a party of Britons emerging from their carriage, with all the impedimenta of travel appropriate to a people accustomed to domestic comfort venturing into an uncertain world. The rash of touring generated a copious literature, but the vast majority of tourists followed a well-trodden path –typically up the Rhine and over the Alps to Italy or through France to Lyons and the Mediterranean coast – so that within a couple of decades of the fall of Napoleon some travel writers were skipping details of the classic Rhineland sights as places now so familiar to their readers that further description would be unnecessarily tedious, a fate that had already befallen the 'fully scripted environment' of Italy.[1] As Thomas Hood observed in his preface to *Up the Rhine*, 'since Byron and the *Dampschiff* there had been quite enough of vapouring, in more senses than one, on the blue and castled river '.[2] The first age of mass tourism in British history was of course modest by modern standards. In the 1830s a contemporary witness was told that some 75,000 Britons had visited the Rhine during a recent season – less than half a per cent of the total population (or 0.3 per cent if Ireland is included) – scarcely an overwhelming figure for the most popular destination on the Continent at the time.[3] It was the novelty of the phenomenon that generated such widespread comment. The stereotypical grand tourist of the previous century – young, male and upper-class – outlived the Napoleonic interlude, but he was joined and indeed soon outnumbered on the most well-trodden routes by a multitude of heterogeneous visitors, of both sexes, often travelling en famille, whose motivations for travel were correspondingly diverse.

Restoration of health had played some part in the eighteenth-century grand tourist's rationale for travel, but it was typically subsumed under a more generalized search for psychological and physiological equilibrium.[4] The perceived health benefits of change of scene, diet and routine were widely acknowledged but travel overseas to enjoy these advantages was necessarily restricted to a small percentage of the population with the means to do so in some comfort, and more especially by the near-wholesale embargo on continental travel between 1793 and 1815. In these circumstances, those motivated to travel primarily for the benefit of health usually did so within their own country, either to visit healthy places such as spas or seaside resorts or to remove themselves from unhealthy ones like disease-ravaged towns or malarial fens. Following the Napoleonic hiatus, the well-established grand tour model, which validated continental travel for purposes of education, cultural development and character formation, was increasingly democratized and diffused in modified form throughout a broad middle-class constituency. The Victorian middle classes represented the first non-elite demographic in British history to enjoy the luxury of leisure. However, as Peter Bailey has pointed out, they 'had only an attenuated leisure tradition to draw upon, so that the new life-space they had won for themselves was something of an embarrassment'; a class bred to the 'virtues of unremitting industry' could not abandon itself to pleasure unreservedly.[5] A more earnest age required additional justification for travel to offset the suspicion of pleasure-seeking that hung about the grand tour model: 'Amusement alone was not an excuse that Victorian society could sanction for leaving home', according to Janet Oppenheim.[6] In the opinion of the young Irish medical practitioner Thomas Madden, 'there was a fear of being thought capable of seeking enjoyment for its own sake peculiar to English professional men'.[7] Consequently the notion of travel as therapy was recruited to bolster the existing claims of education and culture. By the early Victorian period the concept of travel as balm for the mind was commonplace.[8]

If people who were fundamentally well were increasingly disposed to adduce restoration of health as a reason for travelling, it was but a short step for the genuinely ill to begin to view touring as a suitable strategy for recovering their health or at least for combating the gloomy introspection of life as a domestic invalid. When in 1837 Saunderson Walker (1815–1845) of Gateshead, a consumptive patient, completed his fourth continental health tour, he wrote up his journal as a 'memorial of a pilgrimage', dedicating it to his father in gratitude for funding his excursion. The details of his earlier tours are unknown, though the fourth was probably the most extensive, taking Walker by sea from Newcastle to Malta, then to Sicily, Marseilles, Genoa and Livorno, before disembarking and travelling overland via Pisa, Florence, Rome, Venice and Milan, and back home by Switzerland, France and Belgium.[9] That such an extensive and demanding tour itinerary should have been deemed suitable for a consumptive patient might seem surprising. There is no evidence that it was undertaken on professional medical advice, and although Walker claims his earlier excursions had benefitted his health, it is clear that any such improvement was to be anticipated as a welcome by-product of a tour made primarily for cultural purposes. Perhaps the only concession to his compromised health was the decision to travel to Italy by sea rather than risk the rigours of the overland route.[10] Walker's use of the term 'pilgrimage' emulates the many published accounts by continental tourists, whether acknowledged invalids or not, that had become a bookseller's staple. He even prefaces his chapters with epigraphs culled from Byron and other poets.[11] There is no indication that his itinerary was governed by any search for an ideal climate or residence. It was presumably enough to be away from home, travelling in the Mediterranean, refreshed and diverted by immersion in the sights and sounds of Italy. Invalidity provided an opportunity, if not an excuse, to undertake the sort of excursion that would have been equally appropriate for a healthy tourist.

The archetype of the invalid's travelogue was *The Diary of an Invalid*, by Henry Matthews (1789–1828), which recounts a two-year expedition made between 1817 and 1819 by the consumptive Matthews on a continent just emerging from the turmoil of war. There is little in the author's dyspeptic narrative to indicate any therapeutic programme – he does not even name his illness until the account is well advanced; rather his invalidity acts as a cover for a journey of exploration of national identity in the guise of an extended continental tour.[12] Certainly no patient at home could have derived much useful information from the work in relation to his own treatment, even if the author's practical recommendations about roads and inns might have been briefly topical. *The Diary of an Invalid* had five editions by 1835, by which time any practical guidance it contained would have been largely out of date. Its publication history confirms its place as a work of genre literature rather than a guidebook, still less a health manual. Taking their cue from Matthews other writers adduced the search for health as a convenient justification for publishing extensive accounts of continental travels intended primarily for the armchair tourist rather than the intending visitor. Dr James Johnson's *Change of Air* describes an Italian tour undertaken in late 1829 in the ostensible interests of investigating the country's suitability as a destination for health-seekers worn out by that almost uniquely British complaint 'wear and tear'. His alternative title, *Diary of a Philosopher in Pursuit of Health and Recreation*, hints at the work's overriding theme, a digression on the moral implications of residence in Italy, which led the author to conclude that 'it was one of the worst places in the world for an invalid', having 'too much both of moral and physical excitement'.[13]

Walker, Matthews and Johnson were invalid grand tourists, travellers moving by easy stages from one cultural highlight to another, chiefly in Italy, the cynosure of grand touring. Others travelled further afield. The physician William Fullarton Cumming (1804–1892), having suffered severely from 'inflammatory attacks of the chest' while in Paris in the winter of 1835–6, decided to accompany a friend to Italy and Egypt to recover his health. Cumming had been advised to take the waters at Eaux Bonnes and Cauterets in the Pyrenees by his consultant, Gabriel Andral – advice he seems to have ignored in favour of a more interesting opportunity for diversion. From Egypt he returned via Greece, Istanbul and the Black Sea, before heading up the Danube to Germany to join the Rhine at Mainz, and then home by the well-travelled route now so familiar to his readers, having completed a tour of some eighteen months.[14]

Equally ambitious were the continental tour itineraries of William Money-Kyrle (1808–1868), unmarried son of the rector of Yatesbury, Wiltshire, whose infirmity is unspecified in his letters home but whose expatriation was evidently deemed beneficial if not essential for his health. In the autumn of 1843 he travelled through France to Marseilles, then by sea to Genoa and finally to Naples, where he based himself for about five months, before leaving for Sicily,

Malta, Greece and then home via Corfu, Trieste, Switzerland and the Rhine. The following autumn he set out for Italy again, this time crossing the Alps by the Simplon pass to Milan, Florence and Rome, where he spent the winter; in the spring he embarked from Ancona for Corfu, then travelled to Istanbul, St Petersburg, Berlin and back to Istanbul and afterwards winter in Egypt, returning home in spring 1846 via the Holy Land, Istanbul again, Belgrade, Vienna and Munich. Like a good grand tourist Money-Kyrle returned bearing suitable trophies – a chunk of lava from the crater of Vesuvius that had struck him on the head; pictures from Florence to decorate the family home – but he seems rarely to have been free from anxiety about his health, even if it hardly interfered with his activities: he was frequently on horseback and a regular guest at dinners and balls during the season at Rome and Naples.[15] Somewhat later Sir Albert Dennison (1805–1860), later Lord Londesborough, set off with his wife on a tour to convalesce from six weeks' unspecified illness. Like Matthews he began by embarking for Lisbon in November 1848 but took in Malta, Greece, Corfu and Naples, before hurrying back home in May the following year, presumably to avoid the summer heat. He played the stereotypical grand tourist to perfection, spiriting trunks of archaeological finds out of Greece and smuggling Roman coins through customs at Naples by use of judicious bribery. After Naples there is a perfunctory tone to his brief notes on the journey home, for the main business of the tour, collecting antiquities, was done.[16]

The invalid grand tourist need not be male. The London medical practitioner Alexander Morison (1779–1866) was contracted in 1820 as personal physician to accompany two aristocratic women, Lady Bute and Lady Guildford, together with their children and tutor, on a grand tour in the interests of Lady Bute's health; the tour took in Paris, Nice (a sojourn of six months), Switzerland, Rome and Naples, with Morrison only returning home in June 1822.[17] Ann Vavasour recounts in her memoir of her continental tour made in 1840–1 that she had already crossed the Channel or the 'Ocean' (the North Sea) twenty-eight times and was on this occasion making her fifth visit to Rome. She travelled in her own carriage, shipped from Hull to Rotterdam and then onwards by Rhine steamer to Mainz, together with three female companions and two servants. After three months of bathing at the spa of Wildbad in the Black Forest she was ordered to Italy for the winter by her medical advisor and set off in her carriage for Rome, 'the only town in Italy to pass the winter in for those who loved the arts, quiet good society and rational recreation'. The party entered Italy by the Splügen Pass – an unremarkable crossing for a traveller who had already traversed the Alps via the Mont Cenis, Simplon and Brenner on previous occasions. Four months were spent in Rome, 'diligently applying [themselves] to modelling', before a return home in the same carriage via France and Belgium, with a sojourn at the Rippoldsau spa in Baden en route. The tour lasted some fifteen months.[18] Vavasour does not self-identify as an invalid and her account is notably free of reflections on her own medical condition. It is however inconceivable that she would have devoted so much time to spa treatment at two rather unfashionable German watering places if she had been in perfect health. But as with other invalid grand tourists the boundary between the demands of health and recreation was indistinct, and the tourist herself may often have been indifferent as to which call she was responding.

## Diversion and change of air

Foreign travel was considered potentially beneficial in any case of chronic illness. In addition, it might be recommended for those whose family history, habits or professional activities threatened the onset of some debilitating condition, especially mental illness. It was also indicated for recovering convalescents. What was common to all such conditions was that they tended to defy the best efforts of orthodox medicine.[19] The elite London practitioner James Johnson (1777–1845) identified a condition he termed 'wear and tear' that afflicted the professional classes of the metropolis above all, who were worn down by a combination of overwork and competitive pressures. Medicine was useless in face of 'wear and tear'; the antidote was diversion – removal of the invalid from his everyday concerns and distraction by new sights and sensations.[20] 'Wear and tear' was necessarily confined to the male half of the population, but women too could benefit from foreign travel, for a secondary advantage associated with temporary withdrawal from London life was removal to better air: upper-class women spent too much time indoors, for, according to Johnson, 'no mad dog could have a greater dread of water than had a modern fine lady of the solar beams'.[21]

Edwin Lee, a prolific guide to continental health resorts for his invalid compatriots, identified travelling as the best antidote for the sort of 'depressing moral influences' that often led to organic disease if left unchecked: he recommended 'a residence in some locality where the air was pure; the climate such as to admit of daily out-door exercise in winter; when sunshine, the aspect of a cheerful, pleasing country, and agreeable associations tended to divert the mind from sombre thoughts and consequently to strengthen the digestion as well as the other functions of the organism'.[22] For those suffering from inveterate digestive complaints brought on by anxiety it was vital to leave the country, according to the medical climatologist D. J. T. Francis, 'beyond the range of the penny post, and if it were possible the over-stimulating *Times*'.[23]

Belief in the therapeutic value of diversion – removal of the patient from the familiar surroundings, routines and habits that were implicated in his debility – remained largely uncontested throughout the nineteenth century. The sole major exception related to patients who were already fatally afflicted with disease, especially with advanced phthisis – pulmonary consumption – who were by contrast urged to remain among the comforts of home, both to extend their life as far as possible and to soften the pain of their last days. 'I have lived too long', observed James Johnson, 'and seen too much, not to know the errors of discrimination and fallacies of hope that send pulmonary patients from the gloomy skies but comfortable abodes of England to lands where comfort is unknown, even by name, and whose atmospheres cannot work miracles, whatever their saints may do.'[24] With this exception however it was hoped that travel in an interesting country with sunny skies might improve the health of many patients, and plenty of sufferers were consequently 'directed south' by their medical advisors; but such advice was based, in the words of Vladimir Janković, more on a 'stereotypical adulation of the Grand Tour' than any clear hypothesis regarding the therapeutic virtues of the Mediterranean climate.[25]

The Mediterranean basin clearly represented for educated Britons the very definition of an interesting country, but it was much less obvious that Mediterranean air would assist the diversionary benefits of expatriation. Leading eighteenth-century authorities had theorized the benefits of warmth, and in particular recommended escaping the British winter, for the avoidance of 'Fluxes, Quinseys, Pleurisies, Fevers, Agues, Consumptions and other violent and almost incurable diseases'.[26] The influential Edinburgh professor James Gregory (1753–1821) admitted that medicine was in effect powerless in face of the British winter. The meteorological variability, cold and moisture of this season meant that there was no remedy for its attendant afflictions but to wait for summer.[27] Alternatively, of course, the patient could seek 'summer' in the south. Yet reliable first-hand accounts of Mediterranean climates, let alone meteorological statistics, were virtually non-existent at the beginning of the Victorian period so that prospective health-seekers had little more than an idealized picture of the warm south on which to found their plans.

'Change of air', a prescription deriving from the humoral foundations of classical medicine, had become a medical commonplace by the end of the eighteenth century.[28] But there was no agreed definition of what constituted better air, still less any governing conceptual framework to help patients and their advisors select a suitable climate or atmosphere.[29] 'Change of air must ... be said to be prescribed empirically, and not according to any rational principle', remarked one sceptical commentator on the concept.[30] Bad air on the other hand was associated with urban living and especially with fetid indoor spaces.[31] Choosing better air was therefore an aspect of the therapy of diversion: it was not so much the choice of good air but the avoidance of bad that underlay the notion of 'change of air'. The term had long currency, becoming in due course a polite formulation – little more than 'an item of conspicuous consumption'.[32] There was however no implication that better air was to be found abroad. Indeed for most British medical climatologists there was no air more suitable for British patients than that of the home country. According to Edwin Lee, England was the healthiest country in the world, followed by Sweden, Belgium and France; as a rule of thumb, in his opinion, mortality from infectious disease increased in inverse proportion to latitude.[33] This view was a variation on the traditional identification of the tropical zone as the source of epidemic disease.[34]

To seek better air by travelling to the warm south involved therefore a suspension of conventional attitudes to the deficiencies of the Mediterranean climate or at least an acceptance that the advantages of escape from the British winter outweighed the risks of increased exposure to infectious disease and other dangers. Even where it was acceptable as a winter refuge, Italy granted only a temporary, seasonal lease for patients, as almost half the year was generally held to be climatically intolerable. According to Edwin Lee, even the late winter sun of Nice – considered an integral part of Italy until 1860 – was potentially perilous for those of 'an irritable or plethoric habit', who were advised to stay indoors in the middle of the day or carry an umbrella.[35] The Italian summer meanwhile was the supposed source of many long-term medical problems; as Lee noted, 'the foundation of chronic maladies … [was] every summer laid in hundreds of [his] countrymen who wandered about beneath the azure skies of Italy'.[36] The same author identified the Italian summer as the season when 'emanations of all kinds, whether of a putrid or marshy nature, rose into the air, and there acquired a greater intensity from the combined action of heat and humidity'.[37]

Such reservations were not universally held. The British physician Joseph Cox, who practised at Naples, warned against returning home too soon; warmth benefitted patients threatened with tubercular disease, provided care was taken in the hottest months of July and August. The main advantage of uninterrupted residence was however to ensure the patient could spend two consecutive winters in the south and thus better preclude the return of symptoms once back in England.[38] The lay authority Mrs Carleton was also dismissive of the need to leave the peninsula at the onset of summer but nevertheless considered that 'travelling invalids gave themselves a great deal of trouble to go and fetch agues, rheumatisms, apoplexies and bilious fevers'. The climate of Italy was overrated, she concluded: 'The combination of heat with moisture weakened the constitution ultimately'; Italy was a 'land to visit more for pleasure than for health'.[39]

The warm south was at once a source of balm and bane, its two-faced climate seemingly mirroring the ambivalent nature of Mediterranean life, simultaneously seductive and corrupting. It was as if the region were offering its own strong medicine in place of the pharmaceutical regime that patients would have been undergoing at home, a medicine that was to be taken in small doses and then not habitually; Lee considered regular winter visits to Italy to be eventually injurious to health, as 'diminishing the vigour of the body and energy of the mind'.[40] As John Pemble writes, 'For the Victorians [the south] represented both the world they longed to enter and the world they must strive to leave'.[41] Patients were urged to quit their winter quarters before the onset of summer heat in terms that smacked of the direst consequences for disobedience. British visitors to the Riviera took the injunction to heart: the English church at Nice, which depended for its income on pew-rents, took no receipts between May and October.[42] Fear of epidemic disease in Italy meant it took little to persuade visitors to scuttle north on rumours of outbreaks at Naples or Rome. The threat of malaria at Rome to foreign visitors, as of all epidemic diseases, was largely exaggerated, but was securely lodged nonetheless in the Victorian imagination, as illustrated by the exchange between Mrs Proudie and the ointment heiress Miss Dunstable in Trollope's *Dr Thorne*.[43] The pre-Victorian notion that there was something uniquely threatening about the airborne diseases of the Roman environment – so-called Roman fever – ceased to be medically respectable after 1830, but the concept had a healthy afterlife.[44]

If continental travel offered hope of relief from oppression of mind, there was nonetheless a countervailing perception that overexposure to continental, especially Mediterranean, influences carried the risk of permanent moral injury. Just as the meteorological climate of the south held traps for the unwary and the Mediterranean sun – source of that easeful comfort that beguiled northerners – was at once friend and foe, the moral climate of Italy was enticing and perilous in equal measure. Stefania Arcara has stressed the significance of a gendered Italy, symbolized by Bulwer Lytton's reference to 'Circe's spell' in *The Last Days of Pompeii*: 'Italy-Circe offers the voluptuous pleasures of her body in the form of sun, heat and mild skies; in her naked state of nature and timelessness, oblivious of morality, she is both attractive and threatening, casting her spells on the modern English-speaking Ulysses.'[45] For James Johnson, the maxim of the dyspeptic, nervous or hypochondriacal traveller in Italy should be 'that which the Home Secretary had laid down for the guidance of the New Police in England – Keep Moving', as if stasis risked contamination by one or more of the several malign influences that he associated with Italian life, from idleness to immorality.[46]

According to Edwin Lee, the British were particularly liable to moral decay when they had nothing to do, as was frequently the case when they resided overseas, while the Italian by contrast was expert at '*far niente*' (doing nothing).[47] Echoing Lee, the physician Thomas Chambers, who accompanied the Prince of Wales to Spain and Italy in 1859, identified the source of the problem in idleness: 'There could not be a more drear purgatory', he contended, 'than the purposeless existence led by some of [his] countrymen resident abroad without fixed occupation; one almost pardoned them their scandal-mongering or even still worse modes of excitement', he continued, 'when it was remembered that this was all that distinguished their lives from those of the butterfly or the oyster.' For Chambers, a temporary, seasonal residence was therefore preferable to long-term expatriation, although there were some diseases – torpid phthisis, emphysema and Bright's disease, for example – that required permanent exile.[48] Ann Vavasour identified the peril of extended foreign residence in the dislocation of expatriates from their moral bearings. It was healthy for British people to travel abroad but not to reside. The relative ease of personal relations on the Continent disrupted social norms. The young were especially vulnerable, for 'the pleasing, flattering manners of [her] continental neighbours' risked turning a young lady's head, leaving her either 'a confirmed coquette' or 'a sacrifice to some adventurer'.[49]

The only significant exception to the accepted wisdom regarding the inferiority of southern air concerned the island of Madeira. By the early Victorian period, the reputation of Madeira's climate for alleviating respiratory and pulmonary complaints had been built up over generations of medical discourse to become commonplace. So beneficent was its climate for consumptives, it was believed, that a 'Madeira House' had been established in Bristol in 1815 by a local medical practitioner to provide an artificial atmosphere for treating sufferers.[50] The accepted wisdom was reflected by James Clark (1788–1870), doyen of British climate therapists, who rated Madeira in the first place as a destination for consumptives in his influential work on medical climatology of 1830, despite never having visited the island: 'There is no place on the continent of Europe with which I am acquainted', he wrote, 'where the pulmonary invalid could reside with so much advantage during the whole year as in Madeira.'[51] In Madeira, patients could benefit from a warm, relaxing atmosphere without running the risk of miasmatic disease or moral corruption. It could not compete with the Mediterranean in providing cultural or social attractions, but for consumptives these distractions were positively harmful. Madeira was also unique in being the one destination where, according to specialists, invalids could safely reside all year round, although few did. The high standing of Madeira air was gradually undermined as the century advanced as a result of detailed meteorological investigations and analysis of patient outcomes, but for the first three decades or so of the Victorian period it had no equal in professional or lay estimation.

The reputation of Madeira's climate long antedated the Victorian age. The promotion of Pau, in the foothills of the western Pyrenees, was by contrast the work of a diligent campaign of climatological propaganda led by one man, the expatriate physician Alexander Taylor (1802–1879). Clark had given Pau a fair report but was by no means as enthusiastic as he was with respect to Madeira. He tells us that he had only made a short visit to the place, so his views essentially reflected those of his expert informant, Dr Playfair, who had lived at Pau for several years. Pau appeared to be 'one of the most desirable winter residences in the south-west part of France, for invalids labouring under chronic affections of the mucous membranes', but it was no good for rheumatics and the weather too changeable for consumptive diseases. 'According to Dr Playfair, the good qualities of Pau may be summed up as follows', declared Clark: 'calmness, moderate cold, bright sunshine of considerable power even in winter, a dry state of atmosphere and of the soil, and rains of short duration'. On the debit side the weather was changeable, with rapid variations of temperature, and heavy rains were common in spring and autumn.[52]

If this meteorological description seems somewhat contradictory, it doubtless reflects the difficulty of summarizing a climate that was as variable as England's. Publication a decade later of Taylor's seminal work on the climate of Pau propelled the place into the front rank of climatological resorts.[53] As in Madeira, it was the climate of Pau that was deemed to be the patient's physician of first resort, the role of active medical attendance being largely confined to guiding the patient in how best to exploit the climatic opportunity. Indeed, according to Dr Taylor, the soothing, anti-inflammatory qualities of the climate reduced the need for bleeding, purgatives and other pharmaceutical aids: 'These circumstances … are evidently a great gain to invalids suffering under chronic maladies, and enable them, even where a cure is not possible, to linger on the road with more comfort, from the diminished call for active medical interference', he declared.[54]

Another expatriate physician, Dr Drewry Ottley, claimed the Pau climate was better suited to British constitutions than the sunnier skies of Spain and the Mediterranean, as it more closely resembled their own.[55] The best season for visiting was the spring, according to Dr Francis, as it enabled patients to escape the cold air that often blighted other health resorts at that time of year.[56] Frederick Johnson, a medical practitioner who visited during the winter of 1855–6, waxed lyrical in his praise of the climate's therapeutic effects: 'It is in the peculiar stillness and dryness of the atmosphere which exert so powerful an effect over the nervous system, the entire absence of all cold, dry winds, the penetrating warmth of the sun's rays, the rarity of prolonged damp and fog, and the combined advantages of mountain air and the soft, warm breezes that steal from the south,' he warbled, 'that the invalid will find the benefit.' Even lunatics could be cured. The same influence could be detected among the local populace: 'Anger, jealousy, rivalry, grief, political excitement, and enthusiastic outbreaks of excited nervous action were both less frequent and less developed.'[57]

## Climate and disease

Phthisis pulmonalis, or tuberculosis of the lungs, usually designated by the imprecise symptomatic term 'consumption' before the later nineteenth century, in both lay and professional discourse, was a disease so universally associated with British invalids on the Continent that it had come to define them. The lungs were wasted – literally consumed – as a result it seemed of some physiological fault or weakness in the human organism. Tubercles or hard nodules were usually observed post-mortem in the diseased tissues of victims, but what role they played in the development of the disease was unclear. Consumption did not behave like other fevers, being usually chronic or even intermittent rather than acute, with unexplained intermissions and relapses and with other symptoms that were often vague or slow to appear until it was clear that the patient was very seriously ill.[58] There was no suggestion in Britain at least until much later in the century that consumption could be contagious: the tendency of the disease to afflict members of the same family could be easily explained by hereditary or environmental predisposition.[59] James Clark noted in 1820 that the local population of Nice believed phthisis was a contagious disease since it had not existed before the arrival of winter visitors from the north; he remarked that the local landlords disposed of the furniture in lodgings where consumptive patients had died and he cautioned the friends of invalids to avoid discussing the nature of their illness.[60] Advanced pulmonary consumption was not however an easy disease to disguise: although difficult to diagnose in its early stages, the tell-tale symptoms of established phthisis – lethargy, breathlessness, the notorious hacking cough, perhaps bloody expectoration – were only too likely to be present in patients wintering in the south, notwithstanding the developing medical consensus that winter expatriation of advanced cases was useless.[61]

The majority view among specialists in the first half of the nineteenth century was that, whatever the role of hereditary or constitutional predisposition in preparing the ground, pulmonary tuberculosis was a preventable disease brought on a combination of vitiated air, sedentary habits and mental care. The disease once established may have rendered sufferers beyond help, but patients with a predisposition or with incipient consumption could help themselves by adapting their living conditions and lifestyle.[62] Such adaptation was usually facilitated by removal from home and all its customary bad habits and transfer to an environment with purer air and a climate that allowed the patient some prospect of benefiting from it. While it was accepted that the warm south harboured greater danger of infection by acute diseases, chronic chest complaints, especially pulmonary consumption, were apparently comparatively rare in the Mediterranean. To flee a damp and chilly northern winter when threatened or afflicted with pulmonary disease and seek relief or cure in southern Europe at a time when the sun was warming rather than scorching and the risk of miasmatic infection at its lowest thus made perfect sense for those who could afford it.

From quite early in the nineteenth century, however, informed medical opinion began to entertain serious doubts about the suitability of the Mediterranean climate for confirmed phthisical patients, quite apart from the unavoidable physical demands that the journey placed on delicate invalids. In the words of Vladimir Janković, 'with every coffin dispatch the medical south took on a grimmer aspect'.[63] The received opinion of the generalized virtues of an undifferentiated southern climate began to give way to the realization that there was not one southern climate but many and that certain aspects of them in winter as well as summer were distinctly unfavourable for healthy visitors, let alone the sick. Climatotherapists began to categorize health resorts, increasingly basing their conclusions on meteorological data. Resorts were typically assigned a place on the two axes of humidity and temperature, but the practice was hopelessly reductive, and besides there was no stable consensus on what climate suited any particular disease, especially pulmonary consumption.

For James Clark, warm, moist conditions suited consumptives best, but there was plenty of disagreement, amply encouraged by the fact that no one knew the cause of the affliction, whether it was an inflammatory disease as Clark believed, requiring a soothing atmosphere and rest, or a disease of debility and malnutrition, necessitating building up and outdoor exercise.[64] For Julius Jeffreys, inventor of a respirator for consumptive patients, the problem they faced and the cause of much conflicting medical advice was that their lungs required quite different atmospheric conditions (warm and moist) from their general health (dry and bracing): the solution was creation of an artificial, portable climate for the lungs by means of a respirator, so that 'some pulmonary invalids … had sought with benefit the bracing action of even a colder climate than that of England'.[65] This dichotomy was noted by James Pollock, who lauded the palliative qualities of Roman air in alleviating the symptoms of phthisis but admitted that as the disease originated in defective nutrition a more bracing climate was required to meet any hope of cure.[66]

The difficulty in prescribing a suitable climate for consumptives was implied by the practitioner Frederick Johnson, who identified four stages of the disease, each requiring significantly different atmospheric conditions, from tonic in the early stages to sedative towards the end.[67] To complicate matters further there were according to Thomas Madden two distinct forms of consumption, 'requiring climates of a totally opposite character', one marked by a 'dry, irritative cough, hoemoptosis (hemoptysis or coughing blood), and fast, weak pulse' and the other – representing the great majority of cases – by 'excessive secretion from the skin, profuse expectoration and a weak, relaxed habit of body'.[68] Little wonder that patients typically operated by trial and error, sampling one resort after another, if they lived long enough, until perhaps finding one where they could at least be comfortable if not cured. Indeed, even John Thorowgood, physician to the City of London Hospital for Diseases of the Chest, conceded that this was the only sensible approach.[69]

James Pollock estimated in 1850 that 90 per cent of British invalids in Italy were consumptive.[70] This seems implausible. Some fifteen years later Madden advanced the rather more convincing suggestion that two-thirds of British health-seekers wintering in 'southern or eastern countries' were labouring 'under some form of pulmonary disease, or derangement of health, from which mischief to the organs of respiration was apprehended'.[71] It is likely that the term 'consumption' was often used as a catch-all to encompass a range of respiratory diseases, especially as the incidence of pulmonary consumption in Britain seems to have entered a steady decline from the early 1830s.[72] Many whose consumption was suspected rather than confirmed were no doubt included under the label. Diagnosis was largely symptomatic, and symptoms could easily be confused with those of other chest and throat conditions: 'Affections of the bronchia and larynx … were sometimes difficult to [distinguish] from phthisis', observed Edwin Lee.[73] Cases of asthma and chronic bronchitis, which often improved in warm, sedative conditions, were readily misidentified as phthisitic, according to Thorowgood.[74] Madden speculated that 'places like Pau, Mentone, etc. had acquired their unmerited reputation' for alleviating pulmonary disease through such diagnostic confusion.[75]

In the circumstances it is perhaps not surprising that 'consumption' appeared to be so conspicuous a presence in British invalid colonies overseas, long after the consensus among specialists that hibernation in the south was worse than useless in advanced cases had become firmly established. At the same time, there can be no doubt that many confirmed consumptives resisted the medical tide – assuming they were aware of it at all; the popular association of the warm south with restoration of health was just too deep-rooted to be disrupted. Belief in the therapeutic power of climate, 'like other professional errors … had descended to the multitude', averred the Irish physician Henry M'Cormac, 'and one of the first things which non-medical people who had the means thought of, was to send their consumptive relatives to some tepid climate where perchance they languished and decayed with yet greater rapidity than they would have done had they remained at home'.[76]

The value ascribed to warm air in treating consumption took a long time to shift, as even when it became clear that pulmonary affections flourished not only in the north but the Mediterranean too, the region continued to provide better facilities for outdoor exercise in winter than northern Europe. 'If there was a specific for the cure of consumption', wrote Thorowgood, 'it was a life in the open air.'[77] The work of George Boddington, who set out the advantages to consumptive patients of breathing cold, dry air as early as 1840, seems to have had little effect.[78] After all, where should a consumptive patient go to breathe cold, dry air? Thomas Burgess, another early advocate of cold air for consumptives, canvassed Norway and Canada as suitable climates, rather betraying the difficulty of identifying an attractive practical destination.[79] Even discounting the instinctive resistance of specialists, let alone patients and their families, the idea of consumptives being directed to cold winter resorts could only be entertained once suitable resorts in the High Alps had been identified and promoted. At the same time, as much as medical professionals warned against expatriation, improvements in transport, lodgings and other facilities supplied a potent counterweight. Moreover, for people suffering from other conditions, such as nervous or digestive complaints, strictures against expatriation to the medical south hardly applied. Escape had become a necessity 'in the case of many little ailments … which refinement, high civilization, and mental labour, imposed upon the susceptible and the delicate'.[80]

Although consumption had been called the 'English disease' as early as the seventeenth century, there is little firm evidence that it was ever disproportionately prevalent in Britain. The perception had perhaps arisen from the ubiquity of consumptive British travellers abroad compared with the relative invisibility of their continental counterparts. It was also assumed that phthisis, like other chest complaints, thrived in cold, damp climates, which was itself a rationalization of the perception that Britons were especially susceptible. By the mid-nineteenth century, professional opinion was divided. 'In no country are strumous affections and pulmonary consumption, which is very closely related to them, so common as in England', observed Dr Francis, physician to the Dispensary for Consumption and Diseases of the Chest, London; they were caused by the 'chilly, damp atmosphere and clouded sky', as well as 'imperfect ventilation' and 'impediments … to natural outdoor exercise'. On the other hand, Dr Richard Cotton, assistant physician to the Hospital for Consumption and Diseases of the Chest, Brompton, countered that the term was 'completely misapplied' since phthisis was a global disease.[81]

In 1838–9 some 60,000 deaths in England and Wales were officially ascribed to pulmonary consumption, more or less equally divided by sex. However a steady decline in this total had already set in, and an even more marked decrease in the proportion of national deaths assigned to the disease occurred during the following decades. The reasons for the decline are not obvious, in keeping with the intractable nature of a disease that almost uniquely baffled contemporary medical expertise. Pulmonary consumption was only one of a number of diseases caused by the Mycobacterium tuberculosis bacillus, identified as the causal agent in 1882, but it was probably the most common, and crucially the only one that afflicted the upper and middle classes in Britain to any significant degree. It also typically first struck its victims in early adulthood. In other words it impacted just that demographic most inclined and able to travel abroad to seek a cure.[82] At the same time, the soft air and Mediterranean fragrances of the south were deemed especially appropriate environmental conditions for a category of patient that by the early nineteenth century was firmly established as one of unusual sensitivity and refinement.[83] This characterization of consumptives as delicate flowers persisted throughout the nineteenth century, notwithstanding the growing consensus among specialists that the lungs of sufferers needed to be worked rather than mollycoddled.[84]

## Sun, winds and airs of the medical south

The grand tour ideal remained a dominant template for health tourism throughout the nineteenth century. The tension between the promise of foreign travel and the reality of Italian roads, rooms and winds that infuses Johnson's *Change of Air* was mitigated as the century advanced not only by improvements in facilities but also by the introduction of a level of detail and nuance into the description of a hitherto largely undifferentiated atmospheric environment – patients and their advisors were increasingly able to turn to authoritative guidance about where to go and when and crucially what to avoid. James Clark, a specialist in treating pulmonary disease who had practised at Rome from 1819 to 1826 and had briefly ministered to the dying John Keats while there, was the first British physician to make any systematic attempt to analyse and categorize continental health resorts by climate. He shared with Johnson a belief in the therapeutic powers of travel as diversion but, perhaps unsurprisingly in view of his career, held a higher opinion of the virtues of the Italian, especially the Roman, climate. If 'success had not more generally attended the practice of sending invalids abroad', he maintained, the fault lay 'not in the remedy but in the manner in which it had been prescribed'.[85] Ignorant British physicians persisted in sending their patients to unsuitable resorts.

It was convenient that Rome was anyway the destination of choice for most grand tourists. Samuel Rogers estimated in 1820 that there were some two thousand 'English' in Rome when he was there, representing perhaps two-thirds of the total number of his compatriots in Italy.[86] The city was not without dangers: Clark cautioned against exposure to the cold and damp in open carriages and draughty churches, but the moist, sedative air and relative winter warmth of the Roman climate made it, contended Clark, especially suitable for consumptive patients.[87] James Pollock, who practised at Rome during the 1840s, observed that invalids described the air as 'easily breathed' and that consumptives benefited from 'lessened cough, freer secretion, and consequently less frequent occurrence of congestions and the absence of pain'.[88]

Pisa, conveniently located close to Livorno, a major port of disembarkation for tourists travelling south via Marseilles, was also popular with consumptives as a winter station, though it was distinctly inferior to Rome for that purpose according to Clark, the climate being rather oppressively damp. However, since there was little in the way of social life for expatriates it suited 'invalids who [were] confined to the house or whose power of taking exercise [was] much limited'.[89] For Mariana Starke, doyenne of British travel writers on Italy, Rome and Pisa vied for first place for pulmonary patients, provided the lungs were not ulcerated, in which case Pisa was to be preferred.[90] It is difficult to escape the conclusion that its success had more to do with its location than its other attributes. For Clark, one of Pisa's chief advantages was that it was easy to leave with the onset of summer heat, as it was well connected by road.[91] Florence and Naples, by contrast, the two other primary sites of cultural pilgrimage in the peninsula, struggled to find advocates for their qualifications as health resorts. Clark knew of 'no class of invalids for whom Florence [offered] an advisable residence', although Edwin Lee recognized its suitability for 'dyspeptic and nervous patients who sought mental recreation in travelling'.[92] At all events it was too cold for invalids in winter. As for Naples, the best Lee could say for it was that the 'climate [did] not generally disagree with dyspeptic and nervous patients.[93] Clark meanwhile 'had never met one medical man, or consumptive invalid … who [had given] a good report of it.'[94]

There was one region of the warm south above all that British invalids made their own during the course of the nineteenth century until, in the words of John Pemble, 'nowhere, it seemed, was quite free from their sick-room aura and their muted sadness'.[95] Bordering the Mediterranean – *Mare Nostrum* of the Romans – the Riviera was integral to the Victorian mental map of the classical world and like the Italian peninsula proper replete with both the physical remains and topographical reference points of Antiquity, however degraded its current condition might appear to be. Originally the term 'riviera' referred to the Ligurian coastline between La Spezia and Nice, but after the French resorts to the west of Nice began to be developed the designation started to be applied to the entire coastline as far as Hyères.[96] In addition to intimations of the antique, the Riviera possessed other features that few other resorts could match, at least at such relative proximity to Britain. It enjoyed a Mediterranean climate of course – hot, dry summers, that British visitors typically avoided, and temperate winters with plenty of rain but hardly any fog or frost. However variable the weather might prove in any given season, mild air and winter sunshine were more likely to be encountered at Nice than at Pau, for instance, let alone Hastings or Torquay.

A mid-Victorian authority laid out the meteorological offer of the Riviera to the northern winter visitor with impressive clarity:

> Compared with London as a standard, the mean temperature on the Riviera in winter is from eight to ten degrees Fahrenheit higher; the shortest day is about an hour longer as far as actual sunlight is concerned; there are about half as many rainy days and at least four or five times as many bright sunny days; the mean barometrical pressure is higher and subject to less variation; fog and mist are practically unknown; snow, if it falls, as may happen once or twice in exceptional winters, never lies more than a few hours, and prolonged frost, as understood by the inhabitants of northern climates, never occurs.[97]

Perhaps as important as the climate were the flora. It was one thing to discover exotic plants and fruits in subtropical Madeira after a sea voyage of several days or weeks but quite another to suddenly find oneself in a paradise of orange and lemon groves barely three days from home. The cultivation of fruits usually associated with Sicily and North Africa seemed almost miraculous.

Who would not feel that their health and strength must surely benefit from immersion in such an environment?

Professional opinion on the therapeutic virtues of wintering on the Riviera was however decidedly mixed. No medical man, according to James Clark, had ever given a favourable opinion of the climate of Nice in relation to pulmonary consumption. The climate suited patients with rheumatism, gout and nervous affections, but Clark predicted as early as 1820 that 'before very many years the English physician would no more think of sending his consumptive patients to [Nice] than to [Montpellier]'.[98] Ten years later his views had not changed: whatever benefits might accrue to the bronchitic, gouty and dyspeptic from a winter residence there, 'sending patients labouring under confirmed consumption to Nice would in a great majority of cases prove more frequently injurious than beneficial'.[99] The British consul's return of 1829 to the survey by the Royal College of Physicians on global health conditions gave an alarmingly negative picture of local diseases: the worst months were February and March when the winds were at their most severe and affections of the stomach and liver prevailed; but the rest of the year was little better – bilious complaints and dysentery in the summer, tertian and nervous fevers in the autumn and diseases of the air passages such as catarrhs and inflammation of the lungs in winter.[100]

By the start of the Victorian period the lingering therapeutic reputation of the climate of Nice for pulmonary disease had been thoroughly discredited in professional circles. William Farr, an expatriate physician with a practice at Nice, noted in 1841 that every year fewer and fewer consumptive patients arrived, although he advised that the climate remained excellent for those whose phthisis was only incipient.[101] But if pulmonary cases were put off Nice, they do not seem to have avoided the Riviera altogether but merely been relocated. The physician Edward Sparks in the 1870s could still claim that 'the largest contingent of invalids suffering from any one disease which reached the Riviera was certainly the phthisitical'.[102] Besides, there were many others who might benefit from what Dr Farr averred was 'perhaps the finest [climate] in the world', if one discounted the wind. A broad range of diseases could be ameliorated: chronic bronchitis, affections of the larynx, humid asthma, some forms of dyspepsia, hypochondriacal affections, urinary calculi, secondary syphilis, heart diseases, gout, varicose veins, languid circulation and 'coughs of the climacteric period'.[103]

Sir Francis Palgrave, the author of Murray's first handbook to the region, owned that the 'agreeableness and salubrity' of the climate had perhaps been overrated in the past, but the reaction had been excessive: 'The sharp *bise* or west [*sic*] wind is occasionally trying to invalids', he conceded, 'but this inconvenience, to those who seek the indulgence of *comforts*, is counterbalanced by the manner in which the houses and hotels, as well as the people with whom you have to deal, have become adapted to the real or artificial wants of English inhabitants or customers.'[104] The winds contributed to a climate that was classified as tonic or bracing, with a specific benefit for languid patients suffering from atonic indigestion.[105] Despite Nice's former position as 'the burial ground of our consumptive patients', Mrs Carleton considered the air 'excellent wherever it was free from the impertinent intrusion of miasma' but had to admit that it was a puzzle: 'Some are better and some are worse for the air of Nice', she mused, which 'like the Sphinx, as cruel as she is beautiful, demolishes those who do not solve her enigmas'.[106] One person's tonic air was another's irritant. The writer Margaret Brewster described the air of Nice as 'the most curious air that ever anybody inhaled, and … unfavourable for keeping the peace. It is both exciting and depressing', she continued, 'instead of coming in refreshed and soothed, one has a longing to box the ears of all one's friends, and cry for an hour after doing it'.[107]

The atmosphere of the Riviera was governed not only by the prevailing winds but also by the presence of the sea. Clark speculated in 1820 that the unsuitability of the Mediterranean coast for pulmonary complaints had something to do with saline impregnation of the atmosphere, a view that persisted in the literature through subsequent decades. At the same time there were many other health conditions for which sea air clearly was helpful – some like rheumatism and gout that could not be confused with pulmonary disease, but others like asthma, bronchitis and scrofula that seemed to be associated with phthisis, sometimes presaging the onset of that disease, and often difficult to disentangle from it in diagnosis. This may go some way to explain why phthisical cases continued to be despatched to the Riviera despite the settled wisdom of the faculty. It was the very 'emanations from the water such as bromine and iodine' that rendered the sea coast so valuable for the treatment of scrofula, according to Dr Francis.[108] Dr C. T. Williams, assistant physician to the Hospital for Consumption and Diseases of the Chest, Brompton, agreed that it was the combination of 'bright sunshine and saline breezes' that gave Nice its power over 'rheumatic and gouty affections', as well as 'atonic forms of dyspepsia and … many scrofulous complaints'. But even patients suffering from phthisis, asthma, emphysema and chronic bronchitis could enjoy the benefit of the stimulating atmosphere, itself caused by saline breezes and dry air, as it improved digestion and 'assimilation'.[109]

A minority of patients, typically those suffering from neuralgia or who were otherwise of a nervous or irritable disposition, did not thrive by the seashore; they were advised to avoid Menton above all because it was impossible to escape proximity to the shore – life was the equivalent of living 'shipboard'. The lapping of the waves at night might interrupt their sleep, but they usually grew used to this; more damaging, according to local physician Dr Siordet, was some undefined source of irritation arising from the sea itself that frequently gave rise to hysteria.[110] For other invalids though, the surging of the sea on the shingle that diffused health-giving saline particles in the atmosphere ensured the popularity of the benches on the promenade for those keen 'to derive as much benefit as possible from the open air without bodily exertion'.[111] That the sea offered some more or less mysterious quality beyond mere scenery and fresh air seems to have been generally accepted by patients and practitioners alike. Whether this quality was unique to the region or shared by all sea coasts apparently remained unexplored. For Henry M'Cormac, railing against the expatriation of consumptives, one coast was as good as another; not that the sea had any special powers – its benefit was as a source of fresh air, no more, no less.[112]

Patients on the Riviera found an environment that was in several ways more difficult to negotiate than that of Madeira or Pau. Although the entire coast enjoyed a relatively uniform winter temperature, the seasonal variability of the winds and the complicated local topography gave rise to myriad microclimates that challenged the skills even of specialists when prescribing a suitable resort for their patients. In addition, the combination of narrow, medieval streets in almost perpetual shadow, with strong sun even in winter and clear nights, seemed to present a potentially lethal menace to the unwary, especially around dusk. 'To a stranger from a northern region', wrote the Edinburgh publisher William Chambers, 'the striking thing about the climate is, that during the day, while the sun brilliantly shines, there is a feeling of, and a resemblance to, a fine autumn – say the heat of an English September; but no sooner does the sun disappear below the Mediterranean, than we are back in a minute to our old accustomed wintry sensations.'[113] Little wonder that such a contrary region left patients and their carers tossed hither and thither between hopes, doubts and fears and often helplessly dependent on a priesthood of medical specialists to help them propitiate the caprices of the climate.

After several months on the Riviera, Margaret Brewster concluded that 'climate' was a sham: 'I don't believe in a "good climate" myself', she explained; 'in this world we must always have too much sun, or too little sun, or mistrals, or damp, or cold'.[114] The variability of the climate and capriciousness of its winds meant that the air of the Riviera never acquired that reputation, however ill-deserved, as a miracle worker of nature that Madeira's briefly enjoyed in the early nineteenth century. On the contrary, the region's very diversity became one of its strongest selling points as an invalid asylum: if the main benefit of winter expatriation was to escape the northern cold and gloom rather than to embrace any supposed curative qualities of the Mediterranean atmosphere, as most commentators clearly believed by 1850, how much more pleasant to do so on a coast studded with picturesque fishing harbours backed by citrus groves and overlooked by tree-clad mountains, within convenient reach of half the population of Europe, than be confined to a small, dull town on a remote island like Madeira, or locked into a claustrophobic round of mutual visiting, as at Pau. This was a perennial theme in the discourse about the climate of the Riviera; as William Chambers enjoined on his fellow invalids, 'we have to think not so much of what we have enjoyed, as what we have escaped'.[115]

## Britons and the continental spas

Not all health-seekers headed for the warm south when they crossed the Channel. A significant number were destined for Europe's mineral springs, most of which lay north of the Alps. The majority of the patients at watering places were, according to Thomas Madden, suffering from some form of indigestion or from 'diseases occasioned by the gouty and rheumatic diathesis', in other words from stiff and painful joints. Lesser numbers comprised those with 'nervous, cutaneous and scrofulous afflictions'. However, Madden noted, many people at spas were suffering from no particular illness but were merely 'out of health'. For the latter especially it was not the quality of the mineral waters that mattered but the respite from normal life.[116] To a large degree spa-visiting was an example of the strategy of diversion and change of air that we have seen informed the pattern of invalid expatriation. Spas were often in upland regions with unpolluted skies and romantic scenery and even those that were not usually offered the attractions of music, balls and gambling.

A spa cure was not however a means of escaping the British winter since the full therapeutic programme was without exception only available in summer. Some of the larger continental spas such as Baden Baden and Wiesbaden acquired a year-round British expatriate population, attracted by the cultural and economic benefits of permanent residence, but the smaller, more iatrocentric resorts, such as Kissingen and Wildbad, were less hospitable winter locations, where hotels shut their doors out of season and expatriate physicians returned to their usual quarters. Some of the higher Pyrenean spas were virtually deserted in winter, even by their customary summer inhabitants. Climate was not therefore as a rule a prime motivation for continental spa visiting, except in as much as a mountain spa might provide refuge from the summer heat of a place like Pau or Florence. Indeed the Rhine valley, which contained the most popular watering places for Britons, was frequently stiflingly hot in summer. The Anglican chaplain at Wiesbaden appealed for leave to return home for his daughter's health in terms that might have been penned by his fellows in the south of France: he had been advised that 'it would be death to remain in Wiesbaden, and that the changeable and bracing air of England was necessary to life and would certainly restore her energies'.[117]

Although spas had always been rarer in Britain than on the Continent, there had been a boom in British spa development and visiting in the later eighteenth century. Despite an initial check to development following the outbreak of the French war in 1793, the closure of the Continent to British health-seekers after 1803 only amplified the popularity of the country's own resources, with annual visits to Bath at around ten thousand and perhaps half that total at Harrogate and Cheltenham for example during the early years of the new century. Even after the resumption of communication with the Continent, British spas continued to prosper, enjoying their period of greatest expansion during the 1830s.[118] On the other hand, since by 1815 few prospective British spa-goers had first-hand experience of continental watering places, there was an opportunity for evangelists to persuade a perhaps sceptical public of the merits of these unfamiliar therapeutic resources. Augustus Bozzi Granville, self-appointed evangelist-in-chief, lamented the ignorance of and scepticism about continental watering places on the part of the medical profession in England and attempted to leapfrog this impediment by appealing directly to patients in his groundbreaking work of German spa proselytism *Spas of Germany*.[119] The gradual abandonment of English spas for continental ones that occurred during the Victorian decades cannot however be entirely explained by successful propaganda. Ann Vavasour, pondering the recent invasion of German watering places by her compatriots in the early 1840s, suspected that Britain had 'many quite as good'.[120] Propagandists like Granville were preaching to a public already disposed to seek diversion and recreation across the Channel, whether they had particular medical reasons for travelling or not.

Granville was no doubt one of those in James Johnson's sights when he decried the more extravagant claims of enthusiasts: 'The exaggerated accounts that are published respecting the *miraculous* powers of almost every spa in Germany', he declared, 'are quite sufficient to mislead practitioners and patients who have no knowledge of these vaunted springs.'[121] More commonly the exaggerated claims came from the spa authorities themselves: Sir Alexander Downie (1811–1852), who practised at the Rhineland spas from the mid-1830s, urged his readers to beware 'spa quackery', exemplified by the gobbledegook spouted by German spa physicians with a vested interest in promoting the virtues of their own favoured watering place.[122] This tendency was satirized in *Up the Rhine* by Thomas Hood, who ridicules Dr Ganswein's prescription of nothing but '*kalt wasser*' for the ailing Richard Orchard, a reluctant participant in a family excursion up the Rhine ostensibly in the interests of his health: 'He mustn't come again', Orchard protests to his nephew; 'I shall be drowned before I'm cured. Nothing but watering, watering, watering – Egad! He takes me for a sick Hydrangea!'[123]

Furthermore, Johnson maintained, the British constitution was less susceptible to the benefits of mineral waters: 'The digestive organs of our continental neighbours are habitually in a far more tender and excitable condition than those of our countrymen', he contended, 'in consequence of their greasy and sloppy food and the poverty and acidity of their wines and other drink. They cannot therefore bear medicines of any strength, without great suffering.' Foreign physicians therefore, he concluded, found their prescriptions less effective with their British patients, who would be better served by supplementing mineral waters with 'small doses of the blue pill'.[124] Recognizing British exceptionalism was the key to successful spa practice on the Continent, thought F. H. Prytherch, a resident expatriate physician at Homburg: 'The English differ from all others in most respects, and even those who have long resided on the Continent retain to a great extent their native peculiarities; in the invalid these habits are more visible and more clung to, therefore a universal mode of treatment at the spas cannot profitably be adopted for them.'[125]

On the other hand, at a time when patients in Britain were routinely prescribed 'heroic' doses of drugs of dubious composition and efficacy, a spa cure held obvious attractions for those who had grown tired of and disillusioned with the ministrations of orthodox medicine. It also perhaps appealed differentially to those whose social status enabled them to confidently distance themselves from the prescriptions of their physician. The evidence for British curists registering at continental spas shows a markedly aristocratic stamp in the early Victorian period. The Carlsbad bath list for 1840 for example reveals the Duke of Manchester, Marquess of Exeter, Lord William Brougham, later second Baron Brougham and Vaux, and Lord Robert Grosvenor and their families among the British registrations.[126] It was also at the German spas that British visitors were most likely to encounter homeopathic medicine before it crossed the Channel in the 1830s. Homeopathy likewise appealed especially to the upper classes. Lord Robert Grosvenor was chairman of the Homeopathic Association, founded in 1836.[127] Although no expatriate physician practising at the German spas seems to have had any truck with homeopathy in the 1830s and 1840s, by the end of this period significant numbers of homeopathic practitioners were established at British watering places.[128]

If for many British visitors the twin appeal of society and scenery was enough, there is no doubt that the therapeutic virtues of spa waters themselves, whether taken internally by drinking or as baths, represented the core attraction for the chronically ill, despite the best efforts of the faculty to temper expectations. Although spa water was generally thought not to travel well, thousands of gallons were nevertheless exported from sources such as Fachingen and Selters in the duchy of Nassau and Vichy in central France. Artificial mineral waters were even manufactured at the Royal German Spa at Brighton, although spa physicians tended to pooh-pooh this enterprise, arguing that genuine spa water could not be summoned up by mere mimicry, being more than the sum of its chemical parts.[129] Few visitors moreover would have readily submitted to the iatrocratic regime enforced in the Austrian and Bavarian resorts – early rising, spartan fare and relatively few social diversions – without some confidence in the merits of the course. A proportion of chronic invalids would have been persuaded to undergo a cure when all else had failed, especially drug therapy, so they may have been fatalistic rather than expectant participants. One such was the author of *A Hot-Water Cure Sought Out in Germany in the Summer of 1844*, who tells us he decided to try a spa cure for a long-standing digestive complaint that had resisted the best efforts of several doctors at home. A mildly sceptical curist, the author ended his season full of praise for German mineral waters.[130]

Analysis of the constituents of mineral waters and how they might combine in their effect on the human body were matters of fiendish complexity, even before the particular details of an individual patient and his affliction were introduced into the calculation. Specialist knowledge and advice were deemed essential, but most local spa physicians were suspected with some justification of being propagandists for their own source and consequently unable to provide an unbiased opinion on the suitability of different watering places, however expert they might be in the use of their own springs. It was a standard accusation by critics that all continental waters were vaunted as panaceas by their custodians. What was the poor invalid to do, lamented Ann Vavasour, when attempting to select a suitable spa? Trying them in turn took more time and money than most people had available.[131]

Specialists offered classifications of mineral waters based on their chemical composition, although most springs contained a multiplicity of solid or gaseous elements in variable quantities, so that classification had perhaps as much theoretical as practical value. Very crudely the medicinal applicability of waters was a function of the relative presence of salts, iron, sulphur and carbon dioxide. Saline waters were purging and iron or chalybeate waters tonic. It followed that patients suffering from defective function of internal organs might be directed to a saline source, while those in need of strengthening might find themselves at a chalybeate. Of course the same patient could easily be directed to both depending on their condition. Some spas had springs of differing composition that could just about fulfil this requirement, but it was rare. More commonly adjacent watering places performed a sort of double act, chalybeate Schwalbach and Brückenau supporting saline Bad Ems and Kissingen, for example. Waters also varied in natural temperature. Few specialists ascribed any medical significance to this beyond the function of heat in contributing to the efficiency of the chemical action of the water.[132] Nevertheless many thermal springs of virtually pure water provided baths deemed valuable for the relief of skin complaints, stiff joints and nervous affections, as well as general convalescence or after-cure following a course at a more mineralized source. Patients could not of course be expected to follow the arcane intricacies of the virtues of mineral springs and no doubt made their selection as much on the basis of convenience and fashion as on any systematic medical calculation. In practice, although they took professional advice, both before departure and during their course, most British spa-goers seem to have relied above all on their own experience, in the same way that winter expatriates experimented with alternative resorts.

Ultimately however, continental spas could never quite shake off the taint of otherness that clung to them in the British mind, at least until some elite London practitioners began to take continental spa practice seriously in the last decades of the century and started to influence the wider medical profession.[133] For most no doubt this amounted to little more than an amused condescension regarding the gullibility of foreigners. A few however, including medical men, considered some waters potentially harmful, warning against their misuse and readily accepting stories of fatalities resulting from injudicious bathing and drinking. James Johnson counselled his readers to pay attention to their own instincts rather than the reassurance of the spa physician if they suffered persistent adverse symptoms after a regime of warm bathing: 'Giddiness, sleepiness, chilliness, confusion of thought, weariness, head-ache, pains in the limbs, unusual sounds in the ears, sparks before the eyes, loss of appetite, oppression after food, feverishness, thirst, languor, depression of spirits, inability to sleep at the usual hour, malaise, or indeed any uncomfortable feeling not previously felt' were not signs that the cure was working but on the contrary that bathing should immediately cease.[134]

This so-called spa fever or *Badsturm*, which typically arose after about two weeks of the cure, merely indicated that the mineral constituents of the water had thoroughly penetrated the patient's constitution, according to Granville, and certainly did not merit cessation of treatment.[135] On the other hand, he agreed that use of mineral waters without specialist guidance was hazardous, citing the case of the death of two English ladies 'improperly' sent to Carlsbad by consultants at home.[136] The novelist Wilkie Collins (1824–1889) encountered the *Badsturm* halfway through his cure at Wildbad: 'Every lurking ache and pain … had been roused and forced to alert itself', he told his mother; his doctor assured him this was all quite normal, and 'if he didn't go away relieved of his present troubles he would feel a relief a fortnight or three weeks later'.[137]

Saline springs such as Carlsbad, Wiesbaden and Kissingen were especially dangerous, according to Johnson, as the 'saline ingredients acted powerfully on the sentient extremities of the nerves of the skin and too often excited dangerous commotions in the animal economy'.[138] Madden on the other hand considered the chalybeate waters of a spa like Schwalbach especially risky: 'This water is not one of those remedies, which, if it does no great good, can at least do no harm', he maintained; 'on the contrary it often, when improperly used, leads to very injurious results'.[139] As for the sulphurous waters of the Pyrenees, according to Frederick Johnson, 'all recent testimony bore evidence that in the vast majority of cases they were not only inapplicable but … productive of most positive harm'.[140] Some diseases, especially acute inflammatory affections, were simply not suitable for spa treatment. Foremost among these was confirmed phthisis. Mary Eyre recounts the case of a young consumptive patient at Cauterets in the Pyrenees who died spitting blood after taking the waters.[141] This fear of the malign potential of some continental waters, which after all were taken in moderate doses over a long period, sits oddly with the apparent equanimity with which British patients dosed themselves liberally with pharmaceutical remedies at home, including patent medicines of unknown composition. But as Edwin Lee observed, 'English patients … had become accustomed to the speedy action of pharmaceutical preparations',[142] so perhaps the very length of the cure allowed the sensation of self-poisoning to metastasize in a suspicious mind.

## Conclusion

The therapeutic offer of the Continent enticed a wide variety of British health-seekers across the Channel. Some travelled in the mode of grand tourists, and even if they were not themselves experienced tourists, they inherited the inclinations and habits of their forebears. They headed for Italy above all, especially Rome, and merged into and were more or less indistinguishable from the broad mass of their travelling compatriots. Many British visitors to the continental spas, especially the famous resorts of the Rhineland, shared the outlook of invalid grand tourists. They often travelled in some style, accompanied by multiple household members and servants, and regarded a spa visit partly as an extended social call, partly as a means of setting up their jaded health and spirits for the coming London season. For invalid grand tourists the thermometric qualities of any particular resort mattered less, in the words of Vladimir Janković, than 'the advantages of locomotive, sensual, social and peripatetic diversion'.[143]

Such insouciance did not extend to all health-seekers however. Many patients suffering from chronic illness, still more those in an advanced stage of potentially fatal disease, would have been more or less reluctant travellers. They did not set out confidently but hesitantly and anxiously, perhaps finally persuaded to risk extended expatriation among strangers through long experience of disappointed hopes of recovery at home. For such patients, many of whom had no family tradition of grand touring or fashionable spa visiting, help in selecting a destination and preparing for extended residence abroad was obviously at a premium. At the beginning of the Victorian period such help was vanishingly rare. The medical faculty in Britain was largely ignorant of the therapeutic resources of the Continent and moreover had little incentive to prescribe expatriation and thus remove patients from medical supervision and remuneration. Madeira alone seemed to offer a predictably comfortable exile, which was perhaps one reason for its early popularity, despite the challenges of the journey.

As we shall see, in time advice literature for prospective travellers developed to meet the demand. Much of this was written by doctors practising on the Continent, often following a decision to relocate in the interests of their own health. This fact underlines the danger of treating doctors and patients as mutually exclusive protagonists. On the contrary, to a degree they formed part of a single expatriate invalid community. Both had a role in extending the range of potential sites for expatriation through publications and word-of-mouth recommendations, in contributing to the rise and fall in popularity of health resorts and in sustaining the annual exodus of British patients to the south. The next chapter considers the success of their efforts, the consequences for some of their favoured destinations and the available evidence for the size and make-up of the British invalid population.

2

# Destinations

## Authorities and guides

In July 1855 the British consul at Malaga sent a long, plaintive letter to the foreign secretary, Lord Clarendon, detailing the burdens placed on his office by the demands of winter visitors from home, who were turning his town into 'a second Madeira':

> First comes a correspondence, with unavoidable postages, which cannot be recovered, relative to the suitability of climate, convenience of lodging, whether hotels, private houses or floors are to be obtained with relative rates of board and lodging, means of reaching the place, horses and carriages to be obtained, prevailing winds, temperature, barometrical changes, aspects, fireplaces, carpeted rooms, English doctors and apothecaries – whether reading rooms, libraries, chaplaincies and burial grounds exist, if people are safe in their houses and if molested by the traditional *banditti* if they ride out of the town, whether necessary to bring their plate, linen, saddles, ladies maids, couriers and footmen.[1]

Malaga was only just becoming known as a potential destination for winter expatriation at this date and very little reliable information was available for prospective visitors, either in print or from experienced travellers. The range of concerns listed by the exasperated official provides a neat summary of the type of assurances that invalids and their families sought to enable them not only to select a destination but also to anticipate the environment they would be entering and how to prepare for living in it. Medical specialists might pride themselves on their knowledge of continental climates and the diseases for which they were suitable, but equally important from the patient's perspective were the realities of daily existence in a foreign land.

How did an invalid contemplating a season abroad choose a destination? Most prospective exiles probably took medical advice before departure, but it was a standard lay complaint that medical recommendations were often opaque: 'When a medical man … is good enough to express an opinion that the climate of England is no longer suited to his [patient's] ailment, the question is at once asked, "Whither shall I go for a better?"', observed Revd Edward Davies at the start of his account of a journey to Algiers in the winter of 1856–7; 'and then follows a list of Montpelliers and Spas, so numerous, so various, and so opposite, that the inquirer is only perplexed by the answer'.[2] On the other hand, specialists accused their less enlightened colleagues of gross ignorance. D. J. T. Francis, physician to the Dispensary for Consumption and Diseases of the Chest in London, lamented the tendency for the prospective invalid traveller to be 'directed simply to seek a warm climate and left to choose very much for himself whether he should go to Rome or Nice, Pau or Montpellier, Lisbon or Malaga, Madeira or Egypt, localities between which the utmost difference existed as regarded the properties of their climates'; no wonder so many returned disappointed.[3]

At the beginning of the nineteenth century British invalid travel on the Continent was not clearly demarcated from the wider phenomenon of continental touring. It followed the same patterns, obeying the same demands of fashion, and depended on the same range of resources for inspiration and information. Health-seekers followed the crowd and were probably only an obvious presence in a few places that attracted a disproportionate number of British invalids, notably Madeira, Nice and Pisa, as well as at the closest continental mineral springs, especially Spa in the Ardennes and Aix-la-Chapelle (Aachen). There were no dedicated guidebooks for travelling patients before the 1830s, and there was no developed concept of a health resort. It was understood however that invalids had special needs and might benefit from the expertise of experienced tourists. Unfortunately works by invalid travellers were discursive and unsystematic, as likely to dissuade patients from travelling as otherwise, with their disconcerting accounts of the trials of the road, run-ins with the police and thieving inn-keepers.

The earliest published advice for British invalids on the Continent was contained within the appendix to *Letters from Italy* (1800), by Mariana Starke (1762–1838), who was to become the leading British authority on Italian touring. She provided brief notes on climate in Italy, recommendations on suitable places for invalids to spend the winter, and various words of warning about the sun, Italian apartments and local climatic peculiarities. This reflected the medical consensus of the day, especially with regard to consumption, but she cited no professional sources.[4] Starke's fussy directions for timid British travellers became the butt of continental derision, but she evidently fulfilled a need for reassurance for invalids who were taking the bold step of passing beyond the range of English medicine. The first published efforts by doctors were directed above all to members of their own profession and comprised general surveys of continental destinations, their climate and suitability for different categories of disease and patient. James Clark's *Medical Notes on Climate, Diseases, Hospitals and Medical Schools in France, Italy and Switzerland* (1820) was a work of this type, in which Clark, practising at Rome, attempted to assist the faculty at home direct their consumptive patients to an appropriate continental asylum. Clark followed this with *The Influence of Climate in the Prevention and Cure of Chronic Diseases* (1829), a more wide-ranging work that represented the first attempt in print to categorize health resorts climatically.[5]

It is perhaps doubtful whether many patients read Clark's publications, however influential they were in professional circles. The requirement for an authoritative and systematic guide to continental invalid destinations written primarily for a lay readership was supplied by Dr Edwin Lee (d. 1870), a sort of jobbing medical writer and spa doctor whose bewildering array of publications testifies to the needs of a man without a regular income to make a living where he could. Like Clark, Lee was led to climatotherapy through early professional experience on the Continent, but while Clark's first-hand knowledge was largely confined to Italy, Lee spent a significant part of the 1830s travelling, studying and practising in France and Germany, and even after finally settling in England he never enjoyed a secure position in the profession. Lee's *Memoranda on France, Italy and Germany* (1836) established the pattern of a dominant genre in his output, works of synthesis aimed at both practitioner and patient, but primarily the latter, containing a mix of medical advice and touristic directions, informed by the author's own direct experience. The genre reached its mature form in *Continental Travel* (1848), later *Bradshaw's Companion to the Continent* (1851), a work the author claimed was intended to answer the special requirements of invalid travellers rather than merely those of 'pleasure-seeking' tourists, who were already well served by other publications.[6] *Bradshaw's Companion* was the first work for prospective travellers to include meteorological tables for the principal continental destinations.

It is difficult to gauge how influential Lee's works were with the travelling public: there seem to be vanishingly few references to them in surviving letters and journals, in contrast to Murray's handbooks, which began to appear from 1836. The handbooks offered much more practical information on routes and accommodation and went far beyond Lee's somewhat banal efforts in providing details of tourist sights and associated historical and cultural background. Murray also included a good deal of information of particular interest to invalids, especially about watering places, but his handbooks were largely defined by political or broad geographical frontiers. A traveller contemplating a winter on the Riviera, for example, would need two handbooks, to France and northern Italy, to cover the ground, apart from any additional volumes appropriate to the journey there and back.[7] The publisher C. B. Black eventually met this deficiency with *Guide to the South of France and to the North of Italy* (1873), a handbook based like Murray's on routes to the south and between centres of attraction within the region, in other words a guide for travellers rather than those who might be looking for a settled destination. Black later refined this guide to produce *The Riviera: Or the Coast from Marseilles to Leghorn* (1884), which had much more information on the resources available in the individual resorts. However it was Thomas Cook who published the first guide to the region that could be said to be intended for health-seekers rather than tourists. His *Handbook to the Health Resorts of the South of France and Northern Coast of the Mediterranean* (1878) lacked Murray's or Black's depth of detail, but it provided the bare bones of the facilities for invalids in all the obvious resorts between Marseilles and Pisa, with practical advice on the journey through France or Italy, plus a few sightseeing directions; it was in Cook's words a 'reliable, comprehensive and inexpensive Handbook' that would suit the 'traveller who limited his tour to the Mediterranean coast and did not care to burden his pocket with long descriptions of Italian and French cities that he had no intention of visiting'.[8]

Before Cook, general guides to continental health resorts were written exclusively by doctors, even in those instances where they were directed primarily at a lay readership. There was nothing as comprehensive and systematic as *Bradshaw's Companion* until the Edinburgh physician Robert Scoresby-Jackson's *Medical Climatology* was published in 1862. This work surveyed potential invalid destinations worldwide and concentrated heavily on the physical aspects of resorts, but nevertheless strayed far enough onto Dr Lee's chosen terrain to earn its author a mild rebuke for failing to adequately acknowledge his sources.[9] The book's very range necessitated of course wholesale reliance on second-hand knowledge. *Medical Climatology* was intended for practitioners, and although the author anticipated that patients might read the book he hoped they would not be rash enough to select their destination without medical advice.[10] Scoresby-Jackson was immediately followed by the Dublin physician Thomas Madden's *Change of Climate, a Guide for Travellers in Pursuit of Health* (1864), a work that was almost as wide-ranging although it excluded Madeira or any treatment of spas.[11] It was usual for authors to be more selective, whether writing for the profession or invalids directly. Not only was their expertise or experience inevitably limited, but also, as Dr Francis noted in his preface to *Change of Climate* (1853), why include extensive treatment of regions already well covered by others in print.[12]

Relatively few climate specialists claimed expertise in mineral springs, although details of spas and their waters were often included in their works because of the perceived importance of the cure in complementing winter expatriation. Edwin Lee, who practised during the 1830s as a spa physician in the Rhineland, was an exception. Spa guides were already a well-established genre by this date, although they typically covered a single watering place and rarely strayed beyond national boundaries. Lee's early works on the Rhineland spas seem to have been the first original publications in English on these continental resources by a medical professional. His work however was soon eclipsed in range and popularity by *The Spas of Germany* (1837), the first comprehensive survey of central European mineral springs for an English-speaking readership, by the redoubtable Augustus Bozzi Granville (1783–1872), a former naval surgeon turned physician-accoucheur, with a thriving London practice. Granville had travelled extensively on the Continent and was exceptionally well connected both within the medical profession abroad and socially so that his ability to expatiate on the German watering places was facilitated by ready access to local doctors and spa authorities, as well as presumably by introductions from influential contacts. Lee could not compete with this. While *The Spas of Germany* immediately took its place as the British spa-goer's bible, Dr Lee continued to strive for recognition and above all a living in a succession of publications with variant titles but largely recycled content, while adding more and more subjects, not all by any means relating to health resorts, to his lengthening back catalogue.[13]

Part of the agenda of Granville and Lee was to bring to the notice of Britons the wealth of smaller continental watering places that hitherto they had largely ignored. In this they had been anticipated to a degree by publication of *Bubbles from the Brunnens of Nassau, by an Old Man* (1834), a light-hearted account of a visit to the Rhineland spas in 1832 and 1833 by Sir Francis Bond Head (1793–1875), which first drew the attention of English-speaking readers to the attractions of Schwalbach and Schlangenbad, two small resorts a little away from the river valley in the Taunus mountains.[14] The official *Kurlisten* (visitor lists) for these spas, which were appended to those for Bad Ems until 1845, show a remarkable increase in British visitor numbers in the years after the publication of *Bubbles*: in 1833 only about 2 per cent of Schwalbach curists were Britons, but by 1835 the proportion was some 22 per cent. British prominence at Schlangenbad – a spa whose silken water imparted an almost miraculous softness to the skin according to Head – was even more marked, with a rise from less than 10 per cent to about 34 per cent of total visitors over the same period.[15] Murray was in no doubt that *Bubbles* had made Schwalbach's fortune (and had had a correspondingly detrimental impact on the prospects of more familiar British haunts): 'Many thousand English have taken up their summer residence [at Schwalbach]', Murray declared, 'each with the Bubble-blower for his guide, and Spa, Aix-la-Chapelle and other watering places have been comparatively deserted by them in consequence.'[16] Neither Granville nor Lee however considered advocacy by a mere layman sufficient validation of the merits of hitherto unvisited watering places. Indeed Granville went so far as to accuse Head of luring thousands of credulous British visitors to Schwalbach and Schlangenbad on false pretences; the waters might not have done the visitors much good, but Head's book had certainly proved a 'sovereign beautifier' for its author, he joked – 'it had made a young man of him, a knight, an assistant poor-law commissioner, a lieutenant-governor of a colony, and lastly a baronet – authors were not always so lucky'.[17]

Granville's *Spas of Germany* was, according to Sir Alexander Downie, an expatriate physician at Frankfurt, the work that was instrumental in persuading British invalids of the virtues of continental watering places.[18] Its star resort was Wildbad, a small, poor place in the Black Forest, with only just over 900 visitors in the 1836 season; but its spa water, according to the author, had a unique quality of 'caloricity', a mysterious natural heat, distinct from mere temperature, and perhaps, Granville speculated, akin to electricity. At all events, it seemed to be designed for the convenience of the human body, as it required no artificial regulation of temperature, as at Wiesbaden, Baden Baden or Carlsbad for example, before bathing, while the constant replenishment of the baths ensured that the water never cooled.[19] It was necessary to undermine the competition in order to ensure British invalids make the extra effort to reach so relatively inaccessible a place: Schlangenbad water, puffed by Sir Francis Head for its 'milk-like warmth' was in reality 'foul water, drawn from tanks and used in tubs'; far better to trust to the word of a medically qualified guide and essay the baths of Wildbad.[20]

Granville seems to have started directing patients to Wildbad soon after his first visit in 1836. While in 1837 only ten Britons used the Wildbad waters the following year this had increased to 130, according to James Johnson, who visited in 1839.[21] Those suffering from a chronic and intractable condition that had confounded the best efforts of the profession at home found in *The Spas of Germany* the possibility of escape from a tedious round of unsatisfactory consultations and baffling prescriptions. Allan Young (1806–1895) of Orlingbury, Northamptonshire, suffered from an unnamed persistent illness that defied all medical intervention: 'All sorts of medicine I have tried and they only contribute to my disorder', he complained. His brother in London, perusing a copy of *The Spas of Germany*, noticed that Granville reported remarkable recoveries in similar cases by use of German mineral waters. In early 1838 Allan decided that, provided his own doctor agreed, he would let his house and decamp to the Continent for a course of water treatment and a winter in southern Europe.[22] He tried the waters of Bad Ems, Schwalbach and Wiesbaden in turn, but family circumstances prevented his reaching Wildbad before the end of the season. If he had made his final spa destination he would not have been alone: a young English invalid at Wildbad reported the same year that there were between twenty and thirty compatriots staying at his hotel, 'most of them recommended by Granville'.[23]

If it was just about possible for a man of Granville's ambition and connections to write with credible authority about a wide range of health resorts within the single category of German mineral springs, it was beyond the capacity of any specialist to accomplish an equivalent feat for climate stations. The resorts were just too diverse and far-flung, and the time required to assemble meteorological data and other essential information was prohibitive. It was not until the 1870s that Dr Edward Sparks was able to collate the requisite detailed information about the entire Riviera region to enable him to produce the first comprehensive account of its meteorology, natural environment and individual health resorts for the benefit of the British medical profession.[24] Edwin Lee was probably the most well-travelled writer on health resorts of his day, but even he never visited Madeira, Algiers or Egypt, and indeed the range of his coverage came at the expense of depth of engagement. True expertise required extended residence and preferably clinical experience on the spot. In these circumstances authors frequently justified their authority by reference to personal practical knowledge or depended on information provided by local experts. Both cases carried the risk of partiality.

By the middle of the century the existing danger of ignorance on the part of both invalids and their doctors at home was joined by the perceived threat of special pleading so that health guides of the 1860s began to make a virtue of their impartiality. Scoresby-Jackson's *Medical Climatology* had in its author's words 'no particular climate to eulogise above its fellows, no personal interests to serve'.[25] Thomas Madden hoped his wide experience of many resorts would obviate the problem of unconscious bias in authors who 'very often exaggerated the propitious influences of the particular climate of their place of abode'.[26] Thomas Chambers urged his medical colleagues not to collect facts 'in the spirit of an advocate, to praise or to condemn'.[27] Later in the century, as more and more detailed comparative information became available, fear of deception subsided. Furthermore, as increasing numbers of Britons gained personal experience of the Mediterranean resorts and continental spas, the sort of exaggerated claims about climate and cures familiar from earlier in the century became unsustainable. Later guides tended to restrict themselves to practical information about facilities and recommendations concerning travel, diet and regimen without indulging in too much partisanship.

## Winter in the south

Those encouraged to travel abroad for their health fell broadly into two categories: sufferers from chronic organic illness or victims of depression or other forms of psychological stress. The categories were not mutually exclusive, but on the contrary often overlapped, as physical disease took its toll on mental health or conversely depression of spirits led to somatic illness. The form of exile prescribed for each category was however usually mutually antagonistic, providing ample scope for confusion. Sufferers from chronic diseases were typically urged to seek out a favourable climate and live quietly, avoiding excitement and obeying the instructions of qualified advisers concerning diet, regimen, exercise and so forth; conversely, the despondent patient required mental stimulation to lighten his spirits and restore his state of mind. William Money-Kyrle, writing from Naples in 1844, noted that the interest of daily life prevented him falling back into his 'natural habits of inactivity and indolence'.[28] For the latter category of patient, the precise itinerary and destination of travel were less important than the journey itself. Nevertheless, the well-worn routes of the grand tour were clearly more likely to provide the requisite range of distracting stimuli than a less-travelled path through dull country.

James Johnson, recalling his journey in 1829, declared that 'France … presented very few spots indeed compared with her vast extent of surface, on which the eye could rest with either pleasure or admiration'.[29] Apart from Paris, France offered little to detain the traveller, who usually hurried south to the Mediterranean coast to take ship for Italy or cut across from Lyons to Turin via the Mont Cenis pass.[30] Better still was the route via the Rhine and the Swiss Alpine passes. At all events Italy was the prize, at whose borders the traveller moved, at least in his imagination, from an outer zone of secondary sights north and west of the Alps to the Mediterranean core of Classical and Renaissance civilization. In the words of John Pemble, 'at the limit of olive cultivation the British traveller was conscious of crossing a frontier whose significance was far deeper than that of the Channel or the Rhine … He passed from the circumference to the centre of things.'[31]

However, the towns of Italy were hardly conducive to rest and quiet. Dr J. H. Bennet claimed that patients 'ordered south' rarely returned better, as they 'travelled about for pleasure … constantly occupied in sight-seeing rather than health-seeking'.[32] Even those who might benefit from the cultural and social advantages of urban living could not escape the grim reality of Italian domestic life, according to critics. As late as 1865 Thomas Chambers could warn his fellow practitioners against sending patients across the Alps with insufficient means, for Italy was 'not a place for a poor man unless he was strong enough to rough it'.[33] Large southern towns were typically overcrowded and badly ventilated, with narrow fetid streets and open drains; smaller ones often had no sewerage at all beyond cesspits. Few cities could outdo Naples, which according to Chambers sat 'in a pool of its own excrement',[34] but every large town in the Mediterranean was equally ill-equipped for accommodating invalids, thought Dr Bennet: 'In reality it would be as reasonable to send consumptive patients in the summer months to live in the worst parts of Whitechapel, Liverpool or Glasgow as to send them in winter to live in the centre of these unhealthy southern towns', he concluded.[35]

As Edwin Lee recognized, Bennet had a vested interest in disparaging Italian destinations that might lure patients beyond his favoured resort of Menton: visitors did not normally reside in city centres, and Lee had never heard of one who had died from exposure to poor sanitation alone.[36] But it probably took little to persuade a timid invalid to avoid places that he was perhaps already predisposed to distrust from long indoctrination in the horrors of foreign habits. The physician-invalid William Bullar, concluding his Mediterranean health tour in 1860, decided that sanitary conditions in some places were so bad that 'there seemed to be no escape for invalids but flight'. Foreigners were simply dirty: 'The filthy mind of some foreign novelist could only convey a just idea of the nastiness of some foreign carpets', he shuddered – a neat conjunction of stereotypical insular views on continental hygiene and morals.[37]

For patients who required rest and quiet rather than mental stimulation, nowhere in Italy really passed muster. Pisa had a well-established reputation for hosting consumptives in the early nineteenth century and was appropriately socially dull; however it was not a dedicated health resort but a sort of invalid clearing station, where routes from Rome, Florence and Livorno met.[38] Even Nice – 'the great rendez-vous of English invalids', according to James Johnson, at the beginning of our period[39] – was almost as much a fashionable way station for travellers en route to the south as a sanatorium. The local expatriate doctor William Farr lamented that consumptive patients who should have led sequestered lives were fatally attracted to the bright lights of the Croix de Marbre, the British quarter that developed to the west of the old town.[40] All authorities agreed that for pulmonary patients especially the Croix de Marbre was too exposed to the wind, leading to the development of the district below the Cimiez hills, some two to three miles inland. In 1841 Dr Farr listed thirteen furnished houses for let there, offering some eighty beds, besides accommodation for servants, and at a considerable discount in rent, but it was too isolated to be popular.[41] The Italian coast east of Nice, which became such an important site of health tourism in the later nineteenth century, was relatively inaccessible until the 1860s, and the small fishing villages hugging the shore had no adequate facilities for housing visitors. Italian spas popular with Britons, such as Bagni di Lucca, were, like their northern counterparts, summer venues and consequently unsuitable for winter expatriation.

Away from Italy, the two most important winter destinations for consumptive patients in the first half of the nineteenth century were Madeira and Pau, locations whose somnolent social environment matched their mild winter climate. Plenty of other places outside Italy met these desiderata, but Madeira and Pau had the advantage of the presence of British expatriate colonies on which to graft a seasonal influx. Madeira's long-established British community, about three hundred strong in the early Victorian period, mainly comprised wine merchants, hoteliers and medical practitioners and their families, as well as a number of professional exiles. They supported a range of facilities conventionally required by nineteenth-century British residents overseas – Anglican church and burial ground, British shops, club and reading room – but did not provide the social milieu or facilities for entertainment that typically sustained British visitors to the more fashionable continental resorts. For specialists this made Madeira an ideal asylum for patients in need of rest and recuperation, irrespective of the advantages of the climate. Madeira's attractions for healthy visitors at this date were few: even those who took a broader interest in the island were sometimes themselves invalids or companions of invalids exploiting the opportunity of their enforced exile.[42] No other southern resort in the first half of the nineteenth century was so thoroughly given over to the demands of sickness.

Like Madeira, Pau had an established British colony at the start of the Victorian period, but it was of recent formation. Lord Selkirk (1771–1820), the first British invalid known to have wintered at Pau in 1819–20, was only there because of a delay in reaching his intended final destination, Valencia in Spain; twenty years later the choice of Pau as a winter resort was so obvious to Mrs Elllis, recording her journey and residence in 1839–41 for her husband's pulmonary illness, that she did not trouble to explain the decision to her readers. The permanent British residents were already heavily outnumbered during the season by winter visitors, many of whom were health-seekers, and invalids in every stage of illness were conspicuous in the parks and terraces of the town.[43] Pau was no longer the primitive backwater of Lord Selkirk's day, according to Dr Taylor, when 'there was not a house with a carpet, not a carriage to be hired … and not a trottoir in any of the streets'.[44] Pau was not however a sophisticated resort in the 1840s. Taylor might remark on the improvements in the accommodations, streets and amenities that had occurred in the recent past, that had made Pau a town fit for fashionable society, but the writer Louisa Costello, who visited in 1842–3, would not have recognized Taylor's portrayal: 'The less a visitor sees of the town of Pau and the more of the mountains, and *coteaux*, and streams, the less likely is he to be dissatisfied with a residence in this most favoured and misrepresented of all ugly towns', she wrote; she assumed that the resident expatriates must be 'Irish, Scotch or from some distant country towns in England', and thus 'unused to London or Paris', to be content with the lack of amenities.[45] It seems clear however that Taylor's vision was a surer guide to the future, for by the 1850s 'the amount of bustling traffic' in the streets might astonish 'those who expected to find themselves in a mountain town, sighing for the comforts of civilized life', according to Frederick Johnson, while the shops sold 'anything which caprice, comfort, luxury or fashion could require'.[46]

There were two winter destinations in south-east France that might offer equivalent climatic benefits as Nice without the risks associated with living in a busy town. The long-standing reputation of Hyères, a couple of miles inland east of Toulon, as a health resort withstood the reaction against other southern French destinations such as Marseilles and Montpellier that set in after the Napoleonic hiatus. The reason for such durability is a little difficult to understand since British published opinion in the first half of the century was distinctly lukewarm. James Clark in 1820 considered Hyères's winter winds and meagre accommodation ruled it out for consumptive patients.[47] Ten years later he damned it with faint praise as 'the least exceptionable residence for the pulmonary invalid in Provence'; the scenery and vegetation were delightful, and the climate the mildest in south-eastern France, but still fatally compromised by the mistral.[48] Murray was not a fan, considering Hyères 'too much cried up', with 'little beauty in its situation'.[49] Edwin Lee thought Hyères inferior to Nice as the latter was at least partially protected from the mistral by the Maritime Alps.[50]

The other French resort that might provide an alternative to Nice was Cannes, only a day's journey by foot to the south-west and almost the last settlement on the coast before the Italian frontier. Cannes had many natural advantages but virtually no accommodation suitable for discerning visitors before the later 1830s. When Sir Herbert Taylor and family stayed in 1837, at the suggestion of Lord Brougham, Cannes's most notable British resident, hotel and rental facilities were so inadequate that Taylor ended by buying a plot of land to build his own house: 'With the exception of the Rue du Port', he wrote, 'which is open to the sea, Cannes is wretchedly built. The streets are crooked, narrow, dirty and ill-paved, the shops without any appearance, and the houses divested of any regard for comfort.' Already two new hotels were under construction however.[51] Murray's first handbook was more positive, describing Cannes as a 'neat and cheerful small town, finely situated in a mountainous country at the bottom of a beautiful bay'.[52] In 1851 Edwin Lee predicted that Cannes would become a serious competitor to Nice once the accommodations were brought up to scratch.[53] The 1850s seems to have been the decade of take-off as a destination for over-wintering invalids, when a resident British physician, Dr Whiteley, arrived and those other essentials of Victorian expatriate society, an Anglican church and a Scottish Presbyterian chapel, were built by British residents.[54]

## New resorts for old

Spain did not have any significant role as a health destination in the first half of the nineteenth century. It formed no part of James Clark's cognitive landscape of comparative climatology, and there was no place for the Iberian peninsula in *Bradshaw's Companion to the Continent* (1851). It was not however terra incognita for Britons, loaded as it was with historical and cultural associations, quite apart from important commercial and political ties. The 'discovery' of Spain as a health destination in the 1850s was clearly assisted by improved transport options, especially rail links to the south of France and beyond, as well as better connections by sea. Perhaps more important however was the opportunity it seemed to offer for alternative sites for winter expatriation for pulmonary patients, just at the time when dissatisfaction with the traditional destinations was building. The first British medical authority to pay attention to Spain was D. J. T. Francis, who spent three winters there in the early 1850s. His *Change of Climate* (1853) presented Malaga as almost a model resort for consumptives, with a January temperature like London in May or Rome in April, little variation in temperature from day to day or between day and night, and just enough moisture in the atmosphere to ensure comfort. It offered, he hoped, the sort of balanced conditions that patients struggled to find elsewhere, where resorts were either too sedative and oppressive (Madeira) or too tonic and exciting (Nice).[55]

Perhaps suddenly conscious of having neglected an emerging locus of medical climatology, Edwin Lee spent the autumn of 1853 travelling in Spain and the following year published *Notes on Spain*, a work that followed his usual format of combining therapeutic with touristic guidance but with particular emphasis on Malaga.[56] His object however seems to have been not so much to expand his range as to resist the claims made for an insurgent resort, for as he wrote in his preface, 'as regards the choice of winter residence for an invalid, it was not the climate alone which should be considered' but other 'accessory circumstances' that writers on climate often overlooked.[57] Sure enough Malaga was still 'greatly deficient' in accommodation for visitors, and there were many other objections.[58] Spain duly made no appearance in *Bradshaw's Invalid's Companion* in 1861. The British consul had boasted that Malaga had 'the two finest hotels in Spain for Englishmen', the Almeda and Victoria, as well as 'comfortable, well-furnished appartments for winter invalids', and possessed the only Anglican chaplaincy in the country.[59] But after a brief surge in popularity in the late 1850s there is evidence of a subsequent waning of interest. The chaplaincy trustees in the 1860s frequently lamented the decline in winter visitor numbers and its impact on chaplaincy finances.[60] A later visitor expressed surprise that Malaga should attract as many invalids as it did 'when there were so many more attractive places in Spain and elsewhere'.[61]

The other western Mediterranean resort that came into focus during the 1850s was Algiers. The French colonial authorities were in the process of turning this Arab port into a model European city, at least superficially, and Dr Francis, who visited as part of his Spanish tour, was suitably impressed: 'There was perhaps less of what was English in Gibraltar, than of what was French in Algiers', he observed.[62] Francis considered the climate of Algiers, which was similar to Malaga's, eminently suitable for consumptive patients and other chest cases, although there were as yet no British health visitors. Unlike Malaga, there was no settled British community, no resident British physician or clergyman and consequently no familiar social and cultural matrix to receive compatriots. The British consul struggled to appoint a vice-consul in 1851 as he only knew one other British resident, an elderly doctor who lived in the hinterland.[63] Prospective British invalids would therefore have to be prepared for a thoroughly French experience, with a dash of Arab exoticism and all that entailed. On the other hand access to Algiers was relatively easy, with an efficient maritime connection with Marseilles – Algiers was easier and quicker to reach than southern Italy or Spain. In 1862 the requirement for passports was abolished, making a visit to Algiers hardly more difficult for Britons than a visit to metropolitan France.[64] By this date a resident British community had grown up, chiefly associated with infrastructure development in the booming port. In 1868 the British consul reported an expatriate population of two hundred, presumably excluding temporary visitors.[65] However, Algiers never experienced even the brief surge in popularity enjoyed by Malaga. Unlike Madeira, its climate was not deemed sufficiently distinct to encourage development of a sense of exceptionalism, and those few Britons who relished immersion in a French cultural milieu could find the real thing closer to home.

It was not on Spain or North Africa that British invalids increasingly bestowed their favours after 1860 but on the new resorts of the Riviera. Nice was already a large town by this date, with a population approaching fifty thousand. The risks of living in a densely populated location, with carriages raising clouds of dust in the streets and the seductions of dinner parties, dancing and late nights, encouraged a search for alternative winter stations. As we have seen, the Cimiez suburb inland from Nice was originally developed for invalids who needed shelter from wind, but it was also usefully remote from the bright lights. Cecil Monro, a consumptive patient wintering at Cimiez in 1868–9, was safely removed from the fast lane of life down in Nice, where the disgraceful antics of the Duke of Hamilton, fined by the police following an altercation at the races and challenged by officials on departure when trying to smuggle an additional 'lady' into his railway carriage, were merely noises off.[66] The smaller settlements along the Riviera suffered like Nice old town from primitive sanitation. The invalid Lord Harrington always took the same route from his hotel at Cannes on his carriage rides to avoid 'the very unpleasant smell of the town'.[67] East of Nice, however, at Menton and San Remo, for example, human 'manure' was harvested for the olive groves, which reduced offensive smells, provided one steered clear of the peasant women transporting their cargo up the slopes.[68] Indeed the development of new resorts along the coast from the 1860s can be seen in part as a flight from contamination, a process that began with the creation of the Croix de Marbre suburb of Nice itself. The threat was not just cloacal. The monotony of existence in the smaller resorts away from Nice noted by many visitors was the necessary condition for optimizing the health benefits of winter expatriation, according to specialists.

The role of Dr James Henry Bennet (1816–1891) in the promotion of Menton as a health resort mirrored that of Dr Taylor at Pau. Both were influential in advocating for their adopted sanatorium over several decades, but neither created their chosen resort from scratch. As we have seen with Pau, Menton already hosted a sizeable British expatriate population when Dr Bennet arrived. Edwin Lee had recommended Menton to 'those who required tranquillity and a mild climate, and possessed their own resources' in his 1851 edition of *Bradshaw's Companion*, but in 1858 could still claim that the place was 'not much frequented by invalids'.[69] It was however evidently favoured by enough compatriots to have impressed Augustus Hare, author of the first English-language guidebook to Menton, with their villas in the surrounding hills, and it seems clear that the local economy was already heavily reliant on letting apartments to winter visitors, with transactions facilitated by a British agent, Mr Willoughby.[70] Many of these visitors were 'real invalids, rather glad to escape from the gaieties of Nice',[71] a town that by 1860 reminded Hare of Paris, with its river quays, boulevards and stone houses.[72] Despite its tranquillity Menton was not an obviously suitable resort for invalids because food supplies were poor, carriage hire expensive and a railway connection not completed till 1869. Bennet arrived in 1859 as an invalid himself – 'the harassing labours and cares of a London professional life had broken down vital powers' – and after exploring other potential sites in Italy the following season, returned to Menton 'determined to wander no more, and to adopt Mentone as a permanent winter residence'.[73] Soon afterwards he published his favourable review of Menton's climatic and other health benefits in the *Lancet*, reprinted in book form as *Mentone and the Riviera as a Winter Climate* in 1861. The book had three further editions under variant titles and was also translated into German.

Nowhere between Nice and Genoa had much in the way of tourist infrastructure before the middle of the nineteenth century. Moreover, Bennet himself had dismissed the prospects of the coast east of Menton as most of the settlements were built at the mouths of rivers, whose valleys provided a conduit for the wind.[74] The site of San Remo was an exception to this topographical generalization. In 1860 Augustus Hare thought San Remo had potential as a winter resort but had 'not yet been reached by many of the English comforts which [might then] be obtained at Mentone'.[75] According to Bennet, the international frontier marked a boundary not only between two states but between a relatively developed coastline geared to visitors and a zone where the inhabitants 'ignored entirely the multitudinous wants and requirements of [his] difficult-to-please countrymen'.[76] San Remo was the first of the Italian Riviera towns to address this perceived deficiency. A bronchitic invalid who spent the winter of 1857–8 with his family at San Remo, having rejected Menton as too expensive, described an unspoilt and welcoming paradise in a letter to the *Times* but urged his readers to grasp the opportunity while it lasted.[77] An early proselytist for San Remo was a pulmonary patient, W. B. Aspinall, who spent two winters there between 1863 and 1865, having tried several other resorts, including Madeira and Nice. According to Aspinall, San Remo shared the best climatic points of Nice and Menton without their corresponding disadvantages. It enjoyed the protection of encircling mountains like Menton but was less claustrophobic and more invigorating. It was largely free of wind and dust and enjoyed plenty of shade so that he envisaged a potential future as a year-round destination. Although there were already several hotels, as an international resort the place was still in its infancy. Aspinall considered this an advantage: it could be 'modelled into anything', he wrote; 'if an English company would take the whole affair in hand now, it might, at a comparatively light expense, be made at once into the favourite winter residence of the Mediterranean'.[78]

Although Aspinall's fond hope of development under a British monopoly did not come to pass, San Remo nonetheless evolved into a resort that suited British tastes, almost as surely as did Cannes, Menton or Pau. By the end of the 1860s an Anglican church had been built, the shopkeepers were beginning to understand a little English and a British chemist was in the offing. There were already three resident British physicians, one of whom, Dr Rose, who doubled as British vice-consul, had plans to turn his suburban villa, 'Woodlands', into a summer refuge for invalids who did not wish to return home at the end of the season.[79] William Chambers found in 1869 'a dirty, old-fashioned Italian town, which had not even got the length of gas-lighting'.[80] Ten years later San Remo had been transformed, according to Edward Sparks: instead of two there were now nine or ten first-class hotels, besides sixty to seventy villas for rent and several pensions; the place was better paved and the shops were as good as Menton's, even rivalling those of Cannes. San Remo was now also connected by rail to both Genoa and Nice. Unsurprisingly San Remo had become as expensive as Menton and Cannes in consequence, but at least the villas tended to be more modest in size than Menton's and therefore more affordable.[81] Dr Sparks was a little more open-minded as to San Remo's deficiencies than Aspinall had been. The climate was not perfect, as the winds in spring could be very 'rough and unpleasant' and the mistral, rare at Menton, was certainly not uncommon during the winter. At the same time, although San Remo had less rainfall than Menton, its clay soil retained moisture, an obvious drawback for patients. As for facilities for invalids, San Remo lacked a town promenade, and although there were many pleasant walks in the olive groves and donkey excursions in the hills available, there were few carriage roads.[82]

## Trouble in paradise

The rapid development of the Riviera resorts from the 1860s risked undermining the virginal qualities that had attracted foreign visitors to them in the first place. This tendency had been anticipated at Pau, the first continental health resort to undergo a steep increase in visitor numbers earlier in the century. It was all very well for a small number of wealthy foreigners to rough it in an unsophisticated backwater, safe in the knowledge that they could escape to a suburban villa to evade noxious smells and the threat of miasmatic disease, quite another to contemplate a season in a busy hotel or apartment block with rudimentary sanitation overlooking an open sewer. Frederick Johnson, a great admirer of Pau as a health resort, nevertheless admitted that 'the crying evil of the place was the defective arrangements of its sewerage and drainage. The *cloacae* (sewers) were little better than huge cesspools contained in a narrow space left between adjoining houses'.[83]

In September 1858 an unnamed British doctor wrote to the *Times* to announce that he was having doubts about recommending Pau to his patients owing to inadequate sanitary arrangements, as well as high prices. Dr Taylor mounted a stout defence:

> Although Pau will not stand comparison with an English town subjected to a proper system of drainage, still it even now takes rank with most towns on the Continent of the same size on the score of cleanliness. Twenty years ago there were few English in Pau. The houses were badly furnished, no carpets, no *cabinets à l'anglaise* (water closets), no carriage to hire, and not a single yard of foot pavement. Since then 340 houses have been built and furnished with *luxe* and there are *cabinets inodores* (odourless toilets) in almost all of them. There are trottoirs to all the streets; fifty to sixty carriages are to be hired at a moderate rate.

The anonymous doctor's complaint arose from an unusually dry winter season in 1857–8, which deprived the town of its natural drainage, according to Taylor.[84] The geologist and author Elizabeth Carne (1817–1873), who spent the early months of 1859 at Pau, warned against lodging in certain localities in case of offensive smells but added that the open ditch that ran through the middle of town and took the bulk of its refuse was in process of being covered over by the municipality.[85] British complaints about Pau's inadequate drainage fell away after 1860, probably owing to this and other improvements inaugurated by the new mayor elected in that year.[86]

At Menton, the unspoilt hideaway discovered by Dr Bennet and Augustus Hare did not survive the consequences of their advocacy for long. As at Pau a decade earlier, complaints soon arose around those two predictable gravamina of the British visitor experience, prices and stinks. A correspondent brought both together in a letter to the *Times* in June 1868, which attempted to put the authorities of Menton on notice that they risked losing their lucrative invalid trade if they did not reform: prices were not only as high or higher than at Cannes and Nice but even exceeded those at the German spas, while the stench from the cesspits was not to be borne. At Pau such unwelcome exposure in the British press had been countered by Dr Taylor; at Menton the Anglican chaplain Revd Morgan stepped into the breach, ensuring readers and prospective visitors that the June letter, translated into French, had galvanized the local authorities into action: a medical officer had been appointed, a new water supply was planned and a regime of rubbish collection organized for the hotels and pensions along the seashore, hitherto obliged to toss their refuse into the sea.[87]

The cesspits endured but do not seem to have held Menton back. By the 1880s disagreeable smells that 'assaulted the nostrils at every turn' were still a nuisance but not a health menace, according to the visiting British doctor Alfred Drysdale, who claimed Menton was largely free of the threat of typhoid because it had resisted the 'English system' of drainage. The latter was unsuited to the Riviera because it relied on an uninterrupted flow of water to flush faecal matter through the pipes. At Nice by contrast, where English-style sewerage had been introduced, typhoid was on the rise among visitors.[88] The problem was really one of the British visitor's own making, according to a correspondent in the *Times*: 'The sudden accumulation of thousands of English, with their fastidious taste and their wasteful ways, has produced everywhere a problem very hard to deal with', the writer contended; 'we find it hard at our own watering places, where a tidal sea, a shore abounding in streams and a very regular rainfall are at least very great helps'.[89]

The most serious public health crisis arising from unregulated development occurred at Cannes. By the late 1860s Cannes was in the midst of a building boom. The Anglican chaplain reported breathlessly on the hotel expansion underway in June 1868: 'The Beau Site … was being doubled, a new wing [was under construction] at the Pavaillon, a third floor at the Europe, a fresh hotel in front of the Provence.'[90] Cannes soon acquired an unwanted reputation for bad drains. William Miller noticed the sewage outflows near the bathing establishments at Cannes, which must he felt have health consequences,[91] and Cook duly warned intending bathers to 'avoid those stations which were situated near the outfall of the town drainage'.[92] At length a typhoid scare in 1882 led to an enquiry by the British engineer Douglas Galton (1822–1899).[93] His report ascribed Cannes's problems to the building of villas and hotels on the outskirts of the town 'without regularity, and without much care as to the relative positions of the houses, or as to their interference with the wants of neighbouring houses'; consequently 'the fouled water which had been used in villas and hotels at high levels … often found its way into and polluted the subsoil of a neighbour on a lower level'.[94] Although the human waste of the old town was removed manually, the suburban villas and hotels had cesspits that were 'a continual source of danger, difficulty and expense – the retention of a large amount of fecal matter in a putrefying condition in close proximity to houses was most dangerous'.[95]

Galton's recommendations called for the construction of public sewers for receiving domestic wastewater and the gradual elimination of cesspits in favour of mains sewerage, as well as a system of dry refuse collection currently entirely lacking in the suburbs. The pitfalls of the 'English system' identified by Drysdale would be avoided by excluding rainwater from the domestic drainage arrangements, thereby enabling the use of much smaller pipes with consequently faster flow and regular flushing. A new sewer outfall into the sea was already planned by the municipality. By the time Cook's 1893 handbook was published, Cannes 'was well kept, in a sanitary point of view, thanks to a splendid supply of water and a good system of drainage'.[96]

## Winter visitor numbers and profile

Nobody in the nineteenth century knew how many British people wintered abroad. Passports were not required to leave or re-enter the country, and no government agency had any interest in monitoring the traffic. The local authorities in the several destinations that received visitors increasingly attempted to collect and publish statistics, chiefly in the interests of resort promotion, but methodologies differed, and many visitors were excluded or conversely double-counted. Travellers moved about and were likely to be recorded at different resorts during a single season or even re-registered on return to the same place. Local British consuls or other expatriate residents sometimes provided estimates of visitor numbers to the Foreign Office, but they were typically vague and, one suspects, often inflated in the interests of trying to justify a salary increase or government funding for a new church. The best we can hope for from such unpromising raw material is to get a sense of the trajectory in the popularity and relative importance of individual resorts, as well as of the contribution of British people to overall visitor numbers.

If reliable gross numbers are unattainable, it is even more difficult to estimate the proportion of visitors who were invalids. Thomas Madden wrote in the mid-1860s that 'it had been calculated that between seven and eight thousand English invalids … annually spent the winter in the south in pursuit of health'.[97] He gave no source for the claim, which had disappeared twelve years later when he issued his revised work on health resorts, suggesting no very firm foundation for the calculation. Even if remotely accurate, the figure must have been intended to comprise not only patients but their accompanying families and travelling companions as well. Few invalids travelled alone, and it would have been impossible to isolate the patient proportion in any visitor population, however reliably calculated. Only two things can be said with any confidence about overall British invalid numbers – that they increased over the course of the century while at the same time they fell as a proportion of all nationalities.

John Pemble reckoned that Italy received some 5,000 British visitors per annum in the mid-1830s, rising to perhaps double that number fifty years later.[98] How many were invalids is unknowable. At the beginning of the Victorian period the only Italian destination that was first and foremost a health resort was Nice, at that date as we have seen still beyond the French frontier. The Anglican chaplain there reported in 1835 that 'from seventy to 100 English families' wintered there every year, a figure that would represent a total British visitor population in the low to mid-hundreds. The rise in subscriptions for church sittings over the following two and a half decades gives some indication of the growth in visitor numbers: some 63 individuals subscribed in 1837, just over 100 in 1845, about 200 in 1855 and nearly 300 by 1861.[99] The early 1860s seem to have marked a peak in such subscriptions, evidence perhaps of the increasing attraction of rival resorts such as Cannes and Menton in later years. Dr Sparks estimated the annual number of winter visitors at Cannes at about 3,000 at the end of the 1870s, of whom between 500 and 750 families were British (so perhaps between 50 and 75 per cent of the whole), and about 300 British winter visitors to Hyères.[100]

The municipal authorities at Menton collected visitor statistics which British commentators were able to consult. Sparks noted the rise in foreign visitor numbers registered every 15 March – deemed the height of the season – from 14 families in 1856 to 2,180 in 1879; there were 449 families in 1866, 594 in 1870 and after a temporary dip as a result of the Franco-Prussian War a sharp rise to 1,067 families in 1872, coinciding with completion of the rail link between Nice and Genoa. There was also a noteworthy step up between 1878 (1,331 families) and 1879 (2,184 families).[101] Sparks did not give a breakdown by nationality for most of this period, perhaps because it was not compiled by his source, but he did have access to separate statistics for different nationalities for 1876 to 1879; these give the number of 'English' families as 621, 481, 543 and 839 successively,[102] equivalent to perhaps from about 1,500 to 2,500 individuals, roughly the same as British visitor numbers at Pau at the same period. The number of Britons at San Remo was between two and three hundred in 1869 according to a contemporary witness.[103] This may have been an exaggeration as about a decade later the municipality recorded only some seventy British families in residence, representing 167 individuals.[104] Although it is clear that the majority of visitors to the smaller resorts of the Riviera in the 1850s and 1860s were health-seekers, if not genuine invalids, the visibility of the sick declined markedly within a few years. Dr Bennet observed as early as 1870 that 'sun-worshippers' easily outnumbered invalids at Menton, and he predicted that like Nice before it Menton's character as an invalid asylum would be overwhelmed by the influx of healthy 'idlers'.[105]

Madeira was unique among health resorts in posing few problems to recording accurate visitor statistics. There was only one entry point to the island, and all British arrivals seem to have been regularly registered by the consul. British visitors to Madeira numbered perhaps 200 a year in the late 1830s, rising to an average of about 350 during the later 1840s and a peak of 430 in the winter of 1851.[106] For the remainder of the 1850s numbers hovered around 300 a year, apart from 1856 when they dipped to 126 as a result of the Madeira cholera epidemic of that year.[107] Although it is clear that only a proportion of visitors were invalids, it is reasonable to assume that the great majority, at least of those who stayed for more than a week or two, were part of the wider invalid community – family members, nurses and domestics and so on. Invalid statistics acquired by James Clark for the period 1838–40 indicate that 182 British consumptive patients arrived on the island during the two seasons up to mid-1840,[108] which would imply that perhaps half the visitors at that time were patients. A writer in 1859 noted that half of the three hundred or so annual visitors were friends and relatives of the sick, which confirms a fifty-fifty split between patients and companions.[109] British visitor numbers declined in the 1860s[110] as alternative destinations closer to home, such as Menton and San Remo, became available, and doubts about the therapeutic efficacy of Madeira's climate gained strength.

Such adverse factors did not impact Pau's popularity in the same way. The municipal authorities at Pau began compiling foreign visitor statistics in 1844. These show a rise from about 700 per annum to some 1,500 in 1854 and about 2,500 in 1870. The British proportion was about a quarter in 1844, rising to about a half in 1853 and two-thirds by 1858, the apogee of their dominance of the winter influx.[111] From the 1860s the British contribution declined according to Pierre Tucoo-Chala, even though absolute numbers continued to rise. The British vice-consul claimed in 1869 that 'the floating British population' of Pau – that is to say seasonal visitors – for the previous two years was 2,000, clearly an overestimate driven by his attempt to justify the salary for which he was petitioning.[112] A more reliable figure for the 1860s is the 1,162 individuals recorded by the Anglican chaplain for the winter of 1865–6.[113] The proportion who were patients is impossible to gauge. Clearly Dr Thorowgood's claim, citing Alexander Taylor, that Pau received about 2,000 'English' invalids per annum, mostly consumptive, is nonsense.[114] The ratio was obviously much less than the 50 per cent that seems to have obtained in Madeira, since Pau was not merely a sanatorium. As the century advanced even this proportion must have declined as Pau's appeal to invalids increasingly gave way to its attractions as a social and sporting resort.[115]

The number of British winter visitors to Malaga and Algiers never approached the figures for Pau, Madeira or the northern Mediterranean resorts. A visitor in the early 1850s reported that 'four hundred English' were wintering at Malaga for their health, a figure that was certainly a gross exaggeration but indicative nonetheless of increasing popularity.[116] There is some evidence that following a brief flush of enthusiasm, which was presumably responsible for the British consul's complaint that invalids were turning Malaga into a second Madeira, numbers settled down to manageable proportions; he himself reported in 1855 that the usual permanent church congregation of about a hundred was increased to only 180 by winter visitors.[117] At Algiers, it seems clear that visitor numbers remained small, 'not more than fifty or sixty at the very utmost', according to a contemporary witness.[118]

Wintering abroad was never a preoccupation of more than a small minority of the British population. Despite the overall increase in numbers over the century, the expense and time required to support months of winter expatriation restricted its appeal to a relatively shallow pool of prospective exiles: 'The bulk of the colonists are people well to do, who can afford the expense of a winter away from home and of a villa at £150 the season', wrote the historian John Richard Green (1837–1883) of the British expatriates on the Riviera.[119] There was however a growing professional and commercial class in Britain in the nineteenth century, for many of whom foreign travel became as unexceptional as seeking rest and recreation at home, and an increasing tendency for the sick of relatively modest means to see winter abroad as a desirable and realistic means to better health; as Scoresby-Jackson observed in 1862, 'people looked forward to the season when they "went away" to have their mental and physical condition re-invigorated, after nine or ten months of constant toil, [and] invalids too – real invalids – travelled much more than in former times, when the wealthy alone could enjoy the privilege'.[120]

Popular perceptions of the Riviera and Pau make much of the supposed aristocratic stamp of these resorts in the nineteenth century, but in reality the bulk of British visitors were from the middle and upper-middle classes – especially so among the invalid population – and, moreover, individual destinations varied considerably in social flavour. An analysis of the winter visitors to Pau in 1844–5 shows that almost half were from the rentier class or retired, 20 per cent were serving military types and 14 per cent were 'nobility'; in short, according to Tucoo-Chala, the core were middle or upper-middle class.[121] The list of British temporary visitors given in the *Liste des Etrangers* of 1867 seems to broadly confirm this pattern.[122] Nevertheless there was evidently an increase in wealth over time, if not necessarily in social status. The travel writer Henry Blackburn reported in 1867 that 'houses in good situations were let for £200 for the winter season', some four times the rate of thirty years previously.[123] He went on to retail the words of an old resident: 'These thriving millionaires, these *rentiers*, oppress us', his informant grumbled; 'where they come from noone knows; they bring their families, their servants, their horses, and surround themselves with every luxury and comfort, and are to their poorer neighbours like a blight on the land'.[124]

According to J. R. Green, Menton had acquired a distinctly clerical feel by the 1870s: 'The bankrupt element of Boulogne, the half-pay element of Dinan or Avranches is as rare on the Riviera as the loungers who rejoice in the many changing toilets of Arcachon or Biarritz', he declared; 'the humdrum tone of the parson best harmonises with the winter resort and parsons of all sorts abound there'.[125] In fact all the lesser resorts of the Riviera seem to have had their clerical moment at one time or another: Cannes was especially attractive to religious types in the 1850s, according to Margaret Brewster, and had a corresponding reputation for respectability and early nights.[126] The mantle was assumed by Menton as Cannes evolved into a pleasure resort and eventually inherited by San Remo, which was a safer distance from the gaming tables of Monte Carlo.[127] Dr Sparks, writing in the mid-1870s, 'had heard it whispered … that San Remo was rather dull, that dances and lawn tennis were hard to meet with, and that prayer meetings were largely in vogue at some hotels'.[128] Clergy and invalids from clerical families also seem to have been prominent among winter visitors to Madeira. The surviving burial registers for the British cemetery at Funchal provide a serviceable proxy for the complexion of Madeira's invalid population during our period since they are both complete, from 1836 onwards, and give enough personal information about the deceased to enable a fairly confident assignation of visitor status. Fifty out of about 390 visitor burials between 1836 and 1880 (12.75 per cent) relate to clergy or members of clerical families. More broadly something between a quarter and a third of all burials relate to members of the professional classes (clergy, military and naval, medical and legal). There are very few entries for members of titled families.

The gender balance among winter expatriates is difficult to gauge because the visitor statistics we have almost never give breakdowns by sex. It is reasonable to assume that the female proportion of the expatriate invalid population grew over time as travel difficulties eased and facilities and comforts improved. In 1820 James Clark had warned that 'all the inconveniences of travelling fell with double severity' on females.[129] Even healthy women travelling alone or without male companions on the Continent in the first half of the nineteenth century were regarded as eccentric – 'unprotected' in contemporary jargon – and could be objects of curious comment.[130] There was a widespread perception that females were differentially susceptible to consumption, which in other circumstances might have encouraged medical consultants and family members to contemplate a winter in the south for their female patients more readily.[131] This supposed susceptibility was a handy prop for everyone with an opinion on female education, habits and dress to hang their own pet theory: for Revd Edward Davies, wintering in Algiers in 1857, the problem lay in 'the evil of busks and tight corsettes'.[132] Reluctance on the part of female patients themselves, or their carers, to contemplate expatriation was still apparently differentially depressing numbers on the Riviera in the 1870s, despite improved communications: female consumptive patients were significantly outnumbered by male according to Dr Sparks, who ascribed this to their difficulties in travelling; they were also more likely to be hopeless cases, suggesting a hesitancy about leaving home before becoming seriously ill.[133]

There was also a view that females were more prone to certain types of nervous complaint and might therefore benefit particularly from the diversion afforded by continental travel: Edwin Lee described a species of hysteria that typically struck young women between the ages of fifteen and thirty-five, which was brought on but also potentially alleviated by 'moral and mental impression'.[134] Sparks thought the exciting climate of the western Riviera unsuited to nervous cases: he had treated 'cases of hysterical convulsions, hysterical vomiting, nervous headache, insomnia, and neuralgia in females, generally from eighteen to twenty-five years old'.[135] Opponents of winter expatriation naturally had no difficulty in using the supposed susceptibility of females to nervous derangement as an additional reason for keeping them at home: 'Hysterical women should never be sent on tour … without great caution', warned Thomas Chambers, 'or a travelling medical man with them.'[136] The only resort where we have any reliable clue as to gender balance of invalids is Madeira, where the burial records mentioned above show a female ratio of about one in four in the 1840s, rising to perhaps one in three in the following two decades. Madeira however was not a typical resort; not only was it more difficult to reach than almost all others, but also it really only catered for pulmonary cases. It seems likely that the invalid gender balance at the more accessible resorts was closer to fifty-fifty, by the second half of the century at least, especially if we include spas.

Children were often associated with women in the category of delicate invalids, and suitable resorts and therapies recommended accordingly. Thus the equable climate of Pau was especially favourable to the weaker constitutions of women and children according to Dr Taylor, and sea bathing indicated for 'delicate women and girls', in the opinion of the spa authority John Macpherson.[137] Children often accompanied families with an invalid member to the Continent, but they were rarely patients themselves before the teenage years, for obvious reasons. Once into their teens however young people seem to have been despatched to the south with some frequency. Fanny Blathwayt encountered two English brothers aged thirteen and fourteen at Pau, one an invalid under Taylor's care, who had been sent out for the winter accompanied only by a maid.[138] It was more common of course to travel with a senior family member, as in the case of Charles Marling, whose first winter in Madeira at age sixteen was shared with his mother.[139]

Madeira's invalid population seems to have been remarkably young, presumably because it specialized in pulmonary cases, who were typically patients in early adulthood. Over 50 per cent of recorded burials of British visitors between 1836 and 1880 were for deaths under thirty, including almost 12 per cent in their teens. The gender balance among teenaged burials was close to fifty-fifty, consonant with the common contemporary observation that consumption typically struck females at a younger age than males.[140] Other resorts had a quite different invalid demographic by mid-century. Nice gradually lost its pulmonary invalids, so that by 1858 Margaret Brewster, musing among the classical remains at Cimiez, could wonder what the Romans would have made of the current fame of their colony as a 'shelter [for] John Bull's rheumatic gout'.[141] Pulmonary cases migrated to Cannes, Menton and San Remo, leaving Nice with a mixed invalid population whose stereotypical representative was, as Brewster implies, a gentleman of mature years burdened by the infirmities of age. In due course the latter resorts went the same way, in an easterly progression, driven by multiple factors, from the ease of access and departure to the impact of overdevelopment, and perhaps the secular decline in the incidence of pulmonary consumption.

Some sense of the differences in the invalid demographic at various resorts can be gleaned from comparing death notices in the *Times*. During the twenty-five years, 1860–84, that covered Menton's heyday as an asylum for pulmonary patients, some twenty-six of forty-nine notices of deaths at Menton that specified age were for individuals in their twenties and thirties, 53 per cent; the corresponding figure for Cannes for the same period was 35 per cent. Conversely only 14 per cent of Menton's deaths were in the over-sixties (all of them after 1875), compared with almost 30 per cent of Cannes's. Here then we get some intimation of the predominant character of Menton's invalid population under the presiding superintendence of Dr Bennet. Cannes by contrast had already become a place of general refuge, distinguished more by the social status and wealth of its invalid residents and visitors than by their medical profile. By the later 1870s the presence of genuine invalids, menaced by a potentially fatal disease, seems to have become so diluted as to be scarcely visible.

## Summer at the spas

Heading south for winter commanded the attention of climatotherapists and dominated discourse on the benefits or otherwise of travelling for health, but the majority of British tourists who crossed the Channel in the Victorian period, as today, did so in summer. Even those who could be classed as health-seekers were probably more likely to be found heading for a summer spa cure than a winter south of the Alps, until the very end of the century at least. Spa visiting was big business in early-nineteenth-century England, and there was a large potential British clientele for continental watering places, which were much more numerous and varied than those available at home. Before the mid-1830s the only continental spas known to any but a small handful of Britons were a scattering of long-established historic watering places that lay for the most part astride the well-worn tourist trail to the Rhine and southwards towards Switzerland. There were many more mineral springs accessible from the Rhine than these few, but as Sir Francis Head observed, Britons were like locusts, 'they ... were found either eating up a foreign country, or not one of them was to be seen there'.[142]

Spa, near Liège in Belgium, was a resort the English had visited from as early as the sixteenth century, and as soon as the Napoleonic hiatus was over Britons resumed their place as the town's most populous and visible foreign residents.[143] Spa was not of course German, but its location on the route to the Rhine valley meant that it was often included in surveys of the Rhineland mineral springs and indeed regularly visited by British spa-goers travelling to and from that region. By the early Victorian period Spa was still attracting Britons – especially those who wintered at Brussels – but it is clear that its popularity was waning as improving communications drew more and more travellers further south.[144] Spa water was chalybeate, recommended for anaemia and other conditions of general debility, but its action was very similar to the water of Schwalbach, a coming resort near Wiesbaden, that was as reassuringly dull as Spa was racy, so patients and their advisors had a ready-made alternative at no great distance.

The closest German spa to England, Aachen (Aix-la-Chapelle) in the kingdom of Prussia, was also one of the most well-appointed and versatile. The bath facilities were luxurious, bathing in the hot spring water as well as drinking were available, and the establishment was open all year round. The water was sulphurous – unusual for a German watering place – but also contained a quantity of salt, so it was deemed suitable for a wide range of ailments. British people had been visiting the spa at Aachen for centuries, but at the opening of the Victorian period it faced the challenge of newly accessible and recently advertised resorts further south. Aachen was also a town-centre spa, so visitors without an overriding interest in pursuing the cure no doubt missed the scenic and recreational advantages of more sequestered locations. Although gambling flourished and Aachen was by no means an iatrocratic resort where medical superintendence exercised its baleful influence, the place was nevertheless an invalid's spa, in contrast with the more hedonistic Wiesbaden and especially Baden Baden further south. Wilkie Collins visited in 1863 for his 'rheumatic gout' on the recommendation of an experienced spa-goer. He enjoyed his stay: there was no stinting on the good things of life, and his regime was by no means arduous – a tumbler of sulphurous water before breakfast, brought to his bed by his German courier, and a regular douche in the afternoon.[145] By this date the spa was recommended especially for rheumatism and skin problems. Later it developed a specialism in syphilis.[146]

Bad Ems, in the independent duchy of Nassau, close to Koblenz in the scenic valley of one of the Rhine tributaries, had an established reputation for treating respiratory illness with its mild alkaline waters and also provided specialist gynecological treatments, especially for perceived sterility in women, by means of its dedicated fertility spring, the Bubenquelle. In the late 1860s it was still the 'most popular women's bath in Europe' according to John Macpherson.[147] British visitor numbers rose from 272 in 1830 to 833 in 1846, before falling away to a figure in a range of between about 450 and 600 a year in the later 1850s and early 1860s. Numbers were at their highest on either side of the Franco-Prussian War, reaching a peak of 979 in 1869, at a time when Ems was at the height of its popularity, but fell back to the high five hundreds by the mid-1870s.[148] Bad Ems tended to attract a high-class clientele: visitors during 1846 for instance included the earls and countesses of Chichester, Fingal and Northesk, the marquesses of Ely and Londonderry, and the viscountess Hereford.[149] The proportion of British curists who were female rose steadily from about a quarter in 1830 to about a half by the end of our period, though by this date Ems was attracting barely half the number of British guests of a decade before.[150]

Nearby Schwalbach also offered treatment for women's complaints, principally 'chlorosis' or languid anaemia in girls, but its chalybeate waters were generally recommended for cases of debility in both sexes. Schlangenbad, the 'beautifying' spa puffed by Sir Francis Head, maintained its reputation for treating skin complaints, though by the 1860s it chiefly attracted 'hysterical ladies, and ladies suffering from functional derangement of the uterine system'.[151] The evidence we have for the female contribution to British numbers at Schwalbach and Schlangenbad suggests a rough equivalence with Ems for the former and a somewhat higher proportion for the latter, but the evidence is difficult to interpret, and moreover there are no available numbers for the post-1845 period.[152]

Spa, Aachen and Ems had been well known to British spa-goers for decades or more. Knowledge of more remote locations in Germany was, as we have seen, largely the work of Augustus Granville. After a brief flirtation with Wildbad, Dr Granville returned to his usual summer residence at Kissingen, where from the late 1830s till 1868 he regularly advised British patients during the summer season, many of whom had been referred from his London practice. Kissingen, in the far north of the kingdom of Bavaria, was not particularly accessible to Britons before a railway connection was made in the 1870s, so there is no doubt that Granville's active advocacy and presence were responsible for its sudden popularity with British patients. Its springs produced cool, relatively mild saline waters used mainly for drinking, but the resort was also well known for its salt and mud baths. Kissingen also benefitted from a secluded, scenic location and just enough royal patronage to supply a dose of social cachet.

By 1846 Granville had accumulated details of some 700 British cases at Kissingen since 1837, representing a substantial proportion of the British patient population. He categorized the cases into four broad groups of ailments relating to the stomach, nerves, women and the skin, of which the first three were the largest. The most frequent single complaints were constipation (seventy-nine cases) and frequent miscarriage (ninety-three cases), but there was a wide range of other conditions, from 'general debility' to acne, from which it is clear that most patients who came to Granville's notice in London were probably deemed suitable cases for treatment at the spa. Naturally most were reported 'cured'.[153] It is likely that the British presence at Kissingen was never more prominent than when Granville was in his pomp in the 1840s. Surviving evidence of British visitor numbers in subsequent decades suggests an annual total of something below five hundred, a little lower than British numbers at Bad Ems.[154] By 1868 Granville had been consulted by the majority of the 5,400 British patients who had visited Kissingen since 1840, according to his autobiography, a figure that represented just under 17 per cent of the 32,000 patients registered by the bath authorities during the same period. By this date he claimed the spa's fame rested largely on its success in treating female complaints.[155] The proportion of British curists who were female by

1868 might have been about the same as that at Ems – something approaching 40 per cent – but the evidence is meagre. It seems fairly clear however that the proportion rose significantly between the 1840s and 1870s.[156]

Homburg, in the small independent state of Hesse-Homburg, north of Frankfurt, was exceptional among Rhineland spas in being a largely new creation designed to exploit the burgeoning tourist trade of the region. Granville was characteristically sniffy about springs of such obviously parvenu origins: 'The Germans were too fond of discovering mineral waters, where only a little dirty water, with kitchen salt, and some iron and steel, were present', he grumbled. He was especially indignant when Sir Alexander Downie, physician to the British legation at Frankfurt, who began to spend the season at Homburg, compared its Elisabeth source with the famous Rakoczy spring at Kissingen.[157] The Homburg waters, which were comparatively cold, were anyway insufficient to provide much in the way of baths. It was therefore as a drinking spa that Homburg made its name. The main mineral constituent of its principal springs was common salt, and their chief therapeutic value was tonic, valuable for all sorts of congestive complaints from gout to constipation. However, as Dr Prytherch, a resident English physician, assured a visiting medical colleague, chemical constituents alone were unable to account for the differing effects of mineral waters.[158]

The proportion of British water drinkers at Homburg was small in these early years: the author of *A Hot-Water Cure* noticed few fellow countrymen at the table d'hôte of the Hessischer Hof hotel in 1844 among the visiting Germans, French and Russians.[159] Overall visitor numbers in this year were 3,222, according to the official *Kurlisten*, of which the British proportion was about 6 per cent. Homburg subsequently developed into one the most fashionable spas in Europe: by the mid-1860s it probably ranked behind only Baden Baden and Wiesbaden among German spas in popularity.[160] British numbers seem to have overtaken those for Bad Ems in the early 1850s, rising to between three and four times as many by the early 1860s. However, Granville need not have worried about the challenge to Kissingen. Although the chemical constituents of the chief springs in both resorts were similar, the tone of the two places rapidly diverged: Kissingen remained a comparatively dull backwater dominated by the routines of invalidity while at Homburg 'you had leading statemen and capitalists meeting all the black-legs in Europe'.[161]

The number of British visitors to Wildbad may have fallen away a little after the boost provided by Granville's *Spas of Germany* in the late 1830s. Ann Vavasour noted that many British patients had been turned away by the local physicians when she was there, having arrived with unrealistic expectations of cure.[162] Edwin Lee certainly considered his rival's purple prose was tantamount to a deception on the public: Wildbad 'was a mean-looking town in one of the most sombre valleys of the Black Forest', he claimed, 'and offered little or no resources for amusement'. Besides, there was nothing special about the spa water, which was simply thermal, with little chemical content.[163] Wildbad water indeed held no magic powers, but despite this the resort prospered without Granville's continued advocacy. Improved facilities and communication with the outside world, allied to its temperate summer climate and beautiful scenery, provided enough assistance to convert it into the leading German spa for rheumatoid arthritis and a range of other disabling conditions of the joints. Visitor numbers remained modest – 4,782 in 1860 for example, about the same as Schwalbach.[164] Macpherson considered that it had 'almost everything that could recommend a place to the English', but the proportion of British curists is unknown.[165] Wilkie Collins arrived in May 1863, after about four weeks at Aachen. The contrast was marked: not only was the water utterly different but also the place was full of hobbling invalids – 'the only place in which he had not had his felt shoes well stared at'. After a course of twenty-eight baths he returned to London, somewhat more mobile, but perhaps still unable to put on his boots.[166]

It was generally acknowledged in the early Victorian period that French spas did not measure up to German ones in accommodation, facilities or cultural and social attractions. Most of them lay far from the international tourist routes, catered for an exclusively French clientele and made few concessions to English comforts. There was no equivalent in France of the mass influx of Britons to resorts such as Ems or Schwalbach that briefly turned some of the hotels in these places into homes from home for the visitors. Society therefore was unlikely to be much of a draw, especially as, according to Edwin Lee, the French 'associated very little with those whom they had not previously known', an accusation more commonly levelled at the English.[167] Other attractions were required to lure Britons to such unprepossessing places. One was the quality of the waters – the possibility of encountering springs that promised a different therapeutic action from the familiar sources of the Rhineland. Another was scenery. Happily the French Pyrenees fulfilled both criteria.

There was a long history of British exploration of the Pyrenees, reflected in the travel literature: 'The largest group of Pyrenean travel writers came neither from France nor Spain, but from Great Britain', according to a recent authority.[168] Ann Lister was only the most famous of these early British mountaineers. In addition, the Pyrenees contained the most important group of sulphur springs in Western Europe. There was little clarity about exactly what special property sulphurous waters offered the invalid, but at a time when trial and error was the order of the day, there were obvious advantages in having access to springs whose chemical composition differed significantly from most of the Rhineland sources. Alexander Taylor, sounding a little like Dr Granville, claimed a mysterious quality for sulphurous waters that was nevertheless so ephemeral that it was lost by 'agitation, transport and cooling'; consequently the water only had medicinal value at source.[169] This did not prevent however some 50,000 bottles of Eaux Bonnes water from being exported every year.[170] At the same time, the Pyrenean waters were by no means all identical in their action, and like many specialists Taylor regretted the tendency of patients and their advisors to treat them indiscriminately. For instance, Bagnères-de-Bigorre had simple thermal springs for the most part, unlikely to be of much therapeutic benefit alone, but being at a lower altitude the place could be a useful first stop, preparatory to exposure to the stronger, sulphurous springs in the high mountains.[171]

Although every French spa was supervised by a government-appointed director to whom prospective curists needed to apply for appointments at the baths, visitor statistics are elusive, and we usually have impressions rather than tabulated numbers. Most British commentators remarked on the relative scarcity of fellow countrymen at the Pyrenean spas, which were heavily dominated by French and Spanish guests. Eaux Bonnes, the closest spa to Pau, was fashionable as it attracted relatively wealthy visitors and refugees from that place. Its waters, which were largely taken by drinking rather than bathing, were indicated for chronic chest complaints, but its attraction for Britons probably lay more in its cool summer temperatures than the quality of its springs. Taylor quoted a figure of about 2,800 patients taking the waters in 1840, but the British proportion was small, certainly compared with the

Rhineland spas at the same date.[172] At the height of its popularity Eaux Bonnes probably attracted no more than 250 Britons annually: there were 228 in 1861, falling to 129 by 1870 – barely a quarter of the number of British visitors to Kissingen at the same date, despite being a resort of similar size.[173] The decline probably reflects the secular change in the profile of British winter visitors at Pau. Eaux Bonnes was one of those half-dozen formerly significant French spas that saw overall numbers decline in the second half of the nineteenth century as the social attractions of places like Bagnères-de-Bigorre, Luchon and Vichy drew off the fashionable crowd.[174] Like nearby Eaux Chaudes, a simpler sort of place recommended for rheumatism, sciatica and troublesome old wounds, Eaux Bonnes remained primarily a therapeutic resort.

Bagnères-de-Bigorre, lower in altitude than the other resorts, was deemed to have a sedative climate like Pau's. It was larger than the high mountain spas, with more facilities and consequently a pleasant place to stay, but its mild, saline waters, principally recommended for digestive complaints, offered little that could not be found at a spa such as Baden Baden or Bath for that matter.[175] The author Charles Weld praised the 'bathing-rooms and marble baths in the *Thermes* … which possessed all the advantages of a German *Kursaal*, excepting the very disgraceful "Hell", which, greatly to the credit of the French government, was no longer a plague-spot at the spas of France'.[176] Bagnères was the only Pyrenean resort that betrayed much evidence of an English cultural stamp in the style of Pau. Henry Blackburn remarked:

> It is curious to find the English language spoken continually, to hear the click of croquet … to see cricket bats and to be asked in English at the shops if we would buy any Pale Ale. On Sunday morning at the little English church, at the Club, and even in the streets, we might almost fancy ourselves in a country town in England, so familiar and so frequent are the signs of our nationality everywhere.[177]

Cauterets was in Dr Taylor's opinion the most useful spa in the Pyrenees and the one to which he directed more of his patients at Pau than any other. Its principal source, the Raillère, was the most famous spring in the region. The waters were powerful and sometimes mixed with milk to modify their strength, depending on the patient's condition. Like the waters of Eaux Bonnes they were recommended chiefly for respiratory complaints, although Taylor warned that they were likewise useless – indeed positively injurious – in cases of advanced phthisis.[178]

Away from the Pyrenees, British presence at French spas was less visible before the second half of the nineteenth century. Most were difficult to reach before the French railway network – a relatively late-developer in Western Europe – was in place; facilities and social attractions were wanting; and after 1837 gambling was outlawed in French casinos.[179] Unsurprisingly, the numbers of even French curists were low, many Parisians favouring the fashionable Rhineland resorts, which also attracted many visitors from eastern France for reasons of geographical proximity. Vichy, in central France and eventually the country's most popular spa, had just under 7,000 visitors by 1850, roughly the same as Carlsbad or Homburg, but considerably below Wiesbaden or Baden Baden. In the second half of the century Vichy picked up speed; by 1860 it had overtaken Homburg and Carlsbad, and by 1880 was one of the two or three most visited spas in Europe.[180] Before mid-century Vichy was very French: 'We should not, in speaking of Vichy to a friend', explained an anonymous contributor to *Blackwood's Magazine* in 1846, 'ever designate it as a comfortable resort for a family.'[181] Guests put up at second-rate boarding houses and took their meals 'in public', sniffed Murray.[182] The simple alkaline waters were principally indicated for digestive complaints – in the words of Hilary Bonham-Carter, visiting in 1850, it was 'cause [*sic*] of their stomachs and livers that people went there'.[183]

By 1866 still only just under 8 per cent of Vichy's visitors were foreigners, but easily the largest component of these (almost 40 per cent) were British.[184] By 1870 Vichy had an English pharmacy and Anglican services were held in the French Protestant church.[185] But even as more and more Britons came their proportion remained small: the 632 registered British curists in 1866 represented just over 3 per cent of all visitors,[186] not much more than the ratio at Carlsbad and far below that at Ems, Homburg or Kissingen. Murray's handbook reported a figure of 2,000 Britons out of a total visitor population of 28,000 in 1878 – a ratio of 7 per cent, above Kissingen's 5 per cent but still significantly below Homburg's 18 per cent.[187]

The critical factor that turned the tide for French spas as far as British visitors were concerned was the gentrification that progressively modernized them in the second half of the nineteenth century, especially under Napoleon

III.[188] The distance they had to travel to meet the fastidious demands of both British visitors and increasingly those of other nations as well is exemplified by the assurance from Vichy's inspector of mineral water in 1850 that butchers were now prohibited from leaving animal blood, excrement and other rubbish in the streets, farmers had to remove manure, and privies had to be dug and covered.[189] John Macpherson's description of the bath facilities at Plombières in the Vosges – the so-called *Bains Napoléon* – would have been unrecognizible to Edwin Lee.[190] Once French facilities could compete with German the contest for the British pound resolved itself into one of cultural preference as much as therapeutic calculation. After three weeks at Plombières in August 1873, the novelist George Eliot (1819–1880) announced that she was 'in love with the mode of life at the *Eaux* of France, as greatly preferable to the ways of the German *Bad*'.[191] The choice between German and French became more binary after 1870, as French curists largely abandoned the German spas, and Imperial Germany progressively set its stamp on the formerly intermediate Rhineland zone.

## Conclusion

Multiple factors governed the differential appeal of continental health resorts to British visitors, of which their therapeutic promise was only one. The burgeoning advice literature by doctors attended primarily to the climatic advantages of the southern resorts and the medicinal qualities of continental mineral springs, but this advice was frequently opaque, often mutually contradictory, and sometimes suspected of partiality. Besides, health-seekers – especially those whose invalidity demanded the elimination of any unnecessary risk – required more than mere medical advice. They were of course far from indifferent to climatic conditions and the therapeutic action of spa waters, but such considerations alone hardly provided a sufficient basis on which to found satisfactory plans for long-term expatriation. Prospective travellers sought information on routes to the south, accommodation options, availability of provisions and medical services, social conditions and facilities, indeed every conceivable aspect of life that could impinge on the invalid's comfort and prospects for recovery. Medical writers understood that patients needed more than just climatic data and therapeutic injunctions, but hard as they often tried to engage the wider interests of their readers they were rarely able to rise to the occasion. It is surely telling that the only clear evidence we have of publications having an immediate and significant influence on the British patient's choice of resort relates to two works by gifted writers – Granville and Head – whose lively prose contrasts with the turgid output of so much literature for the invalid market.

Drs Taylor and Bennet were undoubtedly influential propagandists for their own resorts, but they were to a large degree preaching to the converted. Neither was essential to the popularity of Pau and Menton, respectively, which had already established a significant reputation with British visitors before the arrival of their celebrated publicists. Like Granville at Kissingen, their ability to propagandize in print and then directly supervise patients on the spot created a closed system that paid handsome dividends to them, if not necessarily to their patients. Each was feted by the municipal authorities of their respective resorts, so their importance in attracting visitors was clearly recognized locally. But to suggest that either was instrumental in creating their favoured resort would be to overstate their role. Rather they rode the wave of visitor preference and fashion, moulding it where they could, defending the reputation of their resorts when necessary, but ultimately the beneficiaries rather than the determinants of patient choice. There is little evidence that patients paid much heed to professional injunctions regarding appropriate destinations, if only because such directions often contradicted one another. Decisions were made largely on the basis of personal and family experience and the recommendations of fellow sufferers. The climatological and therapeutic landscape of the Continent was bafflingly complex and invalids seemed instinctively to understand that pretentions to expertise in such circumstances invited the mockery of disappointed outcomes.

3

# Travelling

## Preparations

It is remarkable that in the early Victorian period families would often head off across Europe with a sick member but no clear idea of their ultimate destination. Published information about hotels and other lodgings was scanty, and even when it became more widely available with the appearance of Murray's handbooks and other guides, the practice of writing to book in advance was slow to catch on.[1] Families relied heavily on word-of-mouth recommendation and the good offices of acquaintances on the spot. Uncertainty about where they would stay did not however mean that travellers were careless of risk. On the contrary it probably only increased their dedication to elaborate preparations for their journey and residence abroad. Invalids were naturally more likely to be among those contemplating extended expatriation, but when travel to resorts was laborious and British medicines and other necessities difficult to obtain, it made sense to create an inventory of desiderata that would usefully serve the needs of patients and healthy tourists alike. Mariana Starke's long catalogue of travelling articles is a case in point, being 'things most requisite for an invalid, and indeed for every family to be provided with on leaving England'. Items ranged from sheets and bedding, to cutlery and napkins, pistols and temporary door locks, kettle and teapot, medicine chest and an array of drugs, with printed dispensary and basic apparatus for preparing medicines, toiletries and more. Mrs Starke's elaborate recommendations were additionally motivated by a desire to make the traveller self-sufficient, for she distrusted foreign couriers; 'I would counsel those who travel by land to dispense with so troublesome a domestic', she advised, 'whose place may always be supplied by a good post-book, some knowledge of French, and an honest active man-servant who understands the management of carriages'. Indeed 'the lower class of Italians always formed a league to pillage travellers'.[2]

In later editions of her guide Starke modified her excoriation of foreign servants to some degree, but there was no reduction in the length of her list of requisites. By the early Victorian period, however, her injunctions were starting to look distinctly out of date. There was no need to travel with such a carriage train of 'necessities', according to Edwin Lee – a large medicine chest, for instance, was surplus to requirements, 'as almost all drugs and medicines of good quality could be obtained in all the towns frequented by invalids'. He suggested a stripped-down inventory comprising a pair of leather sheets to guard against damp beds, a small medicine chest containing essentials for emergencies, and above all black tea, 'one of the most useful articles travellers could be provided with, as it was seldom good in small towns or at inns on the road'.[3] He also recommended that patients with respiratory problems should bring a Jeffrey's respirator, a piece of apparatus newly available for Victorian travellers.[4] This breathing aid was evidently sorely missed by Charles Marling, a sixteen-year-old consumptive patient in Madeira in 1853: 'be sure to bring a respirator for Charlie', his mother urged her husband as they discussed plans for his journey to meet them; 'we needed one on the voyage out and he is more tender now'.[5]

In contrast to Starke, Lee recommended hiring a courier 'to avoid the delays at post-stations, frontiers etc., and to have apartments at the hotels ready prepared'.[6] Couriers could be hired at any stage of the journey but were probably most likely to be engaged at the beginning when the departing traveller needed maximum reassurance. An early-nineteenth century contract for services with a French *voiturier* (coachman for hire) attached to the White Bear Inn, Piccadilly, documenting an agreement to convey a British family from Calais to Nice for £190, for a journey of twenty-three or twenty-four days, survives in the London Metropolitan Archives.[7] The traveller Selina Bunbury thought in the 1840s that couriers were on the way out: 'the glorious days of couriers are nearly over', she announced; 'the English have taught so many people to speak their language … that these polyglot gentlemen are much less in demand'.[8] But couriers were not mere interpreters but factotums. By mid-century courier services, like many other aspects of continental tourist infrastructure, were increasingly mediated through agents: Wilkie Collins hired a German courier through Coutts agency for his visit to Aachen and Wildbad in 1863.[9] The need for such assistance diminished as travel became more regular and predictable, and guidebooks proliferated later in the century. When we hear about them it is usually when they have been found wanting in some way. Cecil Monro heard about two English ladies who arrived to book in at the Hotel d'Ecosse at Menton in December 1866 on the recommendation of an acquaintance of their courier, only to find the same man serving as one of the hotel's waiters. They left almost immediately.[10] Dr Charles Sewell, travelling with his invalid wife in the Pyrenees in 1882, was accompanied by a courier called Horn – presumably an Englishman – but he was useless, and they dispensed with his services at Bagnères-de-Bigorre, subsequently getting on much better without him.[11]

Travellers to the south usually had to make part of their journey by road, even after extensive rail links were developed. Earlier in the century, when continental railways were non-existent or at most largely confined to Belgium and central Europe, British families of means often shipped their own carriage across the Channel, relying on the continental system of posting to provide horses and postilions. Mrs Starke was especially prescriptive about carriages: she recommended a 'strong English carriage, hung rather low, with well-seasoned corded jack-springs, iron axle-trees, and *sous-soupentes* (underside storage cradles) of rope covered with leather'. This was merely the prelude to a host of directions for fitting out the carriage for continental travel, from pitching the underside to make it waterproof to how to fix trunks to the outside of the vehicle to ensure they were stable. Above all everything had to be locked down, with a 'patent chain and padlock for every outside package', and an inviolable cabin. She recommended the coachmaker, Savage, of Queen Street, Long Acre, for the work of fitting out a carriage at a reasonable price. She thought a second-hand carriage preferable to a brand-new one. Technological development is reflected in her recommendation of 'carriages without perches, invented by Elliot [*sic*] and Holbrook, Westminster Road, [which] were particularly well calculated for the Continent, from being suspended on springs without leather (which was a perishable commodity in warm climates); and likewise from being less liable to overturn than were carriages with perches'.[12]

Edwin Lee recommended Turrills of Long Acre for reliable carriages adapted for continental conditions, with a britscka or post-chaise the most suitable designs, particularly for the unforgiving paved roads of France and Belgium.[13] These however had a relatively modest carrying capacity, and British families were notorious for travelling on the Continent with large establishments. The sight of a British household on the move was a standard subject of amused comment. James Johnson's omnibus collided on the bridge at Nice with 'a huge English berline, stuffed, like Noah's Ark, with numerous bipeds and quadrupeds – with parroquets, pug-dogs, ladies' maids, and lazy footmen – together with a quantity of luggage that must have gladdened the heart of every custom-house officer between Dover and Nice'.[14] Hilary Bonham-Carter described the view from her bedroom window at Vichy that greeted her and her companion in July 1850, as a British party arrived: 'we pop out our two heads … to see a Leviathan carriage, covered with maids, couriers, and hat boxes, sweep with five horses into the town', she reported to her mother; 'out tumble two small babies, each with a nurse. These must be English', she concluded.[15] Only the English and Russians journeyed across Europe in such large, heavy carriages, according to Ann Vavasour, although the latter were abandoning them as you could not see out of the windows.[16]

According to James Clark, the best time to leave England for the south was in either early June or early September: 'In setting out at the former period [the invalid] may pass the summer in Germany or Switzerland', he suggested, while 'in September the summer heat will be avoided', for 'the proper time for entering Italy is the end of September or early in October'.[17] The meteorological risks associated with delay in leaving for Italy are brought home in family correspondence. The Baring family, heading for Nice, took the Mont Cenis pass across the Alps in October 1839, intending then to drop directly south to recross the mountains via the Col de Tende. Travelling in their own carriage, heavy rain and the crush of other vehicles slowed their progress south from Geneva. A broken bridge rendered the Tende road impassable so they ended up taking a long, uncomfortable diversion via Genoa and the coast road.[18] The apparently last-minute decision by Joanna Bonham-Carter, travelling home through Switzerland, to despatch her children to Nice for the winter in late October 1843 meant that their first task on arrival was to dry out their wet things as their carriage had been inundated in crossing the Durance.[19] The Fox Talbot family, heading for the Riviera from Switzerland in early October 1867, were trapped by a vicious snowstorm at Berne before they could escape south.[20]

Once the storm relented, the Fox Talbots could at least reach their destination by rail via Lyons and Marseilles. The ease of travel to the Riviera provided by the rail connection that advanced relentlessly down the Rhone valley and through Provence during the 1850s and 1860s increasingly rendered warnings about late departure redundant. On the contrary, Dr Bennet urged his readers not to try to reach Menton before the end of October, as that month was apt to be both hot and humid; he still chose to warn invalids to ensure they got across the Esterel massif before the end of October, however, as at the time of writing the railway still only reached Vidauban.[21]

Just as the railway largely eliminated the Alpine barrier from consideration by prospective invalid travellers to the Riviera, it marginalized the maritime route to Pau. In the early 1840s Alexander Taylor had recommended travelling to Pau by first sailing to Bordeaux, urging a departure not later than 1 September, not only to avoid the danger of autumn gales but also to ensure the best chance of securing good, south-facing apartments, a necessity for patients.[22] Even so early a departure was no guarantee of a comfortable sea passage however: Elizabeth Grant and her family took three days to sail from Southampton to Bordeaux in August 1843 in the small paddle-steamer *Calpe*, which was badly knocked about in the Channel.[23] Only the most devoted disciple of the therapeutic value of sea voyages would continue to approach the Pyrenees through the Bay of Biscay once the railway from Paris to Bordeaux was completed in 1853.

The moment of decision by a patient to leave home is usually hidden from us. Medical consultations are rarely documented and surviving correspondence and diaries notably reticent on clinical matters. Even if not 'ordered south' by his medical consultant, one assumes most patients took medical advice in deciding on treatment abroad, even if they did not necessarily defer to their advisor's choice of destination. There seems to have been some patient scepticism around the qualifications of consultants at home to advise on suitable destinations. Elizabeth Carne criticized the tendency of doctors in England to recommend a favourite health resort regardless of the individual patient's constitution: 'why are first-rate physicians openly quoted as a "Malaga", or "Nice", or "Pau", or "Madeira" doctor?', she protested; 'no one place can possibly suit all cases'. She advised relying on common sense rather than the pronouncements of doctors at home who were afraid to admit their ignorance.[24] Cecil Monro, by 1868 an experienced winter fugitive, objected to a young locum presuming to advise him where to go, 'just as if he had been Walshe or Sir James Clark'.[25] Depreciation of professional ignorance was not confined to patients. Dr Taylor sighed that 'English physicians practising at Pau, Nice, Rome, Naples etc. had patients directed to their care, suffering from maladies which were of the staple of the climate to which they were sent, which were *par excellence* there engendered and which must of consequence have been aggravated by it'.[26]

Patients were urged to obtain a medical case history before travel to facilitate their care abroad. This requirement was deemed especially important if the invalid intended to visit mineral springs, where professional guidance was an essential part of the cure. No spa physician would be in a position to advise a patient appropriately without a statement of his case. How many patients took this advice to heart is doubtful. Besides, there was no substitute for local expertise. Dr Taylor remarked on the absurdity of patients turning up at Pau 'with a plan of treatment all cut and dry' from their doctor at home, which they expected to be carried out without modification.[27]

## Routes

James Clark did not attempt to instruct his readers on the best routes to Italy, presumably because they were already well served by guidebooks, not least Mrs Starke's. She recommended the itinerary via Dijon, Switzerland and the Simplon Pass to Milan if travelling in summer or autumn, despite the alarming lack of parapet walls on the road through the Jura that put a premium on a coachman's skills. However, the Simplon was 'by far the safest and most sheltered' of all the Alpine passes, while the more popular Mont Cenis was liable to avalanches. By the early Victorian years two alternative routes had become available, the first from eastern Switzerland via the Splügen Pass to Milan and the second along the Riviera coast via Nice and Genoa. The Splügen was only practicable in July, August and September, and the new coast road was considerably longer than the Mont Cenis route while suffering additionally from a lack of parapets, despite being 'at the brink of tremendous precipices'.[28] This road was in short 'by no means formed on the

Napoleonic scale' but was safe enough for travellers with 'a careful driver and quiet horses'.[29] It was a slow route however, as every mountain torrent that reached the sea between Nice and Genoa had to be forded. James Johnson encountered a huge English carriage stuck in the riverbed at Port Maurizio; he advised travellers, particularly invalids, to dismount at river crossings and take the footbridge or if the river was in spate to simply wait before attempting to ford.[30] The British preference for large vehicles was an obvious disadvantage on narrow, mountainous roads: Ann Vavasour regretted her choice of carriage when crossing the Splügen Pass in September 1840 – two light vehicles pulled by a pair of horses would have served better.[31]

There were several ways to reach the Riviera from Britain before the completion of the rail link between Paris and Marseilles in the mid-1850s, which effectively funnelled almost all travellers down a single route. The most popular approach was via Burgundy to Lyons, from where the Rhone valley provided a natural, navigable corridor for river traffic to Avignon, where passengers normally disembarked to travel across Provence by road. Even before steam was introduced on the river in the 1820s water transport seems to have been preferred to the road, which according to Mrs Starke was frequently in bad condition.[32] The boats were drawn by horses and tended to put into shore as soon as a stiff breeze arose, so progress could be painfully slow. Although the craft had no cabin on board apart from a rudimentary shelter, passengers would usually travel on their own or in a public vehicle lashed to the deck. Overnight stops were made at waterside inns. The wind and poor quality of inns meant the river route was unsuitable for invalids, according to Clark.[33] The first part of the route to be supplanted by rail was the stretch between Avignon and Marseilles, completed in 1849.[34] By 1856 the entire line from Paris to Marseilles was open, reducing minimum journey times to eighteen hours.[35] Once the railway was available the Rhone became a conduit dedicated to merchandise. Margaret Brewster decided to travel by river rather than rail in October 1856, thinking 'it would be a pleasant variety as the weather was fine' but found it slow, dirty and uncomfortable. She disembarked at Pont St Esprit and made the remainder of the journey by train.[36]

Although it was possible to sail to Nice from Marseilles, most travellers heading for the Riviera went overland via Aix-en-Provence. The road seems to have filled some British commentators with horror, characterized as it was for many by ugly, arid scenery and sometimes despicable inns. The journey from Aix to Nice took about twenty hours by public conveyance, according to Edwin Lee, or an easy two days by private carriage.[37] All travellers seemed to agree that from Fréjus onwards the scenery was beautiful – 'the true garden of Provence' according to Murray[38] – the grim preamble perhaps even emphasizing the impression of the Riviera as a promised land. The railway reached Nice in 1864 (five hours from Marseilles) and Menton in 1869. Notwithstanding advertised minimum times, a journey from Paris would normally last some twenty-eight or nine hours at an unimpressive average speed of about twenty-four miles an hour because even expresses stopped for refreshment breaks. Non-express trains of course were slower.[39] In the meantime the Italian section of the line advanced westwards from Genoa to meet the French, connection being achieved in 1872. The line was not trouble-free. Floods in early 1872 brought down a bridge between Cannes and Nice causing multiple fatalities and leading the *Times* to announce that the bridge over the Var 'was not safe and another disaster might occur at any hour'.[40] Although the accident was reported with horror by Britons on the spot and ghoulishly depicted in the *Illustrated London News*, there is no evidence that it had any impact on British visitor numbers.[41] The opening of the Mont Cenis tunnel in 1871 offered an alternative approach to the Riviera by rail, via Turin, which was a little cheaper for travellers to the Italian resorts, according to Dr Sparks, but relatively slow between Turin and the coast and consequently perhaps less suitable for invalids.[42]

Getting to Pau from England before significant rail links were established usually required a journey of the best part of a week, often longer. As we have seen, Taylor at first recommended the maritime route via Bordeaux: 'The journey is thus performed in four or five days without much fatigue', he declared, 'which if made by land would occupy ten or twelve days.' An additional two or three days were needed for the final leg from Bordeaux to Pau.[43] At this date (1842) the only part of the journey from London that could practicably be made by rail was the first stage to the Channel ports or Southampton. Taylor's estimate of the length of the overland journey was based on travel in easy stages appropriate to a delicate patient; a healthy person could make the journey much more quickly, as indeed could an invalid if he chose to travel by *malle poste* – the equivalent of an English mail coach.[44] Most travellers however journeyed south by *diligence* – the gigantic, heavy omnibus that so amused British visitors – either for reasons of economy or the difficulty of securing a place in the less capacious mail coach, which only took two or three passengers. Private carriages do not seem to have been used much by British travellers to Pau, perhaps because of the scarcity of the sort of convenient river routes that eased the journey to south-east France and Italy.

Systematic extension of rail links south of Paris from 1840 steadily reduced the length of road to be negotiated by coach. By the time Frederick Johnson made the journey to Pau in 1855, the entire route from the Channel to Dax, on the Bordeaux-Bayonne line, could be made by rail, leaving only a final six-hour ordeal by *diligence* to his destination.[45] According to Taylor, writing in 1856, the journey from Boulogne to Pau could by then be accomplished in about thirty hours of actual travelling, leaving the amount of stopping time en route to the discretion of the traveller.[46] By 1863 the line to Pau was complete, and it was consequently possible to travel from Britain to the Pyrenees entirely by rail, with the obvious interruption of the Channel crossing. In 1865 the invalid Fanny Blathwayt anticipated the arrival at Pau of a party of unaccompanied English schoolboys, including her son, for the Christmas holidays. The journey now took only thirty-six hours.[47] By 1867, when Henry Blackburn visited, the *diligence* had become a thing of nostalgic recollection – a contrivance that, however uncomfortable, had given the traveller a supposed connection with the land and its people that rail had obliterated.[48]

Visiting the Rhineland spas usually involved an approach by river. In the 1830s it was common to travel by water for the entire route from the Thames via Rotterdam to Koblenz or the area of Wiesbaden, taking advantage of steamboats or *Dampschiffe* on the Rhine, 'one of the great pavés of the world', in the words of Sir Francis Head.[49] In addition to foot passengers, steamboats carried private carriages. As the Belgian and Prussian railway networks developed in the following decade, this long river route was abandoned by most, but as there was no rail link along the Rhine between Bonn and Wiesbaden until the later 1850s an element of river transport remained an integral part of the package for most visitors, who had not come to Germany only to miss out on its most celebrated tourist attraction. As a traveller explained on returning from Wiesbaden in the 1850s, 'what you gained by steaming rather than posting was seeing those picturesque old towns at the water's edge'.[50] Even after rail was available travellers often preferred a Rhine steamer for the Cologne to Wiesbaden section, though probably few regretted saying farewell to the two-day tedious haul from Rotterdam to Cologne along what was generally agreed to be the dullest stretch of the river.

The rail route through Belgium remained the most popular approach to the Rhine for Britons from the 1840s onwards. The journey from Ostend to Cologne took about thirteen hours.[51] A traveller heading for Wiesbaden in 1849 reported meeting only two Englishmen en route through northern France – had he been travelling 'by the main route he should have seen scores'.[52] Once Calais was connected to the Belgian rail network via Lille in 1848 it became the natural port of disembarkation for British spa-goers, particularly those anxious to minimize seasickness: the crossing from Dover to Calais usually took no more than two hours, compared with five to Ostend. Just as Henry Blackburn lamented the demise of the *diligence*, lumbering through the Landes of south-west France, Thomas Madden thought speed had deprived British travellers to the Rhine of any meaningful contact with Belgium, 'the best governed, and most prosperous, as well as most interesting country in Europe'.

> They take a through ticket from Victoria or Charing Cross to Cologne, enter a first-class carriage at either of these places, are whisked to Dover at a rate of sixty miles an hour, rush on board the steamer, and after forty minutes of misery find themselves in Calais, spend ten minutes in the refreshment room, and are again whirled away through the darkness of night, to Cologne, where they arrive, jaded and fatigued, in nineteen hours from the time they left London.[53]

Once well into Germany however, the pace of travel generally slowed, by necessity as much as choice – no country on the Continent was so 'gridironed' by railways as Belgium. German railways provided Britons with ample opportunity to indulge their fondness for mockery of foreign officialdom. Murray considered 'many of the German rules and regulations … in the highest degree cumbrous, frivolous, vexatious and useless', especially those relating to luggage.[54] Although Britons never got used to German officiousness, the bother of passports eased later in the century. By the 1860s Belgium had ceased to require passports, and German officials rarely demanded them.[55] Madden and his companion crossed several frontiers on their way from London to

Carlsbad in the mid-1860s but had their passports examined for the first time only at the Austrian border.[56]

## Travel for invalids

In the early Victorian period much of the advice to visitors about how to manage their health during their journey was equally applicable to healthy and invalid travellers. Edwin Lee urged his readers to avoid too much meat en route, as it generated heat and flushing, and to limit themselves to a cold evening meal with tea to encourage a good night's sleep. He also advised travellers to ensure regular exercise on the journey by dismounting at post-stations to walk about or even climb the hills on foot when their carriage was labouring up the incline.[57] In his 'directions for invalids making a change of climate', James Clark counselled prospective travellers to guard against overexcitement and concomitant overheating on the journey by various interventions before, during and after travel, such as rest periods, tepid bathing, mild laxatives, even bleeding, to ensure the maintenance of equilibrium. A light diet and avoidance of stimulants were prescribed. Furthermore, the journey was not an ordeal to be accomplished as quickly as possible: 'An invalid can scarcely have too much time for his journey', Clark advised, 'inasmuch as, if conducted with judgement and made at the proper season, it will be more beneficial to his health the more time it occupies, within reasonable limits.'[58]

This was all very well for travellers with their own comfortable carriage, but *diligence* travel, in which the invalid shared a cramped compartment or sat atop a ponderous vehicle moving barely above walking pace, did not encourage such insouciance. *Diligence* travel was especially burdensome in Italy and Spain, according to Dr Francis, because of the likely distances between stops and the poor quality of the roads.[59] But it was bad enough anywhere: 'Nothing knocks me up so much as those long *diligence* journeys', Cecil Monro confided to his father from Milan as he contemplated his return home in May 1860; to shorten the journey he intended to make his way over one of the high Alpine passes, 'walking the most mountainous piece in the middle'. In the event he took the *diligence* via the St Gothard to Luzern, where he arrived 'with cold feet, hot head, burning face and eyes'. His pedestrian plan seems to have been scuppered by the snow – it took three hours for the *diligence* to cross the pass on sledges.[60]

Rail travel increasingly relegated tales of *diligence* misery and frightful inns to the past, but the promise of speed was not an unmixed blessing for invalids. National frontiers, haphazard development of the network and new and unfamiliar arrangements for dealing with luggage, refreshments and other practical matters meant that rail travel could be anything but restful, while at no stage did it offer the autonomy or flexibility of travel by private carriage or hired *voiturier*. Moreover, the increase in speed over road and river transport was more gradual than sudden. The journey from London via Antwerp or Ostend to Mainz still took about sixty hours in the early 1840s, according to a contemporary, only a day's saving of time over the route via Rotterdam.[61] Dr Granville continued to recommend the 'water route' for delicate invalids heading for Kissingen rather than try to reach the spa by rail:

> What with passports and examination of baggage on landing [at Ostend or Antwerp], and again on crossing the frontier between Belgium and Prussia; what with the changing and shifting of trains, and the constant fear of missing them, of getting into the wrong one, or of losing your luggage; what with the flies and the omnibuses that are required to convey you from one terminus to another, or from the landing to the terminus; the trouble, the vexation, the constant worry and bustle, are truly disheartening and not likely to suit invalids.

He calculated that the rail route via Antwerp required ten changes of mode of transport for his putative invalid, while the water route needed only one, from cross-Channel steamer to river steamer at Rotterdam. It was also slightly cheaper.[62]

As a man of an earlier generation, Granville was never reconciled to railways, but to avoid them entirely in travelling to Kissingen would have been eccentric in the extreme by the time Mrs Louisa Wilmot Campbell, wife of Colin Minton Campbell, joint owner of the Minton pottery company in Stoke-on-Trent, headed there for a cure in 1866. She left London at 7.25 am on 29 May 1866, crossed to Calais after some delay caused by a mechanical breakdown and only reached Brussels at 9.00 pm. She rested at the Hotel de Flandres for two nights, bookending a day of shopping and sightseeing, then took a train to Koblenz at 9.20 am on 31 May, arriving at 7.25 in the evening.

For some reason she had been obliged to buy an additional train ticket for her maid, Elise, from the Belgian frontier, first-class as far as Aachen then second-class to Koblenz. After a night at the Hotel Giant, the pair left the next day at 10.00 am on the river steamer for Biebrich, arriving at 5.00 pm, and reached Frankfurt, their night's stop, at 8.00 pm. After a night at the Hotel d'Angleterre they set off at 11.00 am by rail for Gemünden, finally reaching their destination at 7 in the evening of 2 June, after a last leg by carriage via Hammelburg. The entire journey therefore lasted five days with four overnight hotel stops.[63]

The chief objection to rail for invalids was that it threatened to undermine James Clark's prescription for slow travel. For travellers to the Mediterranean a stately progress by road or river allowed the patient to gradually adjust to a new climate, diet and sensations. Patients travelling by rail were therefore advised to proceed cautiously, with plenty of rest stops. The consumptive Lord Harrington, travelling across France in 1865, left London on 11 November but did not reach Cannes till the evening of the 18th, having made overnight stops at Dover, Calais, Paris, Dijon, Lyons (two nights to incorporate a rest day) and Marseilles.[64] Cecil Monro, bound for Menton, made much speedier progress the next year, leaving Paris by the 8.00 pm train on 31 October and travelling overnight to reach Lyons for an early breakfast at 5.00 am and finally an overnight stop at Marseilles, before proceeding to Nice, where at that date the line terminated. The night train from Paris would clearly have taxed the strength of even healthy travellers. The train was warm enough – 'they changed the hot water three or four times', Cecil recorded – but otherwise the journey sounds gruelling: 'We fortified ourselves with some chocolate to eat and half a bottle of St Emilion', Cecil continued; 'at Lyons they allow you a quarter of an hour for café au lait … Some minutes after you are driven up to the train by angry shouts of *En voiture*'.[65] Evidently, the experience did not prevent him repeating it three years later.[66] Notwithstanding his frequent rests, Harrington arrived at Cannes the worse for wear: 'His Lordship was very unwell for a week or more after coming here', noted his doctor; 'the maitre d'hotel said this was the "entrance fee" paid by everybody, even those in health, into the country'.[67]

By the time the railway had reached Menton, Dr Bennet noted that a traveller could 'leave the London Bridge station at 7.40 on Monday morning, by mail train for Paris, and be at Mentone for supper at 9.45 pm the following day, Tuesday'. Invalids should on no account be tempted: 'The transition from the cool, moist climate of England or Paris in autumn, to the dry, sunny, stimulating atmosphere of the north shores of the Mediterranean is too sudden', he contended, 'and develops various forms of liver, intestinal, skin, and head disease.'[68] Bennet advised avoiding travelling at night but making regular overnight hotel stops to ensure healthy sleep and feeding: 'If good nights are secured, and a quiet breakfast is taken at the usual hour, travelling during the day is very easily borne, and the invalid arrives at the journey's end without feeling wearied'; however, he continued, 'for invalids who feel every change from the train as a dreadful fatigue and trial, it may … be as well to pack up comfortably in an invalid carriage, and not to loiter on the way'.[69] William Chambers recommended avoiding the problems with luggage occasioned by detraining by sending it on to one's destination in advance.[70] These problems included the tiresome practice by French railways of collecting 'every box, basket and bag belonging to the whole train' and sorting it 'in the most leisurely manner on a long table' before the disembarking passenger could collect his own.[71]

As for 'invalid carriages', the nearest thing to specialized accommodation for invalids on French trains in 1870 were so-called *coupé-lits* – sections of carriages where three of the four seats in a compartment converted into a bed, with the fourth doubling as a commode. In 1877 *wagon-lits* were introduced on the fastest evening express from Paris to Menton, enabling passengers to reach their destination in about twenty-four hours in unprecedented comfort, but the service was expensive and the chance of sharing a sleeping compartment with strangers was not to everyone's taste. Dr Sparks continued to recommend *coupé-lits* 'for an invalid who required much attention if he travelled by night. By taking the whole compartment he can occupy the bed, while his friend or nurse has the vacant seat', Sparks explained. 'He can be absolutely undisturbed as there is no stranger to get in an out and the windows can be regulated at pleasure.' In addition, the fare from Paris to Menton was only sixteen francs more than a normal first-class ticket while a *wagon-lit* berth commanded a premium of forty-six francs.[72]

Sparks did not however think many invalids could bear lengthy stretches of uninterrupted rail travel. He suggested instead a gentle progress southwards, with overnight stops for the most delicate at Dover, Amiens, Paris (two nights), Dijon, Lyons, Marseilles (two nights) and even possibly Cannes, in order to reach Menton without injury. Frequent overnight stops allowed regular meals, which Sparks considered of utmost importance to invalids; in their absence he advised patients to bring a 'well-cured ox-tongue' from home to see them through the Paris to Lyons stage.[73] Rail travel to and from the Riviera was not problem-free. The journey was never seen as part of the therapeutic package, as for example a calm passage to Madeira might be. Even healthy travellers seemed to consider it a burden to be endured rather than an adventure to be enjoyed. A correspondent in the *Times* in 1875 claimed many invalids 'suffered so much through the journey as to leave little hope of their recovery'.[74] But compared with pre-rail travel, journeys were not only shorter but also more predictable, so that seasonal expatriation became less of a step into the unknown, and consequently much easier to contemplate with some equanimity. It seems unlikely that a family like the home-loving Reckitts, Quaker industrialists from Hull, would have contemplated a season on the Riviera for their health's sake before the coming of the railway.[75]

Non-stop travel to Pau might have been tolerable for schoolboys, but invalids were advised to take it easy. Elizabeth Carne recommended night stops at Amiens, Orleans, Bordeaux and Dax. The last halt could be easily dispensed with by healthy individuals, but invalids were advised to spend the night at Dax to avoid having to 'enter the Pau *diligence* without rest or refreshment [to be] cooped up for six hours in a close little omnibus … not arriving at Pau till ten o'clock at night'. This was 'enough to knock up any invalid, after three previous days of incessant travelling'.[76] Revd Wynter Blathwayt and his wife Fanny, who suffered from chronic asthma and may have been consumptive, spent every winter season from 1864–5 to 1868–9 at Pau, accompanied by a changing cast of family members. They invariably travelled in both directions by train, via Paris and Bordeaux, usually stopping for a day or two in the French capital for a bit of sightseeing and shopping. In 1864 they left Folkestone on 9 November, arriving at Pau on the 16th after extended breaks at Paris and Bordeaux, a journey of over a week. The following year they left Dover on 19 October, took night stops at Calais, Angoulême and Bordeaux as well as Paris, arriving at their destination at 3.00 pm on 23 October. In October 1866 they dispensed with overnight stops after Calais but took a *coupé-lit* from Paris to Bordeaux and arrived at Pau station at 2.00 pm on 17 October, having left Dover on the evening of the 15th, a journey of about forty hours, which they repeated the following year. Perhaps the choice of non-stop travel between Paris and Bordeaux was determined by Fanny's deteriorating condition: the Blathwayts did not return home at all in the summer of 1868 but spent the season in the high Pyrenees.[77]

## Roaming and restlessness

For those suffering from nervous disorders, Edwin Lee advised, 'travelling, and the moving from one place to another without hurry or fatigue, would frequently be more beneficial than residing for several months together in one place'.[78] But many others could benefit from the distraction of travel:

> The cheering influence upon the mind of clear skies and sunshine in winter; the interest excited by scenery of a novel and magnificent character, or by works of art, etc., are powerfully calculated to divert the mind from dwelling upon unpleasant or gloomy ideas, and consequently to procure the removal of many diseases, especially when induced by, or connected with, circumstances of a mental nature.[79]

As we have seen, many British health-seekers on the Continent had no settled destination in mind when they left home. Invalid grand tourists might have had a planned itinerary, but it was far from rigid, being liable to last-minute alteration through a range of contingencies, from exigencies of travel to mere whim. William Money-Kyrle, contemplating his future itinerary at Florence in January 1845, envisaged a journey from Rome, his immediate destination, to Corfu via Ancona, then on to Constantinople and a return home up the Danube via Vienna; in the event he went from Constantinople to Russia and spent most of the following year touring the Near East.[80]

In 1867 the Fox Talbot family of Lacock Abbey embarked on a cultural and sightseeing tour of the Continent, with the aim of restoration of health as integral to the package. The medical condition of the travellers is a little difficult to determine from the surviving family correspondence, but it seems that Constance Fox Talbot and at least one of her three daughters, Ela (b. 1836), were invalids. The family passed through numerous German spas on their way to Switzerland but made no use of their waters, much to the surprise of Constance's Swiss doctor. He recommended the grape-cure at Vevey, a natural remedy that perhaps indicates that Constance was suffering from digestive problems. It seems she was also probably addicted to Chlorydine, an opium-based patent medicine. At first the Fox Talbots had expected to spend the winter in Switzerland but, warned that it was too cold, an alternative was canvassed: 'The choice seems to lie between Hyères and San Remo', Rosamond Fox Talbot reported to her brother at Lacock; 'both enjoy a delightfully warm climate and both have English doctors and other conveniences and good hotels etc.; besides, being less frequented than Cannes, Nice or Mentone, they are much less expensive'.[81] They chose San Remo, spending the winter at the Hotel Victoria. Father, William Henry Fox Talbot (1800–1877), the photographic pioneer, bored and restless, had returned to England from Switzerland, promising to rejoin them in due course. After wintering on the Riviera, the family resumed their tour, returning home via Venice, Milan and the Italian Lakes. As for the health outcomes, these seem to have been positive. Constance never took the grape cure, of which she had entertained no high hopes anyway, but managed to procure enough Chlorodyne from a Lyons chemist on the way south to see her through the winter. Ela too seems to have improved.[82] For Rosamond (b. 1837) the visit to San Remo was the start of a life-long passion for the western Riviera.

When the writer Mary Shelley (1797–1851) headed across the Channel in June 1842 she had no clear idea of where she would go, beyond a determination to winter in Florence. Accompanied by her son, his friend and her maid, she crossed to Antwerp in June 1842, then travelled overland to Cologne, largely by rail. Here, like so many others, she boarded a Rhine steamer for the south, disembarking at Mainz for Frankfurt. At this point Mary decided a German water cure would benefit her health, choosing Kissingen because of its proximity and reputation as a pleasant, quiet place to spend a few weeks. They hired a *voiturier* and, reaching the spa towards the end of June, Mary began her cure almost immediately, following a consultation with a local doctor. The party endured Kissingen for a month before the boredom of the non-invalid members drove them to rebel. Mary considered the drinking and bathing had benefitted her but was likewise glad to leave so dull and depressing a location. The party headed off east towards Leipzig and Berlin. En route they passed the spa at Brückenau, which Mary found much more to her taste than Kissingen but where they were unable to linger, having already made other commitments. But the Shelleys had not done with 'German' baths yet. On the way from Dresden to Prague they stopped at Teplice (Töplitz) at the end of August, where Mary had a delicious bathe 'in water of delightful temperature and pellucid clearness'.[83]

Spas seem to have encouraged peripatetic behaviour. Many were close together but with significant differences in both tone and water quality, so that visitors were tempted to try several in turn. For every determined curist like Ann Vavasour or Wilkie Collins there were probably many who merely sampled the waters in a spirit of curiosity before moving on. The frequency with which names were re-registered in the published *Kurlisten* shows that it was not unusual for visitors to return to the same spa during a season, having spent some weeks away in the meantime. There were also genuine invalids like Fanny Blathwayt, who visited spas but never took the waters at all. Since the season was relatively brief, spas were anyway places of short-term resort. There was no equivalent to the six- to nine-month sojourn that invalids typically made in Madeira, Pau or on the Riviera. A 'cure' would normally last four to six weeks – Ann Vavasour's three-month stint at Wildbad, involving two cures, was exceptionally lengthy. Even short stays were liable to be interrupted by dissatisfaction with the resort, disagreement with the waters or a change of circumstances. The Young family of Northamptonshire left Ems hurriedly in July 1838, driven out by the heat and moved to nearby Schwalbach, which provided welcome relief. After two weeks Allan Young was advised to try the waters at Wildbad, but en route to that spa disaster struck as his youngest child Francis (Frank) sickened and died from whooping cough. Marooned at Wiesbaden throughout August and early September by the grave illness of another child, Lizzy, Allan nonetheless took the opportunity to profit from Wiesbaden's waters. By the time Lizzy was well enough to travel the season was almost over; so abandoning plans for Wildbad the family set off for Nice via the Splügen Pass and Milan, in a second-hand carriage purchased at Frankfurt.[84] Winter on the Riviera was now deemed vital for the recovery of the little girl as well as desirable for the health of the father.

Quite apart from personal preference or force majeure, patients might be advised to combine cures at different watering places for optimal results. Thus a course of saline waters intended to ease congestion might be followed by a strengthening regime of waters at a chalybeate or steel spa. Edwin Lee recommended bathing and drinking at a warm saline spring such as Baden Baden or Ems, followed by 'internal administration of a light chalybeate water', as at Schwalbach or Spa, for certain cases of hysteria.[85] James Johnson considered the waters of Schwalbach a kind of 'finish' after the powerful alterative waters of Wiesbaden and the strong alkaline waters of Ems, 'always remembering that Schlangenbad was to give a polish to the surface at the end of the process'.[86] Hilary Bonham-Carter expected her mother to be prescribed a course of Schwalbach waters 'or some similar dessert to [her] long watery banquet', following her stint at Kissingen.[87] Spa-goers were therefore frequently on the move, privileging their health, escaping heat or crowds, indulging their curiosity. Sir John and Lady Eleanor Naesmyth made annual summer visits to Germany to meet the twin challenge of Sir John's rheumatism and their daughter Ada's education. From the late 1850s they decided to remain permanently. Winter was passed at Bonn, away from the damp of home but with ready access to German tutors for Ada, while the summer and autumn were spent touring various spas in the interests of health and scenery. As Eleanor wrote from Homburg in September 1857, 'Although it is a trial to Sir John to be so long absent from his own dear home, still his health has decidedly benefited by the foreign climate, as well as the waters and baths of which he is able to take advantage whilst so easily within reach.' The family had also visited Schlangenbad, Wildbad and one or more Bohemian watering places during that summer, but Homburg, whose 'waters had a magic charm' for Sir John, was their favourite. Another favoured resort was Bad Godesberg, just south of Bonn, where the Naesmyths sometimes spent the autumn months. It had a mineral spring and congenial hotel, but an additional attraction was proximity to Bonn, enabling Ada's masters to continue their work.[88]

There was another form of restlessness that afflicted many invalids, more unsettling than the desire to head off to the next port of call, experience new sensations or merely escape the inconveniences of the moment. Consumptives were perhaps especially prone to moving about in response to their subjective experience of illness. Uncertainty about the progress of a disease typified by unpredictable maxima and remissions – or even whether they had the disease at all – allied to the bewilderingly contradictory climatic claims of different resorts and specialists encouraged patients in a perpetual merry-go-round of trial and error. As Sheila Rothman has written, 'Since they could not know with assurance when a dry, hacking cough would turn moist and blood-streaked or when an intermittent fever was actually consumptive, they had to make decisions with qualms and misgivings, never confident that they had made the right choice.'[89] For many, expatriation in the south was not the first resort in their search for health but the last. Cecil Monro first displayed unmistakable symptoms of consumption – bloody expectoration – in January or February 1859. From March to May he resided at Hastings, exposed to the sea air and dosing himself with cod liver oil. The following winter he was no better – the 'Hastings project', as he termed it, had failed, so 'he must give himself another chance by a different treatment'. In February 1860 he headed for Rome via Marseilles and spent the next three months touring northern Italy. On the way home through France the scarlet sputum reappeared. The failure of Cecil's mini-grand tour evidently led to the last resort, exile to Madeira in late 1860. For the next decade Cecil spent every winter abroad, five in Madeira, two in Algiers and three on the Riviera. These self-imposed sentences were rarely arduous, but they were all unsatisfactory, which is why the place of exile often changed from year to year. Nowhere ultimately met the conditions to provide a settled winter destination.[90]

Failure to find a satisfactory or even tolerable winter resort drove the restlessness of many invalids. Fanny Blathwayt met the widowed granddaughter of the bishop of Exeter at Pau, who had given up on Nice and Cannes because, 'though brighter and more cheerful for an invalid than Pau yet they did not suit her, for the air was far too exciting and invalids almost all complained of the want of rest and sleep in consequence'.[91] At Hyères in 1869 Cecil Monro was reunited with a family of wandering invalids, the Scotts, whom he had met in Madeira and Nice in former years. They had just returned from Egypt, which had at last proved 'the climate that did agree with Mr Scott' – 'One might ask why they don't stay there' was Cecil's acid comment.[92] His most restless acquaintance was Revd A. H. Hosmer, formerly Anglican chaplain in Madeira, whom Cecil had met there on his first visit in 1860 and whose wife – 'the only handsome women on the island' – became the object of some infatuation.[93] She was also however an invalid and presumably therefore the reason for Hosmer's appointment. After leaving Madeira the Hosmers never settled. They bought a house at Pau, but the climate did not suit Mrs Hosmer. They decamped to Biarritz but after some early good omens it disappointed. Corsica was ruled out because it had no English church. Cimiez was too expensive. 'I am pretty satisfied that no air will do which is not really genuine [*sic*] southern', was Hosmer's mournful conclusion.[94]

Cecil was somewhat contemptuous of the shallow ignorance of fellow invalids who moved from place to place on the flimsiest excuse and without adequate preparation. A man called Watson turned up at his hotel in Algiers in 1864, who had left Malaga because 'the hotels were bad and he had got tired of it'. He had assumed Algiers would be hotter as it was in 'Africa'.[95] Restlessness created a fraternity of nomads whose small numbers ensured there was always a good chance of encountering familiar faces. After five years Cecil Monro was reunited with Sir Archibald and Lady Dunbar at Nice, having shared a hotel with them at Algiers. The Dunbars were inveterate wanderers in search of health, but it seems doubtful that their peregrinations assisted much; Cecil found them looking 'very ill and by no means younger than five years ago'. To add to his disappointment they had come without their daughter.[96]

## Travel by sea

By the beginning of the Victorian period, sea air was prescribed, according to the popular medical writer Dr William Kittoe, 'in a multitude of complaints, viz indigestion, debility from various causes and in other nervous disorders', as well as in incipient consumption.[97] Some might doubt that salt spray had anything useful to offer a patient, but almost all understood that he was more likely to breathe uncorrupted air at the seaside and to fill his lungs more readily with draughts of invigorating oxygen. Sailing also had a venerable therapeutic ancestry; 'medicine … had suffered no small loss', claimed the eighteenth-century Scottish physician Ebenezer Gilchrist, 'by the neglect so much of antient remedies', one of which he attempted to revive for its use in the treatment of consumption, scrofula and asthma.[98] By the early Victorian period the perceived health advantages of sea voyages seem to have been widely shared by professionals and patients alike. Katherine Foxhall has remarked on the tendency of both surgeons and convicts on voyages to Australia to cite health as a justification for embarkation – 'the sick needed to go to sea'.[99] In addition to the tonic of superior air, sea voyages offered the restorative promise of touring that patients looked for in a leisurely excursion on land, without the attendant drawbacks. While at sea the patient was relieved, it was hoped, of the customary burden of his daily preoccupations, could maximize the time he spent out of doors and could enjoy an equable climate without abrupt temperature changes between day and night as he moved in easy stages from the chill of England to the warm south.[100] This promise could not however be redeemed until passenger comforts on ocean-going vessels met the basic requirements of invalids.

It was not common to prescribe sea voyages per se at the beginning of our period because vessels were rarely designed primarily for passenger transport. Even ships that took passengers generally relied mainly on mail contracts for their commercial viability. The exception were private vessels such as Scottish merchant Robert Meiklam's 130-ton steam-yacht *Crusader*, in which he cruised the north-east Atlantic and Mediterranean in the autumn and winter of 1837–8, in an effort to restore his health.[101] *Crusader* was the maritime equivalent of the luxury carriage that rich travellers took to the Continent, 'with all the comforts such a mode of transit could command', in the words of Meiklam's medical attendant. Invalids were frequently recommended to reach their destination by sea, where feasible, but this was usually to avoid the rigours of the road. The young invalid Saunderson Walker of Gateshead travelled to Malta as a passenger on a newly built sailing vessel belonging to one of Newcastle's leading Mediterranean trading houses, 'by which … many of the inhabitants of the town and neighbourhood [had] made excursions to the south of Europe for the recovery of heath'.[102] The diseases for which the climate of Pau was indicated, according to Alexander Taylor, were also often alleviated by sea voyages, but he soon abandoned his recommendation to travel to Pau by sea via Bordeaux once the journey could be made by rail.[103] Sea-cruising for patients without access to their own private yacht developed towards the end of our period. Dr C. B. Faber, former ship's surgeon on a sailing vessel on a round-the-world voyage via Australia in the 1870s, recalled that the ship 'resembled a regular hospital ship for consumptive patients' and later heard of a project to 'fit out a ship exclusively for invalids, and take them to Australia and back again'.[104]

All British travellers to the Continent had to contend with the risk of seasickness. Medical specialists had their own pet remedies. Dr Granville recommended laudanum as a preventive, though thought prussic acid might be even better.[105] Dr Francis preferred dietary measures and 'steadfastly maintaining the recumbent posture, lying with the head as low as can conveniently be borne'.[106] Dr Erasmus Wilson, who was habitually prone to seasickness, tried a new technique to prevent nausea during a crossing to Calais in 1857: he tied a shawl tightly around his midriff, braced his heels against the deck, crossed his arms and did his best to resist all motion of the vessel. The experiment was a success, though he had to admit the crossing was not rough.[107] It was one thing to endure a few brief hours of torture in the Channel, quite another to contemplate days of suffering on the open ocean. Dr Kittoe claimed in the 1840s that 'the comforts of sea travelling had of late been brought to a state of perfection which in former times could scarcely have been contemplated' but had to admit that nothing 'cast such a gloom over a voyage as the fear of sea-sickness'; there were various techniques for mitigation, but the only sure preventive according to Kittoe were the 'patent double or single action sea beds, couches and cots' invented by the ship-cabin furniture manufacturer, Joseph Brown: 'Let the vessel roll or pitch how she may', Kittoe continued, 'the bed will retain its perpendicular gravitation, and the occupant may repose as unconsciously of the vessel's motion as if in a chamber ashore.'[108] The popularity of this contraption is doubtful. Furthermore, the increasing use of screw propellors in place of paddles by steamships for additional speed only added to the discomfort of vulnerable passengers, as it increased the tendency of vessels to roll.

Patients heading for Madeira had of course no choice but to go by sea. The sea route could be shortened by travelling overland to Lisbon or Cadiz, but this offered scant advantage before completion of the rail link between these places and Madrid and onwards to the French border in the 1860s. Otherwise, getting to Madeira at the beginning of the Victorian period required a sea passage of at least eight days, generally more, often under sail. Various vessels took passengers, and though their routes varied, some sailing direct to Madeira as sole destination, others touching there en route for the Americas or the West African coast, usually via Lisbon, they all had to cross the Bay of Biscay, taking their chances with its notoriously capricious seas. Invalids were advised to set off no later than mid-October to avoid late autumn and winter storms, but the experience of passengers at any time of year involved a large slice of luck: nineteen-year-old Emily Shore, a consumptive invalid from Suffolk, had a beautifully calm passage in December 1838 aboard the merchantman *David Lyon*;[109] surgeon William White Cooper by contrast was 'dreadfully knocked about for eight days' aboard the Brazil packet *Alert* in January 1840, with a further week to finally reach the island.[110]

The most comfortable sailing vessels were thought to be the sleek brigs *Dart*, *Comet* and *Eclipse*, that sailed direct to Madeira from London and Southampton. They carried some forty-five passengers 'in family and double-berthed cabins, well ventilated, with good bedding and even the luxury of a bath-cabin'.[111] The passage however could still last two weeks even in fine weather, when time would hang heavy with healthy travellers accompanying invalids. In bad weather these small vessels were not for the faint-hearted. The invalid Elizabeth Wynter recorded the arrival of the *Dart* at Funchal, Madeira's capital and chief port, on 19 September 1839 'after a most boisterous passage':

> It was ten days in reaching Falmouth, during which time a handsome horse on board belonging to a merchant here was so injured that they were forced to throw it overboard, and the greater part of the passengers, alarmed at the unpropitious beginning, landed at Falmouth with the intention of performing the remainder of the voyage in steam vessels via Lisbon.

Elizabeth's own return voyage, which she dreaded, was eventually made via Cadiz in March 1840, presumably to minimize the amount of sea time.[112] It was not generally possible to avoid sail entirely until 1841 when the West Indies service of the newly created Royal Mail Steam Packet Company was inaugurated: the company's paddle steamers called at Lisbon and Madeira every month, en route for Barbados, leaving Southampton on the 9th and arriving at Funchal, all being well, on the 18th.[113]

Whether undertaken under sail or by steam, a voyage to Madeira could under favourable circumstances form an integral part of the patient's regime of recuperation or at least a peaceful intermission between the labour and anxiety of leaving England and full immersion into invalid society in Madeira. Emily Shore never felt better than during her passage: 'I continue to be an excellent sailor', she confessed to her journal, 'my cough is almost gone, and I never wake up feverish and throbbing as I did in England. Really I shall hardly be an invalid when I reach Madeira.'[114] Some physicians regarded sea air as absolutely vital to the recovery of their consumptive patients: the mother of Charles Marling was so impressed by this necessity that she rented a house on the seashore at Funchal for three months in early 1853 and planned to take Charles on a fortnight's sailing cruise to Tenerife in the spring.[115] An expatriate physician, Dr Lund, whose expert opinion was quoted extensively by British resident Robert White, considered the slower passage provided by sailing brig positively beneficial for invalids: 'A passage of from twelve to fourteen days is decidedly preferable; the change is then gradual, and the constitution becomes accustomed to the greater warmth which prevails in Funchal.'[116] Indeed the six days normally required for the voyage by steam by 1870 was too short, according to expatriate physician Dr Grabham.[117]

The sailing brigs were specially adapted for delicate passengers, with numerous stewards and a medicine chest. Whatever vessel was taken, however, the chances of a beneficial sea passage diminished after mid-October as stormy weather became more likely. Cecil Monro's first passage to Madeira was made aboard *Comet* from Southampton in late October 1860 and took twenty-five days, owing to contrary winds, although the voyage did enable him to lose his cough.[118] Apart from the discomfort of the journey itself in heavy seas, passengers disembarking at Funchal were lowered into rowing boats for delivery to the beach, a procedure that must have alarmed many a delicate invalid even in propitious conditions. The *Times* carried an eyewitness report of the disembarkation of fifty-two passengers from the Royal Mail steamer *Dee* during a great storm in late October 1842:

> The sea was so rough that it was not without considerable difficulty that she landed the passengers. All gained the shore with imminent peril; one woman was immersed as she was lowered down the ship's side, and the rest were not less completely drenched in the sea of rain through which they had to wade to the town.[119]

Disembarkation from the steamers was often more hazardous, according to Emmeline Stuart-Wortley, because, governed as they were by stricter sailing schedules, they made only a brief stop at Madeira and could not afford to wait for calm conditions. The sailing brigs by contrast could choose their time to deposit their passengers swiftly and comfortably on the beach.[120]

Reaching Madeira was difficult enough, leaving it more so. Sailings from England to the island, by brig or steamship, were regularly timetabled, even though the date of arrival depended on weather conditions en route. Return sailings by contrast were highly irregular. The sailing brigs that served Madeira exclusively tended to wait in port until they had enough passengers.[121] The steamships of the Royal Mail Steam Packet Company from the Americas (sometimes called 'Brazilians'), or the African Steam Ship Company (known as 'Africans'), founded in 1852, from west Africa, called at Madeira as their last stop before home so were usually already crowded with passengers: 'Persons at Funchal have little chance of obtaining accommodation unless by prevailing on some of the officers to give up their berths', warned a contemporary guide.[122] A correspondent wrote to the *Times* on 12 April 1861 to draw attention to the difficulty of leaving the island: 'It may surprise many of your readers to be told that, in its main feature, there is considerable analogy between the position of the foreigner who has come to Madeira as a refugee from the winter and that of Alexander Selkirk on Juan Fernandez', he began, before claiming that the west African service was the only scheduled direct steam communication with England. This was not in fact the case for very long, as the 'Africans' were soon supplemented by the Union line to and from South Africa, but the complaint spoke to the general truth of the island's isolation and dependence on the vagaries of sailings. If a visitor could reach Lisbon it was then possible to pick up a returning Peninsular line steamer from the Mediterranean: both Cecil Monro in 1861 and Charles Marling in 1862 adopted this course, but reaching Lisbon on the small Portuguese steamer *Lusitania* took several days, and Marling needed a couple of days to recover before proceeding.[123]

Travel by sea remained an important element of the journey to many Mediterranean health resorts into the second half of the century. By the 1830s coastal steamers connected Marseilles with the Riviera, Genoa, Livorno, Civita Vecchia (for Rome) and Naples.[124] In 1837 a regular French government mail service between Marseilles, the Levant and Alexandria via Italy and Malta was inaugurated; there were four classes of accommodation available for passengers and the vessels could also take carriages.[125] William Money-Kyrle might have taken one of these during his 'most agreeable voyage' from Marseilles to Naples in December 1843, at the start of his grand tour.[126] By 1853 this fleet and its associated mail contract had been transferred to the so-called Messageries Impériales, whose sixteen ships formed the core of the maritime services available for passengers who wanted to avoid the land route to Nice and Italy. However there were many other vessels under various flags that plied between Marseilles and the Italian ports, as well as Corsica, Spain, North Africa and Egypt. No British service began or ended at Marseilles, but ships of the Peninsula and Oriental Steam Navigation Company in transit between Southampton and Alexandria called there from 1844 onwards, and other British vessels serving Italy and Sicily occasionally called if they had spare capacity.[127]

British invalids heading for Algiers usually went via Marseilles, from which it was about forty-eight hours sailing time. The perils of deviating from the standard route are illustrated by Cecil Monro's experience in 1864. His first, uneventful, passage to Algiers in October 1863 was via Marseilles. The following year he sailed to Gibraltar, apparently on a P&O steamer, intending to move on to Algiers via Malaga or Oran. Details of sailings were difficult to obtain; his attempts to board first a French vessel for Oran and then a Spanish one for Malaga were rebuffed because he did not have a passport, though he had not needed one the previous year. He finally secured a berth on a Spanish coaster that conveyed him to Marseilles via Malaga and several other intervening ports, a voyage of about ten days. The journey was nonetheless quite restful, perhaps partly because he could understand nothing that was said:

> I listen as far as I can to the table talk, but the captain talks without any consonants, the other officer does not talk at all, and the other passenger has no teeth. Besides, if they were all otherwise perfect in elocution, it is not easy to follow a man with a cigaret [*sic*] in one side of his mouth and a toothpick in the other.[128]

Travellers by sea had a particular grievance against a common practice in many Mediterranean locations, as well as Madeira – the imposition of quarantine in the face of suspected infection. The typical British response to quarantine is captured by Dickens' Mr Meagles, in *Little Dorrit*, detained with his family in the lazaretto at Marseilles on arrival from the east: 'I am like a sane man shut up in a madhouse; I can't stand the suspicion of the thing. I came here as well as ever in my life; but to suspect me of the plague is to give me the plague', he protests.[129] For invalids the greater risk was the last-minute imposition of restrictions on travel from home on the way to health resorts. Civita Vecchia and Naples were notoriously liable to be closed to travellers from England on news of the outbreak of epidemic disease in Britain. Such draconian measures seemed especially perverse to British people, who contrasted the filth of southern Italy with the sanitary condition of their own country. The health authorities at Malaga were also quick to impose quarantine restrictions on travellers, generally on receipt of news of the appearance of cholera in Britain or other parts of Europe through which intending visitors might travel to that resort, such as Marseilles or northern Spain, much to the dismay of the British community. The inconvenience usually amounted to detention at one's intended port of embarkation pending the lifting of the embargo or perhaps a sufficient lapse of time to satisfy the authorities that the intending traveller was no longer a risk. In late 1853 for instance ships at Marseilles bound for southern Italy would not embark British passengers unless they could prove they had been out of England for at least a week.[130]

Imposition of an embargo when one was already in transit was much worse. This was obviously more likely to occur in the case of long sea voyages. In October 1857 the Brazil packet *Tyne* arrived at Funchal from Lisbon, where yellow fever was suspected. In consequence the passengers who landed were detained in the port's lazaretto for an unusually long period of quarantine, leading to a barrage of complaints to the British vice-consul. One invalid clergyman had even expired before release, although the vice-consul reckoned that his detention was not a significant contributing factor since 'he had arrived … in a dying state from pulmonary disease'.[131] The following month the *Medway* was denied permission to land its passengers at Funchal altogether. Fifteen passengers, among them five British subjects, were ordered to proceed to the next port. One of the Britons, John Kennedy, marooned aboard the *Medway*, wrote to the vice-consul in desperation about the fate of his wife, 'a great invalid'; 'should it be that we are not permitted to land', he continued, 'the consequences may be fatal to her; her distress of mind is indescribable and she is frantically praying to be thrown overboard'.[132] The Madeira authorities however were unrelenting – they had received orders from Lisbon to close the lazaretto. The ongoing lack of quarantine facilities at Funchal seems to have been a disincentive to invalid travel: as a correspondent wrote from Madeira in October 1873, 'the visitors for the season were coming in, but very slowly, as the barbarous Portuguese government afforded no lazaretto in which quarantine could be performed and this made it very hazardous for invalids to approach Madeira, with the danger of being carried onto the coast of Africa'.[133]

## Conclusion

Travelling was an inescapable component of the search for better health abroad. The journey south however formed no part of the therapeutic package for genuine invalids, whatever advantages it might hold for those who were merely in search of a constitutional overhaul. For the genuine invalid travelling was a means to an end, not an end in itself. James Clark's prescription for slow travel was designed to minimize fatigue rather than embrace any supposed benefit provided by movement per se. R. L. Stevenson's perception of having his jaded sensibilities enlivened by the rolling rhythm of a moving railway carriage seems to have been a most singular view. No medical specialist identified any therapeutic value in rail travel, any more than in the slower pace of travel by road. Only on water was there any prospect of the journey being anything other than a necessary evil to be endured, and that only in circumstances where almost all sensation of movement could be eliminated. One of the few benefits that Venice offered to consumptives, 'to whom the fatigue of walking and the jolting of a carriage were alike unbearable', according to Scoresby Jackson, was 'the soft, gliding motion of the gondola'.[134]

On the other hand it would surely be unwise to mistake the horror stories of continental travel for the common experience of invalid travel abroad. Discomfort and setbacks are after all more readily retailed both in print and in private correspondence than routine accounts of uneventful journeys. Most patients no doubt reached their destination safely and unremarkably, their condition on arrival governed more by their state of health on departure than any effects of the journey. The hazards of travel, such as they were, undoubtedly diminished over the period. Roads and inns improved; frontier examination of documents and luggage became less irksome; vehicles became more comfortable; above all, information and guidance proliferated. Was anything lost from these developments? For the healthy traveller perhaps, but for the sick they offered only unmitigated benefits.

4

# Living and spending

## Hotels and boarding houses

British travellers on the Continent could insulate themselves from the perils of the road to some extent by judicious preparations, careful route-planning and a sensible regime of diet and exercise while on the move, but none could avoid their inevitable assignation with foreign rooms and meals. 'To an invalid', remarked Lady Georgina Chatterton, an inveterate continental tourist, 'almost the entire pleasure of travelling depends upon the look of the rooms, and the view from them.'[1] Chatterton was unusual in preferring continental hotels and continental food to British; most of her compatriots approached both with a degree of trepidation ranging from mild anxiety to downright alarm. Putting up at loathsome roadside inns was one thing; much more important was to ensure suitable accommodation at one's destination, where long weeks were to be passed at the mercy of foreign landlords or hotel managers.

At the beginning of the Victorian period, there were few continental destinations with hotels suitable for long-term residence. Most British winter expatriates put up in rented apartments or villas. As a long-established destination, Nice was something of an exception. It was close enough to the summer resorts of central Europe to enable professional staff, usually Germans or Swiss, to migrate with the seasons between the two. Whether this cosmopolitan element improved quality was a matter of opinion; Sir Francis Palgrave thought that 'the principal [hotels were] so good that it was difficult to say which ought to have the preference', although his successor as editor of Murray's guide was critical of their state of cleanliness and quality of furnishings.[2] There seems to have been a marked fall in reported quality and value for money around the turn of the 1850s and 1860s. In 1857

Margaret Brewster thought the hotels at Nice were comfortable enough and not exorbitantly priced, while Joseph Pentland, author of *Murray's Guide to Northern Italy* (1858), deemed several very good, with moderate charges.[3] Yet by 1864 Murray himself reported that 'the hotels at Nice had become of late years as expensive as those in the largest capitals in Europe':

> Complaints have been universal, not only as regards the high charges, the attempts at extortion even in some of the first-class houses, the want of attention and ordinary civility, the inadequacy, little variety in, and bad quality of the food at the tables d'hôte, even where prices higher than those in Paris, Florence and Rome are charged; the unfortunate foreigner is screwed without mercy.[4]

The complaints perhaps suggest that a rise in visitor numbers was putting pressure on hotel capacity.

Elsewhere on the Riviera, hotels suitable for British families were rare until after 1870. At the beginning of our period they were likely to share the repellent characteristics of the generality of French provincial hostelries: the Taylor family stayed at Pinchinat's hotel at Cannes for twelve days in November 1837, on the recommendation of Lord Brougham, but found it 'one of the worst … they had seen'.[5] Murray in 1844 pronounced the one hotel he mentioned at Hyères, the Hotel de L'Europe, 'good', and Pinshinat's at Cannes, scene of the Taylor family's misery, 'excellent',[6] but by 1852, although the 'very good' Hotel des Iles d'Or had joined the Hotel de L'Europe at Hyères, the inns of Cannes received a collective thumbs-down ('none good').[7] Menton had only one decent inn, Albergo Torino, until the opening of the Hotel Vittoria, described by Pentland in 1854 as 'a new and excellent hotel, kept by Camillo Passaglia, who had lived long with English families, and had an English wife'[8] – an intimation of things to come. San Remo was even worse off, though its one hotel, La Palma, formerly dismissed as 'not over clean', had at least 'improved' by 1858.[9] By 1870 the Hotel des Iles d'Or at Hyères and the Hotel Bellevue at Cannes seem to have established precedence in their respective localities. Lord Harrington lived and died in the latter in 1865, perhaps confirmation that it had achieved this rank by that date. Whatever the improvement in quality over time it seems that the Riviera's hotels in general were deemed to offer poor value for money. According to Dr Sparks the problem lay partly in the need to generate income from a relatively short season, added to the impact of local taxation; how much the fault was due in addition to grasping hoteliers he could not possibly say.[10]

The distinction between a pension or boarding house and a hotel was largely a matter of degree rather than kind – both might offer a range of rooms and suites to suit differing tastes and pockets, together with dining and other public spaces. Perhaps the most salient difference was in tone: pensions were usually run by the proprietor, often operating from his own house, with a small dining room offering meals as it were en famille; hotels were usually larger, increasingly purpose-built, with a professional, often foreign manager, who may or may not have been the owner. A peculiarity of the hotels of Nice, according to Murray, was that in contrast to pensions they did not offer common sitting rooms, 'the inmates being obliged to remain in their apartments – the evident object of the landlords being to necessitate a greater consumption of fuel and lights'.[11] Such an arrangement clearly did not suit single travellers and those on restricted budgets, and even delicate invalids might prefer the distraction of company to brooding alone on their health in their room. The domestic ambience of a pension was therefore often more suitable for a range of clients, and the number of these establishments on the Riviera grew to meet demand.

By 1864 Murray was able to list several pensions at Cannes, Nice and Menton, most apparently run by women. The modest flavour of such establishments is captured in Ann Reckitt's description of Miss Stafford's pension at Menton in 1861: 'We have a two-bedded room,' she began, 'as usual a marble mantelpiece, but only two dogs in the hearth for the woodfire, no fender and great common tongs for the wood.' There were thirteen guests, the majority women. 'We have no private room', Ann continued, 'the drawing room is a pretty room but too small for so many.' The staff consisted of three female servants and a footman.[12] An added dose of familiarity was provided by management by a compatriot or at least a domestic regime that pandered to British tastes: a number of so-called *pensions anglaises* sprang up, first at Nice, later at Cannes, Menton, Cimiez, Hyères, San Remo and even Nervi, near Genoa, while other pensions were favoured by different nationalities.[13] The term *Pension Anglaise* implied, if not British management, then a level of conviviality absent from the large hotels. Cecil Monro, investigating hotel options along the coast in 1868, found a *Pension Anglaise* at San Remo, kept by an Englishwoman, that he thought might suit his mother as 'there would be sitting rooms'.[14] Guests were presumably also less likely to be inconvenienced by declining standards of service that characterized the Riviera's hotels as they prepared to shut down for the summer. Cecil Monro reported on this phenomenon from Hyères in early May 1870:

> There are signs already of that retrenching which I expect in these places at this time. We have not come to anything like the failure to provide us with meat which Charlie will remember at Mentone … but Mme Suzanne took advantage of a frivolous excuse to send away a waiter the other day and the waiting is very bad.[15]

Later refinements to Menton's accommodation offer included 'one or two pensions kept by English ladies exclusively for ladies', such as Miss Newland's Villa Farraldo, situated away from the sea north of the railway line, with 'the shelter of a large olive wood in its rear, where invalids could find level walks and plenty of shade'.[16] Whether this was the same establishment as the 'home for reduced gentlewomen', noted by Murray's handbook (1875), is unclear.[17] Some years later a masculine analogue was founded, St John's House of Rest, 'for clergy and other professional men'.[18]

*Pensions anglaises* were designed, as we have seen, to meet insular tastes, but they were not dedicated exclusively to the invalid trade, although the Pension Anglaise at Menton, where Dr Bennet held court, approximated to such status. It was established in 1860 in a house belonging to a Monsieur Clerici. Rates were eight francs a day, and the place evidently often oversubscribed.[19] Cecil Monro referred disparagingly to 'the Bennet clique system' that operated there, perhaps indicating that Bennet's patients from England enjoyed preferential terms.[20] Cecil booked in in November 1866 but did not remain long, complaining that the meals were 'a great offence'. He moved to the newer Hotel d'Ecosse, an improvement in itself but like all the Menton houses more east than south-facing and consequently deprived of late-afternoon sunshine. Indeed, the fact that the most sheltered part of the bay at Menton faced east might be considered a design fault.[21]

Whatever the limitations of its kitchen, however, it is unlikely that any British invalid guest at Menton's Pension Anglaise felt unwelcome. Patients often made additional demands on hotel management and staff: they might have special dietary requirements, be unable to move about unaided or in the worst case even die on site. Cecil Monro was quite ill at the Hotel d'Ecosse by spring 1867, and Dr Siordet unwisely instructed the staff to carry him upstairs when he returned to his room: 'Being carried up three pair [of stairs] in a house where the attendance was sulky already was an idea no one could entertain', Cecil recorded. He was moved to the ground floor.[22] Earlier at Algiers he had witnessed the reluctance of his hotel's staff to keep a seriously ill consumptive in residence, regarding him 'chiefly as a nuisance to be got rid of'.[23] Rumours circulated among nervous invalids about horrible crimes: a waiter at a hotel at Hyères was said to have hurled a paralytic guest out of a window 'because invalids were found to be such a nuisance'.[24]

One way to avoid such dangers was to book into dedicated invalid accommodation. This was not easy to find and anyway unlikely to suit patients uncomfortable living in continual proximity with fellow sufferers. A Dr Clement, who called on Cecil Monro at Cimiez in 1869, had opened an establishment for invalid boarders.[25] Other expatriate practitioners, such as Drs Daubeny and Rose at San Remo, took boarders into their houses, pending development of suitable hotel accommodation.[26] Nice even had a pension, Pension Finella, owned by a homeopathic physician, who was on hand to advise his guests, though it is doubtful many of these were British.[27] Alexander Brown, who wintered at Menton in 1871–2, thought the biggest drawback for invalids of modest means was the lack of suitable accommodation designed with the needs of the patient in mind; he had heard that a theatre was proposed for the town when what was really required was a sanatorium 'where the invalid in every stage of phthisis might find a home, the requisite attendance, be constantly under the eyes of a judicious medical adviser, and free from the bustle of change inseparable from the more public pension hotel, no matter how select'.[28]

At Cimiez, Cecil Monro spent the winter of 1868–9 at the Pension Anglaise at the Villa Garin, run by two Englishwomen, the Misses Smithers. They had opened a small pension in the Villa Visconti at Cimiez, a location 'recommended by medical men for delicate persons', in the 1850s, together with another at number 69 Promenade des Anglais, which they called Marine Villa, 'for those who preferred the sea'. With thirty beds each, both were advertised as 'pensions anglaises'. During the 1860s, the Smithers sisters relocated the Pension Anglaise at Cimiez from Villa Visconti into a seventeenth-century mansion belonging to the Garin family.[29] The place had been described in a recent local guide as '*pension anglaise de troisième ordre*', a put-down explained by the proprietors as the result of their refusal to advertise in the publication.[30] In many ways it was an ideal invalid asylum, 'nice and clean, facing south, [with] an excellent terrace in front of the windows to get a walk in the sun when it was cold and a garden of which the chief attractions were its Roman antiquities', as Cecil told his mother. But his father, who was accompanying him, was nevertheless annoyed by noisy children.[31]

In Madeira visitors usually lodged at boarding houses, if they lacked the means or desire to rent privately, for hotels were rare. Most, whether hotels or boarding houses, were run by British expatriates: a flavour of their domesticity is captured by their names – Hollway's, Maguinn's, Miles's, Neal's, Reid's, Wardrop's. The chief distinction between the two was that boarding houses offered dining in common, something that William Wilde, a visiting doctor, thought would not suit ladies or families.[32] Rates at the better boarding houses were about ten pounds a month in the 1860s – perhaps a little higher than pension prices on the Riviera – but cheaper places were available.[33] Pau by contrast had few pensions. British visitors typically rented apartments for the season, though they might spend a few days in one of Pau's rather expensive hotels on arrival. Frederick Johnson found a town with some elegant furnished apartments to rent for the season, but a distinct lack of 'lodging or boarding houses where temporary accommodation might be had on such terms as would open out the advantages of the climate to those sufferers who are unable to afford a style of living at least equal to that of the most fashionable of our English watering places'.[34] Single patients and those of limited means, faced with a choice of luxury apartments or unsuitable and expensive hotels, were ill-served. Pau did however possess one boarding house – Maison Planté (named after the family who owned it), in the main thoroughfare of Pau – a place sufficiently unusual to be named by both Frederick Johnson and Elizabeth Carne. By the later 1870s Pau had two 'English' pensions, the Colbert and the Hattersley, the former kept by two English ladies, the Misses Finch, which provided the sort of facilities that British people demanded, such as billiard and smoking rooms. Advertised rates for a good pension at that date were from seven to ten francs a day, roughly commensurate with the Pension Anglaise at Menton.[35]

Most visitors to German spas lived in hotels or boarding houses, which were more convenient for relatively short stays than rented accommodation.

Inns ranged from large commercial establishments with big dining rooms and occasionally their own bathing facilities to small *gasthauser* run by local townspeople from their own homes. Although several spa hotels referenced Great Britain in their names – König von England, Stadt London, Englischer Hof, Victoria and so forth – there was no equivalent to the *pensions anglaises* that proliferated on the Riviera, still less hotels owned or managed by British people, although Granville claimed that there were plans for an English boarding house at Kissingen.[36] Like Nice, the cosmopolitan German spas had established hotels of proven quality. Opinions likewise differed on their value for money. Granville calculated that a four-week cure at Kissingen would cost £11 13s. 0d. per person at a first-class hotel such as the Kursaal or the Russie, exclusive of tips, washing and doctor's fees; a small family could expect to pay five pounds per week. He considered this expensive and advised families to look for private rental accommodation.[37] The author of *A Hot-Water Cure* paid 17s. 6d. per week for his room at the Hotel d'Angleterre (Englische Hof) at Wiesbaden, a second-level establishment without dining facilities, which represented about half the figure quoted by Granville for a second-rate hotel at Kissingen at the same date, but of course it did not include meals.[38] Family apartments at Nice and Pau in the 1840s seem to have been rented out at a rate of about eighty pounds per season, so when we consider that the hotel charges included meals they do not appear unreasonable. Macpherson later reckoned prices at the best hotels were considerably lower than those at second-rate ones at home.[39] By the 1860s formerly unremarkable German watering places boasted luxury hotels. Wilkie Collins found the Hotel de l'Ours (Der Bär) at Wildbad a place of 'gorgeous drawing rooms, accomplished French cooks, banquets, and ornamental bills of fare'.[40]

Charges for accommodation at French spas might have been lower than German on the whole, until the great growth in their international popularity after 1870. Vichy in the early Victorian period had no large hotels – 'the very finest hotels look countrytown like', wrote Hilary Bonham-Carter – and Murray noted that 'everyone lived in boarding houses' in which 'in none was the accommodation first-rate'.[41] The paucity of Vichy's hotel offer was embarrassingly brought home by the lack of suitable accommodation for Napoleon III when he first visited the spa in 1861. Subsequently the offer improved, tellingly led by Swiss entrepreneurs.[42] In 1866 Edwin Lee observed that there were over seventy hotels, including several that had been enlarged or newly opened, including the luxurious Hotel du Parc (1864), one of three hotels most frequently used by British visitors.[43] Murray could still claim in 1864 that Vichy's hotels, though 'fair, were not equal to those in the German watering places', but this reservation had disappeared by 1870.[44] Prices rose in step with quality, and Madden thought Vichy was 'extremely expensive'.[45]

Hotels at the Pyrenean spas received a fairly favourable report from British travellers, apart from the standard complaints about dirty floors and lack of washing facilities that applied to most French inns before the later part of the century. Both Charles Weld and Mary Eyre, travelling modestly through the Pyrenees, lodged at Mlle Jalon's boarding house at Bagnères-de-Bigorre, which was 'greatly resorted to by English families ... as the apartments were regularly waxed, so there were no fleas'.[46] By the 1870s the daily rates quoted by Murray for good hotels at Eaux Bonnes, Bagnères-de-Bigorre and Luchon – about ten francs (7s. 6d.) for bed and board – were about three times the bill paid by the author of *A Hot-Water Cure* at Wiesbaden, but he had no meals.[47] By the mid-1870s Pyrenean spa accommodation received high marks on the whole in Murray's handbook,[48] but only Bagnères-de-Luchon ever approached the luxurious level of Vichy, where the best hotels seem to have been some 50 per cent dearer than at most Pyrenean spas.[49]

## Independent living

The alternative to hotel or boarding house living was to rent a villa or apartment and thus escape the lottery of unwanted company and the tyranny of the table d'hôte. However, patients had special needs and were particularly vulnerable to what James Clark termed 'the inconveniences which to an English family were inseparable from all foreign houses'.[50] Clark warned his readers that Italian – and by extension Riviera – houses were relatively colder in winter than those at home, and visitors should dress indoors accordingly.[51] Floors were tiled rather than boarded. Chimneys were few, and where fireplaces existed they were designed for burning logs, not coal. 'In southern countries the traveller would meet with houses that were built not so much with a view of being warm in winter as of being cool in summer', explained Scorseby-Jackson.[52]

Since British invalids were invariably winter residents this posed an obvious problem. The perennial challenge was to maximize sunlight while eliminating damp and ensuring free circulation of fresh air. Specialists all agreed that rooms with a southerly aspect were vital to the health of pulmonary patients. Clark recommended that apartments should be dried and ventilated before invalids moved in; William Farr advised against occupying new-builds, which were likely to still be drying out.[53] Scorseby-Jackson warned against 'close stoves, hot air, or hot-water pipes and every variety of *chauffage*, excepting that effected by means of an open grate'. Furthermore this grate should preferably burn coal, 'a more wholesome fuel than wood'.[54]

How far invalids could hope to meet such strict directions is doubtful. Although Dr Francis maintained that in Spain he had often seen fireplaces 'extemporised at a small cost by some constructive artizan',[55] most visitors surely had to make the best of what they were offered. The Baring family arrived at Nice in October 1839 and began a search for accommodation among the 'cold and wretched' houses and apartments, with 'neither doors nor windows shutting as to keep out the wind', before abandoning their attempts to find suitable lodgings for the invalid Mrs Baring and booking into a hotel.[56] At Pau, apartments predominated. They were a novelty for most English people, and for Elizabeth Carne their existence in those countries where they were common could only be explained by 'prevalent out-of-door engagements, as on the Continent, or by a lower standard of indoor comfort and cleanliness as in Scotland'. Her peace and comfort were disturbed by the smell of garlic that permeated the vestibule from the floor below and the singing and stomping feet of late-night returnees to the floor above.[57]

In Madeira, accommodation for visitors who wished to live apart or en famille ranged from furnished houses and apartments in the town to country villas – *quintas* – in the surrounding hills. William Wilde in the early 1840s quotes seasonal rentals for quintas of between sixty and two hundred pounds, according to quality, a relatively high figure compared with rates for villas on the Riviera, although for a somewhat longer season.[58] Many visitors who remained on the island for a lengthy period or made repeated visits seem typically to have sampled a variety of houses according to their changing tastes and circumstances. The Marling family took a villa above Funchal in autumn 1852 – quinta d'Andrade – but moved in February 1853 to a location by the sea, with a garden overlooking the shore, to provide better facilities for their invalid member; in addition the new house – so-called Pontinha Cottage – was owned by a Briton, Mr Grant, and consequently full of 'little English comforts which were indeed highly desirable for such an invalid as Charlie was'.[59]

For whatever reason, this sort of flexibility does not seem to have been commonly available in other resorts. At Pau and Nice landlords usually insisted that properties be taken for an entire season, typically seven full months from mid-October to mid-May – a daunting obstacle for those unwilling to commit to such an investment of time and money, which must have kept many cautious visitors in their hotels. Nevertheless Allan Young reported in November 1838 that his was one of eighty-nine 'English' families who had taken houses at Nice for the winter; their house suited them very well, and although we do not know how much he paid he was not extravagant in his spending.[60] In February 1857 Margaret Brewster and her husband managed to rent a small house on a short-term lease in the Cimiez district of Nice in order to escape the noise and dust of town. This house provided drawing and dining rooms, three bedrooms, a kitchen, a pantry and a garden for a modest eighty francs (about three pounds) a month.[61] This district was evidently considerably cheaper than Nice proper where, according to Murray's handbook, 'bachelors' apartments, consisting of a small sitting room and bedroom with a south aspect' were available for from forty to sixty francs a month, plus fifteen francs for 'attendance'.[62] Augustus Hare and his family rented a first-floor apartment at Menton in 1860–1, comprising a salon giving on to a balcony, dining room, three bedrooms and kitchen, all the rooms but one overlooking the sea, which probably cost the equivalent of about 250 francs or ten pounds a month, roughly the same rate as the Pension Anglaise, but without meals and other provisions of course.[63]

Rents on the Riviera clearly rose considerably around the turn of the 1850s and 1860s, as did hotel rates. A price of at least 2,000 francs for the season for lodgings for the Bonham-Carter family had seemed steep in 1843, although it was roughly equivalent to the rental of the Grant family's three-bedroomed apartment at Pau at the same time.[64] Joseph Pentland in the late 1850s claimed that 'very comfortable' lodgings for smaller families were available at Nice from 800 to 1,200 francs, but no such tantalizing promise featured in Murray's handbook of 1864, which reported that 'prices had been carried to an exorbitant extent'.[65] Chambers quotes rates of 1,500 to 5,000 francs for detached villas and from 800 to 2,000 for apartments at Menton at the end of the 1860s.[66] Miller reckoned a small family house at Menton could be had for 4,000 to 5,000 francs for the season by the later 1870s.[67] By this date apartments at Pau were advertised at between 2,000 and 3,000 francs per season, with villas ranging from 4,000 to 10,000.[68]

Although British visitors often complained about the cost of hotels, it was in the rental market that disputes between landlords and clients more frequently arose. The Young family's dispute with their landlord at Wiesbaden only increased Eliza Young's disaffection with Germany. It seems he insisted on full payment despite the family's wish to leave early, leading them to seek the assistance of a local English banker: 'In every dealing with Germans which we have had', wailed Eliza, 'we have found them most infamous cheats.'[69] Mary Shelley, who sought out a house for rent soon after arriving at Kissingen in 1842, had difficulty persuading her landlord, Herr Friess, that their contract was for only four weeks, not four months.[70] From 1856 the Bad Ems *Kurlisten* carried a regular trilingual announcement from the 'Intendant of the Baths' advising private rental guests to make written agreements with their landlords in advance.[71] Those who rented apartments at Pau were strongly advised not only to settle the amount of rent in advance but also to agree on an inventory with the landlord to avoid subsequent arguments. When the Wrottesley family prepared to leave Pau in spring 1862, their landlady – 'a great cheat' – accused them of having substituted earthenware crockery for some of the original porcelain.[72]

Some of these misunderstandings no doubt arose from the widespread expectation on the Continent that Britons could and should pay more. Murray counselled his readers against protesting vehemently about this; after all 'something more was expected of them, especially as they often gave much more trouble to the servants than the natives.'[73] Even those who chose to rough it – a phrase commonly used at the time for economy travel – could not escape the ubiquitous surcharge levied on British travellers. Mary Eyre, a lone woman travelling in the Pyrenees with her dog on a modest budget, was continuously imposed upon according to her account: 'Everywhere and in everything an English person must expect to be charged twice as much as a Frenchwoman', she concluded.[74] For this she blamed rich British tourists, who had foolishly dispensed largesse for the sake of appearances, for which modest travellers like herself bore the baleful consequences.[75]

Independent living meant embracing the additional burdens of feeding oneself and the hire of servants, unless they had been brought from home. Meals in hotels and pensions were normally taken communally, à *table d'hôte*. Independent living by contrast required self-catering, either by employing a cook or buying in meals. Some British visitors evidently brought their own cook from home, but it was more common to employ a local one. The Youngs brought two household servants from England in 1838 but employed a local woman as a cook and kitchen maid.[76] The Brewsters at Cimiez ordered meals from the nearest restaurant, two miles away, but they were poor fare, and the cooking of their *fille de chambre*, Marie, execrable; they were saved by Achilles, 'a very fat, kind Italian man-cook, belonging to an English neighbour'.[77] The Hares struggled to hire good cooks at Menton and ended by buying in meals from a local restaurant and getting their other locally recruited servants to give the food a bit of extra cooking to suit their insular tastes.[78] The Stevenson family also had their dinners delivered by a local caterer while renting the Villa Bosano at Menton in 1863, although their Scottish nanny cooked the vegetables; she was assisted in the kitchen by a teenage girl who alarmed the family by carrying trays of dishes on her head, according to the local habit of female porterage.[79]

Murray recommended buying in meals from a restauranteur at Nice rather than employing cooks, 'who were not there remarkable for their honesty', while at the same time dismissing the town's restaurants with the words 'none very good'.[80] Elizabeth Carne warned 'no one [at Pau to] be tempted by any persuasion to hire a cook, for they were apt to be troublesome and extremely dishonest … a party of three or four may have a comfortable dinner (not including wine) for five or six francs [from a local restaurant]', she continued, 'with enough left for their French servant'.[81] 'A man who went abroad for his health ought to take his own cook with him', was the advice of a family friend of the Monros, which led Cecil Munro to wryly imagine despatching Mrs Sheffield, the family cook, to Menton, for the benefit of its distressed invalids.[82] The only health resort where local cooks seem to have passed muster was Madeira, perhaps because they were so used to pandering to British tastes.

If good cooks were difficult to find, hiring local servants as market intermediaries was nonetheless unavoidable. British servants brought from home were useless for this purpose, however trustworthy and diligent they might be, because they lacked language skills. Besides, many health resorts were in places where the local dialect was quite impenetrable to even competent linguists. Louisa Costello and her party at Pau depended on their girl Jeannotte for communicating with the mountain shepherd who brought cheese into town but spoke little French.[83] Furthermore, as William Farr reminded his readers, however good one's own French, locals would always secure better prices.[84] Elizabeth Carne advised her readers to accept that their French servant would make a percentage on the side in all her transactions on their behalf, for if they insisted on shopping themselves they would merely end by paying the equivalent mark-up at source.[85] After all, as Frederick Johnson playfully riffed about the market, 'the British costume springs the market at least ten per cent, bad French ten more, and an apparent ignorance of both market and language cannot be let off at less than thirty or forty'.[86]

All in all foreign servants got a mixed report. British visitors throughout Europe found the relative lack of instinctive deference that they were used to in the servant class at home surprising.[87] In France, according to Margaret Brewster, 'there was a great deal of *Liberté, Egalité et Fraternité* in the manners of the peasantry'.[88] Locally recruited servants at Pau were generally honest, according to Mrs Ellis, though 'it was customary … to keep such things as sugar and coffee out of their reach'.[89] Even the usually grudging Costello admitted the local servants seemed 'good, industrious, honest and very civil'.[90] William Farr reckoned 'the male servants bore a much better reputation than the females for general honesty' at Nice.[91] Margaret Brewster pronounced 'the native female servants [at Cannes] … stupid, ignorant, and far from cleanly'; as a result she employed a single Italian manservant, Odoni, at sixty francs a month plus fifteen for wine, who did all the shopping and cooking and accompanied the Brewsters when they moved to Nice.[92] It was almost impossible to hire local female servants at San Remo, according to Dr Hill Hassall, who urged that 'the Italian ladies should set on foot an institution for the training of young women in the duties of domestic service'.[93]

Many British families brought domestic servants from home – a habit that was almost universally deplored by authorities, except in limited circumstances: 'If you have a good faithful servant attached to your family', advised an anonymous author writing about Madeira, 'bring him or her, but do not commit the indiscretion of bringing an establishment of English footmen and ladies' maids; they are as a rule discontented and troublesome, complaining of everything because it is not English, and always at war with the Portuguese servants.'[94] The Marlings brought an old female family servant, probably a lady's maid, called only by her surname – Wheeler – in their letters, who died from unspecified causes around Christmas 1852. Samuel Marling offered to send a replacement from home, but his wife reckoned she could 'manage well with the Portuguese'.[95] It is clear however that many British families travelling and resident on the Continent included sizeable complements of support staff, especially if there were children. The Bonham-Carter family left Nice for Kissingen in April 1844, where they were registered as a party of nine, including a governess and other servants.[96] Analysis of a sample of surviving *Kurlisten* from Carlsbad and Kissingen for the early to mid-Victorian period shows that British parties registered by the bath authorities were on average substantially larger than the mean.[97] Large travelling parties seem to have become less common later in the century, perhaps as a result of shorter journeys and improved resources at resorts enabling visitors to dispense with their customary support network.

The Hanburys of Warwickshire were exceptional in bringing out all their domestic servants for the 1868–9 season at Menton. The unsuspecting household was astonished to discover that one of their number, a nineteen-year-old kitchen maid, had been pregnant when her dead child was found in a drawer in her bedroom. The French authorities initially prepared a murder charge against the unfortunate girl, but her employers stood by her, succeeding with the help of the British consul at Nice in obtaining reduction of the charge to involuntary manslaughter and ultimately an Imperial pardon. Far from passing moral judgement on the erring servant, the British expatriate ladies of Nice seem to have taken her under their wing and were conspicuous in visiting her in the local hospital, where she was confined pending determination of her sentence.[98]

## Eating, drinking and exercise

British visitors to southern Europe in the nineteenth century were not led to expect a land of culinary delights. On the contrary, one of the drawbacks of wintering on the Riviera was deemed to be the inferior diet that had to be endured, and one of the attractions of returning north in the summer was the opportunity to recover the nutritious fare of home.[99] The concept of the health-giving Mediterranean diet was unknown. Since one of the few things specialists agreed on in relation to the treatment of pulmonary consumption was the importance of restoring the patient's appetite and improving digestion, the prospects of an inadequate diet were clearly problematic. The country round Nice was highly cultivated, 'like a garden', according to Clark, and provisions were good and abundant,[100] but those provisions were largely vegetable – red meat and dairy produce were difficult to come by. The British consul reckoned the local population consumed about a third less meat than their counterparts in a northern country, and a correspondingly greater proportion of vegetables, and ate frugally as a whole anyway, though this frugality did not extend to their consumption of wine.[101] 'Eatables are cheap', reported Allan Young from Nice in 1838, 'but meat very bad'; fish meanwhile was interestingly varied and exotic in appearance but bore little resemblance to the specimens deemed suitable for the table at home.[102]

Fortunately the dietary challenge was mitigated by the injunction on visitors from the north in their turn to eat less and generally adapt their eating habits to local circumstances: 'At Nice', advised Farr, 'if health be an object, [diet] should partake more of vegetable than animal. Man must assimilate himself to the particular climate which his pleasure or health induces him to inhabit.'[103] This advice was rationalized in terms of physiology rather than the availability of produce. The 'sensibility of the system' increased as one travelled southwards, according to Clark, so that a diet suitable in England became over-stimulating, requiring moderation of intake; fish, milk and even vegetables were 'more apt to disagree in the south' and should be used sparingly by delicate invalids.[104] Olive oil was a particular bugbear. However much British visitors admired olive trees for their beauty and their shade, they generally wanted nothing to do with their fruit.[105] 'Oleaginous ingredients' were 'almost always injurious to persons of weak digestive powers', according to Scoresby-Jackson.[106] Moreover, consumptive patients were often prescribed cod liver oil so that oily food threatened overload.[107]

When Augustus Hare visited Menton in 1860–1 he reported that foodstuffs were of poor quality, the meat bad and butter – a particular British obsession – only fitfully available. Meals supplied by a local restaurant were made palatable by being stripped of their oil and garlic.[108] But local shortages were speedily sidestepped by imports direct from home: within a couple of years Mr Willoughby, Menton's British grocer, could offer everything an expatriate invalid could desire, from 'prepared cocoa' to 'calves' feet jelly and tins of preserved meats', while the local chemists obtained 'the best cod-liver oil direct from England'.[109] Margaret Brewster at Cannes averred that there were plenty of excellent foodstuffs about, including northern European favourites like butter and cream, but they needed to be sought out; people complained about the food because the local servants had no idea how to shop or cook.[110] East of Menton, meanwhile, 'the inhabitants were still thoroughly Italian', living on 'macaroni, olive-oil soup, and bread', according to Dr Bennet.[111] In the contest between Farr's advice to adapt and the natural inclination of visitors to pine for what they were used to, the latter won out. As late as 1880, to judge from Adolphe Smith's remarks, the typical British visitor had yet to be weaned from his insular tastes:

> Let his diet in Provence resemble, at least to some extent, the diet of the Provençal; the heavy English cooking and above all the strong alcohols consumed at home, must be vigorously abjured. The inhabitants of a country invariably know best what is best suited to their climate; it is because the English too often fail to carry out this maxim that they find their digestive faculties impaired and the cost of living dearer than they had anticipated.[112]

Away from the Mediterranean the problem of oily ingredients and lack of dairy produce receded. Madeira was 'a land of eggs, milk and fresh butter', Dr Grabham assured his readers, while Madeiran cooking was 'fortunately exempt from the objection of greasiness so often to be encountered in foreign towns'.[113] Madeiran cooks were long accustomed to catering to British tastes. Elsewhere, even where the basic produce was available it was not always prepared to British standards. Elizabeth Grant at Pau found the local bread 'not very white and very sour', so 'paid high for rolls, called there English bread'.[114] Pau was at least a resort where Britons usually self-catered and could increasingly buy English produce in the shops. Eating at the German spas generally allowed no such latitude. Complaints about German food arose more from the style of cooking and serving than the quality of the basic foodstuffs: 'We should all rejoice to see a nice, plain joint of English meat', moaned Eliza Young, soon after arrival at Ems, 'for the cooking is most disagreeable.'[115] Granville dismissed British prejudice against German food as of a piece with the unreasonable suspicion of German medicine.[116] Dr Erasmus Wilson, touring in 1858, considered German spa hotel food eminently suitable for health-seekers – a light breakfast of coffee and bread rolls, followed by a one o'clock dinner, 'light and sufficient, without trespassing too much on the powers of digestion' and finally a tea or supper of maybe a cutlet or eggs.[117] The problem was that too few spa-goers observed such moderation.

Dietary negligence was a charge frequently levelled at invalids. Spa-goers, who imbibed copious quantities of mineral water, needed to be especially careful at table. Granville advised avoiding 'fruit, raw vegetables, and many of the flatulent legumes, particularly potatoes', for fear of the inevitable consequences.[118] Green vegetables 'kept up in the larger intestines a perpetual borborigmal commotion, quarrelling … with the water, and rendering [the patient] unfit to go into society'.[119] Overeating was also likely to interfere with a bathing regime. It was in order to maximize the therapeutic benefits of their waters that some continental spa physicians succeeded in persuading the authorities to award them extraordinary powers of control. At Carlsbad, according to Granville, the chief physician, Dr de Carro, exercised a 'tyrannical vigilance' over the restaurant menus, and 'were he to see a *gasthof*-keeper daring so much as to offer a salad to his guests, a denunciation to the police … would immediately follow'.[120] De Carro's writ presumably did not extend to The English Coffee House, an establishment run by an Englishman, Mr Harrison, with an 'excellent' restaurant, according to Murray.[121]

At the less iatrocratic spas dining was obviously less circumscribed. Murray described the table d'hôte at the Kursaal at Wiesbaden as 'a most excellent dinner, comprising all the delicacies of the season, even ice', an additive that spa physicians deprecated as stimulating perspiration.[122] However, patients were still advised to take care of their diet, and some hotels made a virtue of their invalid-friendly catering: the Panorama *gasthaus* at Ems for example, a new place built on the shaded south bank of the river Lahn, advertised a 'table d'hôte where only dishes sanctioned by medical men were served, simple but tasty dishes sympathetic to the spa waters'.[123] Few British people appear to have stayed at the Panorama, and the impression gleaned from visitor accounts is that away from the highly medicalized spas Britons did not visit watering places with any serious intention of stinting themselves. Wilkie Collins, a notable bon viveur, delighted in the food and wines available at his hotels at Aachen and Wildbad.

According to Dr Prytherch, continental dining habits were not designed to maximize the good effects of mineral waters in British patients, who were used to plainer food and might benefit from the substitution of English table beer for the local wines.[124] Dr Hoeber, a German practitioner at the same resort, indulged to an extent the insular exceptionalism that several British spa physicians claimed to be key to the successful management of their compatriots at continental watering places: he allowed his British patients a hearty breakfast of toast, eggs and lean meat, as well as tea throughout the day, though this would never do for his German patients. One British habit he did frown upon was the tendency to gulp their wine – good wine should be 'taken in very small draughts'.[125] Indeed the supply of alcoholic beverages seems to have been a topic of equal if not greater importance to British spa-goers as the quality and quantity of the food. The only regular advertisements in English in the Ems *Kurlisten* in the era of its greatest popularity with British visitors were for wines and spirits. 'It is a delightful country', announced the author of *A Hot-Water Cure* on returning from Germany, 'and I know not which most to praise, the wines or the waters'.[126] Wine does not seem to have been prohibited at even the strictest tables, and as a rule physicians did not consider the consumption of moderate quantities of light wine incompatible with a regime of water drinking or bathing. Wilkie Collins's physician at Aachen allowed him 'all wines, provided they were the best vintages'.[127] But heavy drinking was another matter. The British upper classes consumed too much wine, thought Madden; it did not assist digestion, but at the same time to deny drink entirely to spa-goers made as much sense as denying them razors lest they cut their throat.[128]

German concessions to the peculiarities of British taste, such as they were, remained a world away from the efforts made by landlords at the more Anglocentric resorts to pander to the eccentricities of insular dining. In Madeira, the most thorough-going Anglocentric health colony in Europe in the early Victorian years, Elizabeth Wynter had 'to beg now and then to have a few things after the fashion of the country at table' to temper the predictably familiar bill of fare.[129] Continental hotels with large British clienteles made valiant if sometimes unappreciated attempts to humour their guests with a taste of home: Cecil Monro remarked on a 'grotesque attempt' at a plum pudding at the Hotel des Ambassadeurs at Hyères at Christmas 1869.[130] Even at Algiers Christmas dinner at his hotel had comprised roast beef, turkey and '*le plum pudding anglais*'.[131] The so-called *pensions anglaises* scattered along the Riviera promised, in the words of a local advisor to the British community, '*la vie anglaise dans toute sa rigeur*.'[132] These and other hotels and pensions under British ownership or management, of which there were several by 1870, could be expected to provide a familiar regime for British guests, such as eggs for breakfast rather than just bread and butter and a regular tea slot after dinner. By 1875 Murray's handbook could report that the Hotel des Anglais at Nice, owned by 'an English joint stock company', offered 'good draught Bass's ale' for forty cents the bock.[133]

If food in the south was a difficulty to be carefully negotiated by the invalid, exercise was also not without its complications. In contrast to diet, which was rarely an incentive for expatriation for the Victorians, exercise was a positive inducement. All medical authorities emphasized the importance of suitable exercise in the open air for patients of all categories, and the greater facility of managing this under the winter sun of the Mediterranean than at home was one of the chief benefits of exile. 'Exercise in the open air', noted Edwin Lee, 'is perhaps the most effectual means of combating the predisposition to tubercular cachexy, and of remedying it when already existing'.[134] However, patients required guidance as to the correct form of exercise appropriate to their circumstances as well as the relative merits of the various health resorts for pursuing it. Early-stage consumptives should seek exercise that privileged the upper body and increased lung action, according to Dr C. T. Williams – examples included 'rowing, use of alpenstock in mountaineering, swinging from a horizontal bar, climbing ladders or trees'; suitable gymnastic apparatus could be obtained from Mr Hodges of Southampton Row. Walking was suitable for patients in all stages of phthisis, while the 'weak and delicate' would benefit from 'open carriage exercise, sailing or being rowed in a boat'.[135] Even this was not always without peril: Augustus Hare recounted the adventures of two ladies from the Pension Anglaise at Menton, saved from drowning by their crinolines after their boat capsized.[136] Although the life-preserving qualities of crinolines were a happy accident, invalids were encouraged to dress appropriately for their health while out and about. Williams recommended 'flannel or merino underdress' at all times and 'light-coloured suits of thick texture' that did not show the dust. He also urged men to set aside their fear of being thought effeminate by carrying a parasol.[137]

On the Riviera, opportunities for carriage exercise were limited by the state of the roads away from Nice. Menton in particular, hemmed in by mountains, was a place for those who could do little but sit or who were strong enough to scramble up the hills, but it was ill-suited for moderate exercise.[138] Dr Bennet noted that some consumptive patients literally 'walked themselves to death' in an attempt to regain strength.[139] Apart from pulling carriages horses were not much used on the Riviera, but donkeys were ubiquitous. The example of Lord Harrington at Cannes, who had his own carriage horses shipped out from England, was very far from the typical invalid experience.[140] Excursions into the hills or to remote coastal locations were invariably made by donkey. The animals stood about at Nice with their attendants awaiting hire. Competition seems to have improved the price and quality of the animals here compared with elsewhere on the Riviera, where they were more likely to be the same beasts that would otherwise be humping panniers of fruit down from the olive groves.[141] Consequently, at Menton at least, their attendants were likely to be women, who did the bulk of the manual labour. Donkeys were particularly suitable as transport for invalids and other timid or unenergetic visitors, but they were not risk-free. Margaret Brewster had what she described as many 'donkey distresses', including hiring one at Cannes so small that it was scarcely visible beneath her crinoline when mounted.[142] Cecil Monro was intrigued by the 'agreeable amble' of the Mentonese donkey, which 'was an excellent beast, his movement … just as good as a horse's on the hills, and on the road not bad', but his experience at Hyères some years later was less happy: on a donkey excursion with fellow invalids 'Mrs Ross's donkey kicked her on the foot and Miss Ross's pitched her off on her head, or rather rubbed her off against a tree'; the greater embarrassment for Cecil was that he had been helping Mrs Ross mount her donkey at the time.[143]

Carriage exercise in Madeira was impossible as there were hardly any roads suitable for wheeled transport. Apart from travelling by foot – an activity that Elizabeth Wynter considered 'more of a penance than a pleasure' owing to the state of the paths[144] – moving about depended on horses or boats. Horseback riding was clearly not suitable for very delicate or elderly individuals. For those unable to ride, palanquins (a sort of curtained settee) and hammocks, both suspended from a long pole carried by two men, were available. Visitors rarely failed to remark on the sight of corpse-like invalids borne at funereal pace in these contrivances through the streets of Funchal.[145] Sixteen-year-old Charles Marling would love to have ridden but had to make do with a hammock: 'We have bought a hammock for Charlie's use', reported his brother William, 'as he is not allowed horse exercise, and he really likes it very well though of course he would greatly prefer a pony.'[146] Cecil Monro was less keen on riding – 'you can't see a country except on foot', he reported, but 'walking was prohibited to invalids'. He therefore hired a horse during his first stay on the island, at five to six pounds a month.[147] He also rode in Algeria in 1864.[148] Pau by contrast was made for carriages. The roads were good, and apart from scenery there were many attractive destinations, including the Hippodrome, hunt meetings and cricket matches. So-called chair walks were available at the nearby spas, a form of exercise that Fanny Blathwayt decided was a 'cruelty to animals (human)'.[149]

The beach on the Riviera played relatively little part in invalid life. This was not because the majority of invalids were there during the cooler months – British people were used to a cool seaside and summer water temperature at home that was similar to winter values in the Mediterranean[150] – but because the Riviera's beaches were not generally set up for respectable bathing, even if a significant number of invalids had been interested. There was no established tradition of bathing on the Riviera, beyond the splashing about by naked youths, in contrast to Biarritz, for example, where mixed bathing under some semblance of decorum was practised.[151] Sea-bathing was recommended, with caution, to many patients for its tonic effects, such as those 'who were overworked by any kind of business and needed setting up'.[152] Care was required in selecting a suitable time for bathing: Dr Whiteley reported that one of the fatal cases at Cannes during his residence was 'attributed to bathing in the sea after a copious dinner'.[153] The locals bathed in the summer and anyway had no use for bathing huts and other beachside paraphernalia. Bathing at both Nice and Cannes was extolled in Murray's handbooks, but although Murray noted the presence of changing huts at both resorts, Dr Lee missed them at Cannes.[154] Nor were they available at San Remo at about the same date, the mid-1860s, where 'the more primitive method of retiring to dress in the shade of the olive trees' was practised.[155] Rudimentary changing huts were evident when William Miller visited Cannes in 1876–7, but he rarely saw anyone bathing.[156] Cannes was known for its sand baths. Dr William Bullar described the procedure: 'The patient is buried in the sand, which is heated by the sun; he sweats profusely … and in addition to the benefit arising from this, much salutary action is attributed to the saline qualities of the sand, both in its effect on the skin and on the general system.'[157] It was something of a quack remedy invented, according to Margaret Brewster, by a Piedmontese peasant, but responsible it was said for successfully treating cases of rheumatism, inflammation, neuralgia and spinal complaints.[158] However it was only practised in the summer so would have been unavailable to most British visitors.

## Doctors and patients

Only the very wealthiest British invalids took a personal or family physician with them to the Continent. The vast majority depended on foreign practitioners or on expatriate faculty who were either permanently resident abroad or, like the travelling patients themselves, seasonal visitors. British invalids usually preferred to consult doctors of their own nationality and were increasingly able to do so as their number multiplied to meet consumer demand. There were differences in medical culture and practice between Britain and her neighbours that led British patients to seek out compatriots if they could; according to Mrs Carleton, 'foreign physicians were apt to lose their English patients owing to their fondness for bleeding and their dread of powerful drugs'.[159] Probably more important was the simple reassurance of familiarity, for few subjects are more difficult to discuss satisfactorily in a foreign language than one's health. Allan Young, wintering with his family at Nice in 1838–9, was happy enough to call on a local doctor to bleed an ailing British manservant one night, apparently with conspicuous success, but this was clearly an emergency.[160] Edwin Lee could warn his readers to be wary of British practitioners abroad, for 'the title of doctor of medicine (which did not confer the right to practise) could be obtained with very little trouble from certain foreign universities, requiring little else than the payment of the fees', but there is no evidence of widespread dissatisfaction with their ministrations.[161] On the contrary, many appear to have been highly valued consultants and friends in adversity, whatever the occasional deficiency in their formal qualifications. One charge that could reasonably be laid against British practitioners on the Continent was that of touting for business, both in the sense of plugging the climatic and other benefits of their chosen resort and direct marketing to potential patients. But it is not obvious that these defects were any more egregious than those of their professional colleagues at home.

As a body, British physicians on the Riviera received good marks in the early Victorian period. Murray was generally complimentary. Margaret Brewster, ill at Nice, wrote of 'Dr G[urney lightening] illness even to a stranger in a strange land' and the 'great satisfaction' given to his patients by Dr Whiteley at Cannes.[162] Some became fixtures, such as Dr Nathaniel Allan Travis, who practised at Nice from 1841 to about 1872, Dr James Henry Bennet (1816–1891), who served the British colony at Menton from 1860 till about 1887,[163] and Dr Henry Daubeny, who practised at San Remo from 1864 till his death in 1887.[164] There were plenty of British physicians available by 1865, when the subscribers to the English church at Nice, for example, included eight MDs.[165] The Riviera was clearly a region where an enterprising British doctor with the requisite attributes could make a handsome living. The Anglican chaplain at Cannes reported in 1868 that a new doctor, formerly personal physician to the late Lord Brownlow at Menton, had recently set up in business near the Hotel de Provence and looked set 'to carry all before him as far as the fashionable world went'.[166]

Medical fees at Nice tended to track the secular inflation in hotel and other charges. They were generally higher than at home, twenty francs (a little under a pound) a visit by 1870, with patients at Cimiez or other locations at some distance from town charged double.[167] Excessive fees encouraged some, like Alexander Brown, to dismiss medical provision at Menton as a racket – the town was 'the Eldorado of hotel proprietors and expensive medical attendants'.[168] Dr Bennet was probably the most successful British doctor of his day on the Continent. Once established at Menton Bennet was able to charge London fees, twenty-five francs a visit, according to Pentland, and only made night calls in extremis.[169] Ann Reckitt, ill with a feverish cold, called Bennet in on Christmas Day 1861; 'he, overflowing with urbanity, prescribed a gargle and a cough mixture and charged two napoleons (forty francs) with such courtly grace that she almost believed it was cheap'.[170] William Chambers described Bennet's idyllic lifestyle at Menton, 'lolling in his hammock on the cliffs of Grimaldi, enjoying the pure air and sunshine in a little garden of Eden', while his London brethren laboured through the London fog and drizzle to see their patients.[171] Cecil Monro evidently considered Bennet's domination of Menton problematic – 'Mentone is a *trade* with Bennet', he complained[172] – but there were three other expatriate doctors practising there during the season by 1870, Siordet, Bagshaw and Marriot, so Bennet enjoyed no monopoly. Moreover, aside from the well-known names, one is aware of a penumbra of lesser men struggling for an opening, whether the presumably respectable Drs Clement and Beattie, who separately presented cards to Cecil Monro fairly soon after his arrival at Cimiez in 1868, or Dr Duncan from Kilkenny, described by Dr Griffiths of Hyères as 'a disgrace to his country'.[173]

At Pau, Alexander Taylor MD (1802–1879), the Scot who dominated medical attendance on British expatriates by the middle of the century, did not reach his commanding position without effort. When he opened his practice at Pau in October 1838 he found himself in competition with Dr Hazelwood, a long-established expatriate practitioner who enjoyed the official sanction of the local authorities and a loyal circle of patients.[174] Taylor evidently came to suspect before long that Hazelwood was an imposter who claimed medical qualifications he did not possess; despite efforts by eminent Britons at Pau to arrange a peace between the two doctors, Taylor was relentless – pursuing a 'war to the knife', in Elizabeth Grant's phrase – and eventually succeeded in driving Hazelwood from town in May 1844 for fear of exposure. Lord Cowley, British ambassador in Paris, apprised by the University of Edinburgh that there was no record of the award of a medical diploma to Hazelwood, as he claimed, decided to let the matter drop rather than report the impostor to the French authorities, in view of Hazelwood's speedy surrender of his official permission to practice in France, claiming ill health, and representations in his favour from several of his distinguished patients at Pau.[175] Despite Hazelwood's guilt, Elizabeth Grant took a dim view of Taylor's conduct, which she clearly considered self-serving and vindictive:

> As I collect from this gentleman's friends, who or what he was originally he don't [*sic*] appear to be the least anxious to say; he was one of the common

> herd of Edinburgh medical students for some time; then in the 'Spanish Legion' during part of the war; he came here in a very *seedy* condition, made his own way, procured for himself a rich and a well-connected wife, and then commenced his campaign against the poor doctor he found here and who had been settled here fully twenty years, with permission from the French Government to practise, who is really half worshipped by his patients.[176]

She predicted that Taylor would be the loser as Hazelwood's patients would turn to Dr Smythe, another hated rival, who would also attract some of Taylor's own, disgusted like herself with his conduct. His greed would be his undoing.[177]

In the longer term this proved so much wishful thinking. Taylor prospered to the extent that he was able to invest 10,000 francs (about £400) as a partner in the Société des Anglais, an enterprise responsible for much of Pau's property development in the 1860s.[178] By this time his position was unassailable; for Fanny Blathwayt in 1865 he was a paragon of medical consultants – 'I *do* like Dr Taylor, he is very sensible and very kind and comes in the shortest possible time when he is sent for.'[179] The British consul at Bayonne, recommending Taylor for the vice-consulship of Pau in 1864, described him as 'a man quite at the head of his profession … and held in the greatest estimation both as a medical man and as a friend of his countrymen.'[180] Although the application was unsuccessful, Taylor was knighted the following year for services to the British community at Pau, cementing his status as the colony's leading member. Fanny Blathwayt's diaries reveal Taylor as not only a regular caller at her lodgings to administer medical injunctions and prescribe blisters and pills but also an ornament of the expatriate community, host of society dinners and owner of one of the few private carriages available for excursions. The list of foreign residents in 1867 shows two other British practitioners, Drs Bagnell and Ottley, with whom Sir Alexander Taylor presumably had perfectly cordial relations, now that his pre-eminence was assured.[181] He died in 1879, full of honours.

The civil authorities in continental health resorts were usually content to allow accredited expatriate doctors to practice freely, especially if they confined their activities to their own compatriots. Accreditation varied from country to country. On the Riviera, for example, prospective practitioners in the French resorts required a diploma, which was only issued on examination, whereas in Italy no restrictions applied.[182] Superintendence, where it existed, was light-touch, but on rare occasions the full weight of official inquisition was brought to bear. The French authorities might not have troubled to enquire too closely into the formal qualifications of the hapless Hazelwood, but when a patient died in suspicious circumstances there could be no such indifference. At Nice in early 1847 an autopsy conducted on the body of a young British patient of Dr Cecil Gurney, a practitioner who had recently established himself in the town, revealed traces of enough morphia and prussic acid to arouse suspicions of poisoning. Although the Sardinian authorities exonerated Gurney on that charge, he was reprimanded for injudicious administration of drugs, despite continuing to enjoy the full confidence of his former patient's family. Rumours continued to circulate to the extent that in 1851 Gurney was moved to petition Lord Palmerston for support in clearing his name: 'The false and scandalous story has been again renewed, almost to the complete ruin of my practice', he protested. In particular he urged the foreign secretary to instruct a hesitant British consul to sign the public statement in his favour: 'As the visitors here change every season your Lordship will see the importance it is to my complete justification that the only English authority resident at Nice should not be allowed to interpose a barrier.' Gurney's petition failed to move Palmerston, who did not consider it the duty of a British consul to take sides in a local spat outwith his responsibilities. Gurney's practice survived for many years notwithstanding.[183]

Local medical faculty seem likewise to have had little difficulty for the most part in accommodating expatriate doctors into their ranks, in view of the special demands of British patients. The popular German spas, where early attempts by British practitioners to intrude themselves were resisted, were an exception. Edwin Lee was one of a number of British doctors at Wiesbaden in the late 1830s whose freedom to practice was temporarily threatened by police action in response to complaints by a local doctor who seems to have been anxious to protect his monopoly.[184] Augustus Granville's status as Kissingen's pre-eminent expatriate consultant was hard won in the face of opposition from the local German spa physicians, according to Mary Shelley.[185] Granville's privileged position was also resented by plenty of his compatriots. Dr Prytherch, a resident British physician at Homburg, published a translation of Granville's licence from the Bavarian authorities, in an attempt to portray his rival as enjoying an undeserved monopoly in treating British patients at Kissingen and thereby denying them the benefits of choice of medical adviser.[186] In fact the licence granted Granville no monopoly rights but merely permission to practice, and the celebrated doyen of British bath doctors had no difficulty in batting off such slights: Prytherch, he revealed, had an agenda, as he had been denied permission to practice at Kissingen himself in 1843 and had repaired to Homburg in frustration. Two other attempts by Homburg-based practitioners had been made to injure his reputation, Granville claimed, one by Sir Alexander Downie, who had falsely accused him of demanding a £500 bribe from the lessees of the Homburg springs to sing their praises, another by a German physician, Dr Wetzler, also denied permission to practice at Kissingen, and like Prytherch condemned to settle for second best at Homburg, 'that refuge ... of all disappointed practitioners'.[187] Granville's so-called monopoly was finally broken in 1845 when Dr Nathaniel Travis was granted a licence after several years of trying and henceforth was able to combine his winter practice at Nice with a seasonal stint at the Bavarian spa.[188]

In due course many British doctors established themselves at Belgian and German spas, usually with the sanction of the local authorities. Long-serving expatriate practitioners included Downie at Wiesbaden and Homburg (*c.* 1836–1852), Prytherch at Homburg (*c.* 1841–*c.* 1858), Thomas Cutler at Ems and later Spa (*c.* 1842-*c.* 1858), and Granville (*c.* 1840-*c.* 1866) and Travis (1844–*c.* 1866) at Kissingen. Edwin Lee never settled at a single resort for very long, but he spent several consecutive years in the late 1830s and 1840s practising at the Nassau spas.[189] The French spas did not acquire a significant British medical presence until later in the century, reflecting the evolution of their visitor demographic. Alexander Taylor and later Drewry Ottley and W. Bagnell from Pau advised British patients at the nearby Pyrenean resorts during the season. In some contrast to the climatic resorts, however, British patients were always more likely to consult local doctors at spas because the peculiar characteristics of the action of their waters required expert mediation. Frustrated British rivals might complain about the limitations of local spa physicians – Fenner of Schwalbach was an 'ignoramus' according to Granville, while Lee's foe at Wiesbaden 'did not understand English and his French was not very intelligible'[190] – but there is plenty of evidence of successful relations between local physicians and British patients at the German spas at least. Dr

Heinrich Welsch of Kissingen, 'a gentleman-like and skilful physician who spoke English' according to Murray, regularly put up a proportion of British curists in his house.[191] This was the specialist consulted by Louisa Campbell in 1866, for whom Granville by contrast was 'a stupid old man'.[192] Wilkie Collins had nothing but praise for his German doctors at Aachen and Wildbad in 1863.[193] In 1869–70 two British patients at Wildbad were happy to entrust their winter care at Nice to the German doctor who had been advising one of them at the spa during the summer.[194] By the later years of the century British patients were travelling to the Continent to seek out German specialists, such as the ophthalmologist Alexander Pagenstecher at Wiesbaden.

The British expatriate practitioners who provided medical care in Madeira during the period of its ascendency as a health resort had nothing to fear from native rivals. There is no evidence of any British invalid on the island during this period consulting a Portuguese physician. Like Taylor at Pau or Bennet at Menton, expatriate doctors frequently arrived as invalids themselves or had family reasons for seeking a warm climate. Several put down roots and spent decades serving the British community. In the late 1830s the field was dominated by Dr J. W. Broughton (fl. 1838–1859), Dr Alexander Renton (*c.* 1793–1848) and former convict-ship surgeon Archibald Ross (*c.* 1810–1856).[195] These were soon joined by Dr Dugald McKellar (1797–1849), Dr George Lund (1809–1888) and Dr Thomas Gillham (*c.* 1816–1849), as well as two medical missionaries, Robert Reid Kalley (1809–1888) and his brother-in-law John Miller. Although the latter's activities should have been – and no doubt largely were – directed towards the Portuguese population, it is possible that by the mid-1840s an excess of supply of medical services was disrupting the market. In early 1847 Ross charged Gillham with unprofessional conduct by interfering in the management of one of his patients some two years before. The delayed charge strongly hints at a recent history of mounting mutual antagonism arising from competition for patients. Gillham refuted the charge and countered with several examples of similar alleged malpractice by his accuser and others, including Kalley. A committee comprising Broughton, McKellar, Lund and Miller upheld the charge however and decided to refer the matter to higher authority at home.[196] Gillham died in July 1849, leaving the field free for his chief accuser, who however fell victim a few years later to the Madeira cholera outbreak.[197] The second half of the century was dominated by Lund (till 1863, when he left for home) and later Dr Michael Grabham (1840–1935), who arrived in 1861, married a daughter of one of the established British wine merchants and spent the rest of his life on the island.[198]

When British visitors did consult foreign doctors abroad it was usually from necessity rather than choice or because they offered specialist expertise that could not be easily substituted. Frances Bonham-Carter, suffering from an undisclosed condition that had caused her great pain on the journey south, began a course of bathing on arrival at Nice in November 1843, under the supervision of Dr Prevôt, although this was suspended in December by a relapse.[199] The family's principal adviser during their stay was however Dr Travis. Few British practitioners set up in business at the less favoured resorts, such as Algiers, where Cecil Monro for example saw two French doctors, Bodichon and Périer.[200] British patients seem to have been liable to the usual national premium when consulting foreign – or at least French – doctors. Revd Davies reported that the practitioners of Algiers charged French people three francs a visit, Britons five.[201] Revd Mason, travelling in the Pyrenees, was outraged at Dr Dulac's account for his treatment at Luchon, amounting to 200 francs (£8), 'a most amazing attempt at swindling' according to his wife; Mason wrote back declining to pay the full amount and, leaving 100 francs with his landlord, he and his wife departed.[202] The default assumption among most lay people, and probably many professionals as well, seems to have been that continental medicine was antiquated and hidebound; Mrs Carleton advised visitors to seek out a foreign doctor who had lost his prejudices by travelling, when no compatriot physician was available.[203] Edwin Lee thought he knew better, considering English medicine often irrational: cod liver oil, for example, 'appeared to have no special action in preventing or in procuring the removal of tuberculous deposits', but 'this remedy, though still in great vogue in England, where empirical modes of treatment found most favour, and where one panacea was rapidly superseded by some other, was … much less thought of on the Continent'.[204] Notwithstanding Lee's strictures, cod liver oil remained the stand-by treatment for British consumptive patients, and when it was unavailable or of poor quality, as at Algiers, the perceived inadequacies of the standard Mediterranean diet seemed all the more worrying.[205]

It seems clear that the majority of genuine invalids at health resorts consulted medical practitioners routinely. Many no doubt came with a letter of introduction from their adviser at home, perhaps addressed to a named specialist. A minority arrived to find their consultant in place waiting for them, such as patients of Drs Granville and Bennet. Although at the Mediterranean resorts, as well as at Pau and Madeira, the climate was deemed by both patient and practitioner to be the invalid's ultimate doctor, the medical expert on-site still had an important role in advising and admonishing patients on lifestyle and behaviour, as well as in providing psychological support. Private correspondence reveals patients and their carers often pathetically dependant on their medical advisors, if not for cure, then at least for direction or reassurance. J. R. Green's ironic depiction of the dictatorial status of the Riviera doctor, demanding the 'awful submission' of his patients, the 'most refractory [of whom] trembled at the threat of his case being abandoned', is, like all good satire, founded on a bed of truth.[206] Responsibility for failure to recover or otherwise make progress was rarely laid at the door of the doctor. Yet this is surely because patients recognized that illness was mysterious and intractable. So many variables were in play that trial and error was the only and inevitable approach to care, however dogmatic some climate or disease specialists undoubtedly were.

Writing to Charles Marling's father Samuel in June 1853 Archibald Ross, his doctor in Madeira, regretted that his 'interesting young patient had not gained the benefit which was so fondly anticipated for him'; he had however at least been more comfortable than he would have been under an English winter, and perhaps the voyage home would do him good, for 'the sea air and a change of climate often revived most wonderfully very great invalids'.[207] The claim that an invalid had at least escaped the British winter, however little progress he had made in regaining health, was a standard fall-back justification for seasonal expatriation. When Dr Travis at Nice was challenged by the Bonham-Carter family that they had expected more improvement in Frances's condition after four months, Travis had responded: 'You may be perfectly assured that she has been better here than she could have been in England.'[208]

Young men may have been exceptional in being more likely to doubt the competence of their medical advisers. Charles Marling seems to have had little time for Dr Lund, who succeeded Ross as his doctor in Madeira when he returned to the island as an adult patient: 'I never saw such a man for so making out a bad case', he protested in March 1861, annoyed that Lund had contacted his father in England behind his back. Relations did not improve the following season: Lund was forever trying to prevent Charlie from doing things, while 'the amount of medicine [he] had pitched into [him] was frightful'.[209] Cecil Monro was always sceptical of medical pretensions. He quickly concluded at Menton that he had the measure of the sainted Dr Bennet. He decided towards the end of his third successive season in Madeira that 'the advantages of the climate seemed so doubtful and the inconveniences so great' that he would disregard Dr Lund's advice to remain beyond May.[210] When he returned after two seasons' absence in 1865 Cecil consulted Dr Grabham, who also failed to impress: 'Grabham's merits are weakened by a certain weakness of a moral kind', he declared: 'a want of straightforwardness which would be more lamentable if it were more uncommon in doctors, and a fear of being supposed ignorant of this or that'.[211] Before his final visit in 1867 Cecil took the precaution of obtaining the prescriptions for two of the medicines prepared by his family physician in England.[212]

Dr Sparks wrote from the heart when protesting that patients 'would get on much better if they did not regard their doctor – "old So and so" they called him – as their sworn enemy, instead of their best friend, and his injunctions as "all bosh" '.[213] By the 1870s at the latest there was an unmistakable undercurrent of cynicism about the Mediterranean invalid trade, by no means exclusively confined to the laity. Dr Macpherson was amused to see a spoof brochure at Cannes advertising the delights of the fictional winter station of 'Doux Repos', where Dr Anglicide had successfully treated pulmonary cases using the 'fine calcareous dust' of the place, by means of 'pulverizing and inhaling apparatuses'; the brochure told, in Macpherson's words, 'many unpleasant truths, for instance of the doctors often playing into the hands of the lodging-house keepers'.[214]

## Life in the sickroom

James Clark summarized the mistakes invalids commonly made during their winter expatriation as 'errors of diet, exposure to cold, over-fatigue and excitement in what is called "sight-seeing", frequenting crowded and overheated rooms, keeping late hours etc'. To avoid such pitfalls they should eat moderately, dress as warmly as at home, beware of excessive exposure to the sun and above all live quietly.[215] Surviving testimony from genuine invalids would seem to indicate that few required such reminders. Although Dr Bennet remarked on the deceptive energy that consumptive patients sometimes exhibited in the early stages of disease – akin to the delirium of fever[216] – the accounts of living with illness in winter exile that have come down to us typically reveal an existence of numbing monotony, often bounded by the four walls of the sickroom. Whether as a result of such false physiological signals, or more commonly merely by being led astray by friends and acquaintances, the alleged tendency for patients to ignore the recommendation of their professional advisers to avoid excitement was routinely deplored. In the context of the mysteries of disease and uncertainty in regaining health (or otherwise), not to mention the vagaries of the weather and the other conditions of exile, it was natural for doctors to focus on the one aspect of invalid existence that they could at least hope to control. Patients for their part – and the more enlightened doctors recognized this – could not live by medicine alone but required some psychological sustenance to progress. The tension between medical injunction and invalid preference might appear from surviving patient testimony to have been usually resolved in the doctor's favour; but patients who kept to their rooms almost certainly did so by choice rather than instruction, and those so disposed may have been more inclined to confide their feelings to diaries and journals.

The invalid Elizabeth Wynter reported to her brother soon after arrival in Madeira in December 1838:

> Our days pass uniformly but to me very pleasantly; indeed it is a long time since I have felt so equable in spirits and free from care. I find enough to occupy me what with reading and practising the guitar and writing during the morning, and then there are visits to receive and pay. We generally ride in the afternoons and dine at five.[217]

It was common for patients in Madeira to enjoy an elevation in morale for some days after arrival, especially if they coincided with fine weather. Disembarkation alone often provided relief after a rough passage, while the beauty and novelty of the place, and the diversion involved in finding lodgings and meeting new faces and perhaps old friends supplied some distraction from the introspective gloom so characteristic of chronic illness. It did not take long for Emily Shore, another consumptive patient, to sink into the depression she knew so well, especially when left on her own indoors: 'I sank into a long, melancholy reverie on subjects that *will* intrude themselves whenever I am alone, now that the busy excitement of our voyage and arrival is over', she confided to her journal soon after arrival in the island. Nineteen-year-old Emily understood from her earliest days in Madeira that she would never leave: 'I could with happiness and enjoyment live in Madeira for even two or three years, if I could feel that I should then return to the same home I left. But this can never be', she admitted. The period between this confession in January 1839 and her death in July was interspersed with occasional intrusions of optimism – 'I really almost begin to think I *am* making some progress towards health' – but her journal is infused with an overwhelming sense of melancholy, informed not only by her premonition of death but also by the pain of exile.[218] Emily Shore did not however suffer and die alone but in the bosom of her family. Elizabeth Wynter recalled Emily's last days in a letter to her brother:

> I have been much grieved lately at witnessing the sufferings of a very clever, amiable and attractive girl on whose account principally her family came to settle here in the winter. Her troubles however, great as they were, are now over. She expired the other evening, shortly after we had left the house.[219]

Whatever supposed advantages consumption may have offered early Victorian patients to achieve a 'good' death, by ensuring a slow but more or less equable route to the grave, they are not obvious from such accounts.[220] As Nan McMurry observes, in challenging the fictional depictions of consumptive death in Victorian novels, 'real-life consumptives whose thoughts have been preserved were neither ready and welcoming nor blissfully unsuspecting of their own deaths. Instead, uncertainty and apprehension characterize their feelings.'[221] Patients wanted to get well, and if they did not the fact of exile only increased their psychological pain. Death was neither beautiful nor painless: as Sheila Rothman writes, 'The incessant coughs made talking and eating almost impossible and breathing, painful; the swelling of the joints and the loss of weight precluded walking; and the dying often subsisted on opium and whiskey [*sic*]. By the time death was at hand, emaciation was so complete that it appeared as if a cadaver had already replaced the human form.'[222]

Madeira propagandists did their best to counter the perception among visitors that the island was little more than a grim sanatorium, but it is clear that they were struggling against the facts. The tendency of pulmonary consumption to afflict siblings – a pattern of which contemporaries were well aware and was often ascribed to hereditary predisposition – meant that death stalked whole families and encouraged a sort of quiet resignation in face of the inevitable. Elizabeth Wynter recalled meeting 'two very agreeable people, sister and brother, offspring of the vicar of Harrow … neither of them so ill yet as to prevent their being very cheerful companions, but they have lost two sisters within the last five months, and the brother I know looks on his sister as doomed'.[223] Death of course might be – usually was – held at bay until after departure from the island, but the sense that exile in Madeira had been a mere intermission in the trajectory of inexorable decline was pervasive. Elizabeth Wynter remained in continuous residence in Madeira from December 1838 till March 1840, during which time her mood veered between happy relief to have avoided the English winter to despondent realization that she was gaining no sustained benefit to her health through exile. She apparently derived no advantage from remaining throughout the summer, a prescription favoured by Madeira's doctors but rarely observed by patients. Her health shortly before departure was if anything worse than it had been on arrival – 'I shall feel like a bad penny returned', she feared, 'for I am just what I was only perhaps thinner and weaker'.[224] By 1843 she was dead.

The Marling family arrived in Madeira in late 1852 still in shock at the sudden and recent decline in sixteen-year-old Charlie's health. 'It wrings my heart to think how changed he is in one short year', wrote his brother, 'a twelvemonth ago he was the most active of the active, carpentering, climbing, riding'; now he was 'but just able to leave his room'.[225] After some hopeful signs in the early days ashore, Charlie Marling's condition deteriorated. On examining the patient on 26 January 1853, Dr Ross found his left lung to be severely wasted – in a poorer state than when Charlie had left England, with a cavity completely penetrating the organ – and he feared for his life. Margaret Marling prepared for the end and advised her husband to hurry out to the island without delay, 'to share', in her words, 'these precious though most painful days of watching'. On coming to Madeira she had not expected Charlie's complete recovery, she told her husband, but had 'looked forward to two or three years even of life for him with care and every possible expedient we could resort to for healing the lungs and saving what remained'.[226] Happily the crisis passed, allowing Margaret to hope that after all the Madeira air would do its work: 'Really one does see such amazing prolongations of consumptive life here that I cannot feel hopeless', she informed her husband. The family moved into a new house on the seashore in February where a large carpeted dining room on the ground floor was converted into a bedroom for the patient and his mother.

In the event Charles Marling recovered sufficiently to accompany his family back home in June 1853. However he was not cured. He returned to Madeira in 1858 and again in 1860. On arrival in October 1860 he was in good spirits. Dr Lund examined his lungs and found the 'seeds of disorder' in the right still present but 'quiescent'. Charlie spent his days reading, learning Portuguese, watercolour-painting and sketching, playing billiards and riding.[227] The good news did not last. His landlady wrote to his mother in England in alarm at his symptoms: 'He does not rise to breakfast as he has always done up to within a few weeks and he does not like to be asked about himself although I am certain he feels very unwell and has very sleepless nights', she reported.[228] However he rallied, dismissing the fuss made over a fortnight's poor health.[229] When Charlie returned for the following season in October 1861 he was apparently in excellent health. In December he could report that he rode every day and occasionally went out to lunch or early dinner. As ever Dr Lund was more pessimistic, warning that his patient had been 'going out too much, too late at night'. Charlie's plans for a return home in the spring through Portugal and Spain alarmed even his fellow invalid Henry Gedge, who had accompanied him to Madeira.[230] These plans were never realized, but his voyage home via Lisbon was arduous nonetheless. He was dead within the year.

Revd Charles Baring (1807–1879), later bishop of Durham, arrived at Nice with his family in the autumn of 1839, hoping to find relief for his invalid wife. Mary Baring seems to have been suffering from a neurological complaint, rendering her unable to stand and causing partial paralysis of the upper body. Some improvement in her condition was evident by the new year, coinciding with fine January weather, but Baring remained unsure whether the climate of Nice was quite what she needed: 'It is quite extraordinary', he wrote to his brother, 'how at times, and especially towards evening, the whole of the nerves of the body from head to foot are in a state of excitement and fidget so that she cannot sit still, and yet obtains no relief from moving.' Nonetheless, Mr Bowling, the expatriate surgeon advising the family, assured them that 'Nice was just the air for Mary *now*'. Charles Baring was evidently quite happy with Mr Bowling as a medical attendant but would have liked a second opinion on the 'effects of this kind of climate on a nervous constitution'.[231] By early April Mary Baring was worse – 'the difficulty in breathing had increased much in violence and in the length of the attack' – and Bowling had evidently given up, advising that the only remedy he could suggest was a change of climate. The family would be heading home once the bad weather relented. A stop-off at Bad Ems had been recommended by another doctor, but Charles Baring was at a loss to decide whether to adopt this course.[232] We do not know whether the Barings returned via Ems or directly through France, but not long after their season at Nice had come to an end Mary Baring was dead.

Elizabeth Grant was rather contemptuous of the behaviour of her invalid sister Mary at Pau, spending all her money on luxuries rather than the education of her children or 'the necessary requirements of an invalid'. Mary was no malingerer however, but suffering from an acute dropsical condition. When Elizabeth first saw her on arrival at Pau in September 1843 she was shocked: 'There was not remaining one trace of beautiful Mary, her whole features were changed, lengthened, drawn, her eyes staring from her head … her form wasted quite away.' The purgative natural medicine she was prescribed for her dropsy, elaterium, had such serious side effects that it risked becoming as fatal as her disease. The doctors agreed her case was almost hopeless, but she was unable to alter the habits of a lifetime. She tried to drown her sorrows in alcohol and continued to eat sweets rather than wholesome food, being inclined to 'only do just what the whim of the moment suggested'. When she moved to Avranches in Normandy for better air her condition and inclinations remained unchanged, for she was 'slave to those luxurious habits of every kind so long indulged', in her sister's words. But she was so ill Elizabeth could not sustain her annoyance at her perversities. When she finally died Elizabeth was devastated. As she looked at her body, 'stretched on a narrow mattress laid upon the floor in her nightdress with a muslin handkerchief over her face', she recalled a sister 'full of faults, for she was human' but 'pure and innocent and lovely compared with herself who judged her'.[233]

As an invalid Fanny Blathwayt's life at Pau was lived chiefly indoors, at the Hotel de la Poste during her first season (1864–5), subsequently at the Maison Planté. Here the Blathwayts occupied a suite of rooms, including their own drawing room, where Fanny was able to install her hired piano – a must-have for every season – and she and the family could receive guests, take music and drawing lessons and perhaps even have their meals. When her health permitted her days were filled with social calls; and when the weather allowed there were walks in the park, carriage excursions into the surrounding countryside and occasional sporting occasions to observe – meetings of hounds, steeplechases, cricket matches. Fanny was an observer of rather than participant in the social whirl: 'I have no news as I don't go out and the endless train of balls etc. are the chief charge one hears of. Every night until the 26th is taken up', she wrote in early February 1868.[234] Much of her time however was devoted to fulfilling social obligations, all the more demanding on account of her husband's position as a leading member of the expatriate visitor community and enthusiastic sponsor of its activities. As Fanny's health deteriorated the demands of social obligation grew tiresome: 'Several people called but I forget who; I only know I set out my drawing and had to put it by', she noted on 12 November 1867. Her habit of recording her visitors became wearisome: 'As I am quite kept in two rooms and only have change by the people I see I shall take no further trouble writing a journal till I am able to go about a little more – as it is too *stupid*', she determined on 29 February 1868. When her journal entries resume it is to record '*shoals* of callers all afternoon' on 23 April. On 16 May she 'tried hard to do some drawing but was prevented by a good many callers during the afternoon'.[235] Fanny's last diary entry is dated 20 September 1868, and she died at Pau on 22 February 1869, aged thirty-eight.[236]

There is little evidence of hope in these dark accounts of suffering and no suggestion of romanticism attending the last days of consumptive patients. On the contrary, chronic illness is overwhelmingly oppressive, limiting and tedious. The most isolated and pitiable invalids were those who, unlike the examples described above, were unaccompanied by family members or friends and often too ill to benefit from any social support available at their lodgings; patients such as the Mr Dunn who arrived at Cecil Monro's hotel at Hyères in January 1870 in a delicate condition only to die within days, exhausted by the journey.[237] Cecil himself was never more miserable than when left alone at the Villa Garin at Cimiez, depressed by the gloomy autumn weather and largely confined to his room, battling the mosquitoes with a moist sponge.[238] Even in fine weather, once the initial elation of arrival in the warm south had passed, the very beauty of the scene might seem to mock the invalid. As R. L. Stevenson wrote about his return to Menton as an adult patient,

> He recognises with his intelligence that this thing and that thing is beautiful, while in his heart of hearts he has to confess that it is not beautiful for him … The world is disenchanted for him. He seems to himself to touch things with muffled hands, and to see them through a veil. His life becomes a palsied fumbling after notes that are silent when he has found and struck them. He cannot recognise that this phlegmatic and unimpressionable body with which he now goes burthened, is the same that he knew heretofore so quick and delicate and alive.[239]

The Riviera probably harboured more unaccompanied refugees than the more distant resorts, patients for whom the fashionable life of Nice and Monte Carlo must have seemed like another world, however geographically proximate. Genuine invalids on the Riviera – certainly hopeless cases – seem to have been largely out of sight by the later nineteenth century, if not before. William Miller assured his readers that invalids did not predominate at Menton, and although one did see the occasional hopeless case in the streets, most seriously ill people kept to their rooms.[240] Even before the development of specialist sanatoria therefore, the sick were confined, isolated and increasingly invisible. Doubtless this was largely by necessity and patient preference, but there may also have been an element of self-confinement. Conspicuously sick and disabled people could be upsetting. Elizabeth Grant herself, visiting the Pyrenean spa Barèges from Pau, found it 'full of disgusting invalids'.[241] Seriously ill patients might have felt increasingly under psychological pressure to keep out of sight in an environment that was evolving into a place of play.[242]

## Conclusion

The additional challenges for a patient living abroad appear to validate the critique of several medical authorities who, as we have seen, decried the practice of invalid expatriation. Doctors at health resorts clearly had a vested interest in talking up the advantages of winter in the south and evidently had a standard justification for the practice even when a patient did not progress – remaining at home would have been even worse. Patients and their families and friends – even their medical advisers at home – had no particular reason to agree. Why then did the sick acquiesce in what a critic writing in the *Pall Mall Gazette* termed 'transportation by order of medicine'.[243] The testimony of several patients betrays some scepticism at least regarding the supposed benefits of winter exile. Many therefore had mixed feelings, no doubt anxious for relief or cure and prepared, at least initially, to allow 'medicine' the benefit of the doubt, but rarely sustaining any great confidence in the prescription in light of disappointed hopes.

Perhaps though the sentence of 'transportation' had less to do with medical injunction than the demands of family. Loving parents of teenaged consumptives such as Emily Shore or Charlie Marling hastened to Madeira with their charges, desperate to stave off the seemingly inevitable; families such as the Bonham Carters, keen to avoid the gloom of a British winter, headed south with an invalid member as much to address their craving for escape as to benefit the health of the patient. Reading Fanny Blathwayt's diaries from Pau is to be struck by how fully the family was involved in the expatriate life of the resort and to conclude that the motivation for exile must have been quite as much to do with the attractions of sociability and play for the healthy family members as the putative benefits of expatriation for the patient. How many patients who travelled abroad would have done so if left to their own devices is of course unknowable. But it is arguable that the pressures on them to conform to the standard prescription for treatment came not so much from professional medical direction as from the hopes, fears and expectations of relatives and friends, motivated by a broad spectrum of concerns, from an agonized attempt to rescue a loved one from death to downright self-interest.

# 5

# Meeting and mixing

## Home from home

The southern health resorts that British people visited in the Victorian period were almost all in foreign countries – the principal exceptions being Malta and (until 1864) Corfu – but all nevertheless acquired something of the character of colonies. In 1861 the British consul at Nice wrote to the Foreign Office seeking guidance on how to respond to local complaints about British residents ostentatiously flying the Union flag from their houses and in other conspicuous locations: 'No other foreign residents at Nice ever presumed to hoist a flag', he noted.[1] Nice was one of those resorts with a long-established British presence, which inevitably encouraged colonialist tendencies. Other places already had a significant permanent expatriate community, such as Madeira, or, like Pau and Cannes, acquired a body of British property owners or long-term residents on the back of their growing reputation as winter refuges. These settled communities supplied the essential substrate on which the seasonal visitors relied, even if they comprised little more than the British consul and Anglican chaplain and their families, as at Algiers and Malaga. For the most part it was they who lobbied the local authorities for civic improvements, provided the medical services, built and maintained the churches, supervised the burial grounds, sometimes even owned and ran the hotels and boarding houses.

No health resort was so thoroughly colonized as Madeira, which, owing to the prominence of British expatriates in the life of the island, its underdevelopment and its relative isolation, appears to have been viewed by many British visitors as essentially indistinguishable from other outposts of empire. In the words of the British consul in 1835, 'Englishmen felt themselves as much at home in the island as if they were in England, and the police laws and formalities on entry and departure were a dead letter as far as Englishmen were concerned.'[2] The Portuguese authorities periodically asserted their rights, as in 1841 when an invalid, Mrs Serle, 'hurried off to Madeira by the physicians who had attended her', arrived without a passport and was consequently, in the words of the Foreign Office official handling her complaint, 'subjected to inconvenience'.[3] Almost all foreign visitors to Madeira before the middle of the century were British, apart from a few Americans. There was no regular, direct communication between the island and the European Continent outside Portugal, so any prospective visitor from northern Europe had to come to England to take a ship or make their way across the Continent to Lisbon. However in the late 1850s a small number of German invalids began to arrive, numbering perhaps thirty to forty annually by 1860, and as many as sixty by the winter of 1867–8.[4] From the late 1860s onwards non-British visitors may even have begun to predominate, although no significant permanent non-British expatriate population was established.[5] Madeira retained therefore its overwhelmingly anglocentric flavour as a visitor destination well into the later Victorian decades.

Pau also had an established British community by the 1830s, although it was not commercial but largely made up of expatriate members of the rentier class, retired army officers and others with private means. Its size at this date is unknown, but it was certainly smaller than the British colony on Madeira and less prominent in local affairs. Most winter visitors at the opening of our period – so-called *hivernants* – were not British but incomers from other parts of France. Yet already by the time of Louisa Costello's visit in 1842, Pau was well on the way to becoming *ville anglaise*. The British had 'so usurped the place of its original inhabitants', she claimed, 'that only a very few French were left'; she saw no point in healthy people coming: 'Almost all advantages … to be derived from foreign society were denied, and the frequent parties at Pau were nearly exclusively English.' The place was only fit for invalids.[6] By the 1850s and 1860s, Britons dominated the winter trade, and despite the gradual reduction in their relative contribution to the total of seasonal visitors in subsequent decades, their mid-century dominance set the tone for the resort for the remainder of the century. The British had planted the deepest roots; even as late as 1878–9 they contributed the largest component of what the *Journal des Etrangers* called '*anciens résidants*', in other words habitual visitors who typically arrived early in the season.[7] Statistics for the previous season (1877–8), when political instability in France had led to a severe drop in the overall visitor total, which had barely reached 2000 for the season, show nevertheless that the *anciens résidants* were unaffected – they had come in their accustomed numbers.[8]

Costello had evidently misunderstood the motivations for expatriation for the majority of her compatriots. Far from embracing exposure to French influences British visitors drove a relentless anglicization of the commercial fabric of the town: by the 1860s, Cazaux frères, promoting themselves as 'English chemists', issued their bills in English; F. Soennen and company's *Pharmacie Française et Anglaise* in rue Serviez advertised '*médecines patentes anglaises*' and '*thés divers*'; the London Pharmacy in rue Henri IV supplied 'English drugs and patent medicines', while the grocer J. Favre, purveyor of teas and marmalades, advertised '*biscuits anglais*' and '*fruits secs*', Cheyrouze in rue Gassion proudly declared itself a '*Dépôt de Bière Anglaise*', and A. Simonet, on rue Préfecture, was an 'English grocery and general provision warehouse'.[9] By the later 1870s Pau had three Anglican and one Scottish church and facilities for a range of British games and pastimes, from tennis to roller skating. Most emblematic of colonization was the prominence of fox hunting in the social life of the town, with districts in the neighbouring hills given nicknames redolent of home – 'Home Circuit', 'Hill District', 'Leicestershire', 'Old England'.[10] The comic writer and illustrator C-A d'Arnoux Bertall, who visited Pau in 1875, described a town that 'belonged to England': fox hunting and polo, dancing the Lancers at the Hotel Gassion, the garrison band as likely to provide a rendition of God Save the Queen as the Marseillaise.[11]

No Mediterranean resort submitted quite so comprehensively as Pau to British colonization. Cannes probably came nearest to rivalling it. Unlike Pau, Cannes had no national significance before its 'discovery' by the British in the nineteenth century and no expatriate population. It was 'a pure creation of the health-seekers'.[12] The example of Lord Brougham, the first Briton to build a house there, in which he wintered every year till 1868, was followed by others, and there were 'several English villas' by the early 1850s, according to Dr Francis.[13] By the late 1870s there were 'over 500 villas, chiefly inhabited by English families', according to Cook, and 'during the season many hundreds of English lived in the hotels, pensions, and villas in the new town'. There were three Anglican churches and one Scottish. A flavour of the British imprint is conveyed by Cook's description of an excursion down the road towards Fréjus: '*On the left*, the English church. Villa Victoria, English style of fifteenth century, Mr Woolfield's. *On the right*, Castle of the Duc de Vallambrosa, formerly Lord Londesborough's "Château Ste Ursule", English style; Villa Eléonore-Louis, Italian style, Lord Brougham's. *Left*, Villa St George's, Italian style, M. Grandval's, formerly Sir Herbert Taylor's; fine gardens.'[14] The pulmonary specialist, Dr C. J. B. Williams, who moved to Cannes on retirement from practice in London in 1875, found a resort where 'there was such an abundance of agreeable and friendly English society … that [he] hardly seemed to be abroad'.[15] But as in all the Riviera resorts, the British property owners were, like almost all the visitors, chiefly seasonal residents. Both Cannes and Pau were equally desolate in the summer months, abandoned by their winter visitors, but while Cannes' expatriate residents had either returned home or were ensconced at a German spa, Pau's were hunkered down in their suburban chateaux or close at hand at a Pyrenean watering place or Biarritz, primed to return for the season at a moment's notice.

As at Pau, the Riviera resorts attracted an increasing number of other foreigners as the century advanced. Already by the winter of 1870–1, according to the British consul at Nice, Americans made up the largest foreign contingent of seasonal visitors at the Riviera's largest resort.[16] A correspondent writing from Nice in February 1872 reported that her hotel was full of Americans.[17] Away from Cannes Britons were rarely in an absolute majority among foreign visitors, at least after the mid-1860s. During the winter of 1863–4 there were about five hundred British visitors at Menton, according to the consul at Nice, perhaps about 40 per cent of the town's visitor total.[18] This proportion accords broadly with the national proportions provided by Chambers for 1870 and Sparks for the last four years of the 1870s. The next largest contributors, apart from the French, were Germans, Russians and Americans.[19] The British proportion at San Remo was a little lower – about 33 per cent; here the British and German visitor population had a rough equivalence by the later 1870s, as the latter found France a less welcoming destination following the Franco-Prussian War.[20]

The Riviera resorts were more accessible to the populations of central and eastern Europe than Pau, and doubtless more attractive too, not least owing to the proximity of fashionable German and Alpine watering places. Even for Britons, the Riviera remained a region to visit rather than inhabit permanently, as exemplified by the differing patterns of residence of Drs Bennet and Taylor. The British residents never obtained – nor indeed sought – a significant role in civic administration or municipal development, as at Pau, but remained guests in a foreign land. Of course they still imported many of their indispensable foodstuffs and medicines, and even British turf for lawns; they built Anglican and Presbyterian churches; and founded clubs where they could play billiards and read the *Times*. But they did not seek to create a little patch of England, as at Pau, partly because the climate and topography did not permit it but chiefly because most came to the Riviera in the first place precisely because it looked and felt different from home.

British visitors to Madeira and Pau, or Cannes and Menton, in the mid-nineteenth century found themselves in health resorts that their compatriots had been instrumental in founding and where their desires were indulged as far as local circumstances allowed. True, the sanitation might be defective or the local fare deficient in some particular, but there was a good chance that representations for improvement would be heard and addressed by municipal authorities and local entrepreneurs, who after all depended on the British pound for their prosperity. The continental spas were different. Most European watering places had roots in the previous century or earlier, long before the mass penetration of the Continent by British health-seekers. Rarely in this world were British visitors in a majority, even if they briefly made up the largest foreign complement at various resorts at different times. The spending power of British visitors doubtless had an influence in driving improvements in accommodation and sanitation, especially in the early Victorian period, just as it was reflected in the nomenclature of hotels, and contemporary fashion encouraged the development of such features as 'English' gardens. But the continental spas remained fundamentally resistant to anglicization, evolving in response to the exigencies primarily of the domestic consumer or, in the case of the more fashionable resorts, to the demands of an increasingly international clientele. The British never set their stamp on any of these places. The cultural disjunction is encapsulated in the opening chapter of Wilkie Collins's novel *Armadale*, as taciturn Scotsman Mr Neal, arriving at Wildbad in the Black Forest, bids the town's mayor 'shorten the performances of his town band' in deference to his irritable nerves.[21] A German watering place was not somewhere to escape booming music in the open air, itself only one of the distinguishing features of German spa life that received a mixed reception from British visitors.

Like the Riviera resorts, the German spas became increasingly international in flavour over the course of the second half of the nineteenth century – by 1858 for example Bad Ems was already drawing over 60 per cent of its registered visitors from outside Germany. In the early Victorian period Britons often comprised the largest non-German contingent of curists at the Rhineland spas, representing over a third of the total on average at Ems until 1847.[22] British prominence at Schwalbach seems to have broadly tracked the popularity of Ems during the years up to 1845, not unexpectedly since many curists spent time at both spas during a single season, while Schlangenbad continued to benefit from Sir Francis Head's promotion for at least the following decade.[23] However by the 1850s and 1860s Britons were significantly outnumbered at Ems by French and Russians. As the French largely abandoned the Rhineland spas after the Franco-Prussian War British visibility was temporarily magnified – in 1877 Britons accounted for about a quarter of all non-German visitors to Ems – but it was not sustained, and by the 1880s British numbers were usually under five hundred per annum, representing under 5 per cent of total registered visitors and something between 14 and 18 per cent of foreigners.[24]

From about 1860 onwards between 15 and 20 per cent of Homburg's clientele were British. Until the Franco-Prussian War their contribution to foreign visitor numbers was matched only by the French, and it reached a peak of well over 3,000 visitors in 1872. This figure was never approached again in later years even though the 15 to 20 per cent ratio was broadly maintained as overall visitor numbers settled around the 10,000 per annum mark.[25] At Kissingen the number of registered bath visitors more than doubled in the two decades between 1858 and 1878, although the British proportion was a diminishing figure: in 1858 it was about 9.25 per cent, falling to 7 per cent by 1869; by 1878 it was only 5 per cent. The overwhelming majority of water drinkers at Kissingen during this period were Germans, with Russians making up the largest foreign component (11.6 per cent in 1858, 5.4 per cent in 1878).[26] At Carlsbad the bath authorities began publishing a breakdown by nationality in 1856, when only 234 British visitors were registered. Henceforth the annual number of British curists followed a general upward trend to reach a maximum of 506 in 1882. However, since overall registrations also rose during the period, the British proportion rarely exceeded 2.5 per cent.[27]

## Compatriots

Mixing in company was never part of an invalid's care regime. On the contrary, specialists were often vociferous in warning patients against excessive socializing. Nevertheless, it was recognized that invalids would not thrive in isolation but would need some 'society' to see them safely through their lengthy exile. It was invariably presumed that this would comprise the company of compatriots. Dr William Marcet, reviewing his years of experience as an expatriate physician on the Riviera, imagined a reluctant patient, ordered south for the winter, worrying among other things about the want of company in a land where he did not understand the language.[28] In reality an invalid rarely lacked for English-speaking society in the southern health resorts or continental spas. Few British visitors to the Continent looked forward to socializing with the local inhabitants, and genuine invalids would doubtless be even less inclined to seek out foreign company. British visitors tended to flock together, turning individual hotels or districts into monoglot oases. Over two-thirds of British registered visitors to Bad Ems between 1835 and 1852, for example, stayed in only half a dozen hotels and between a third and a half in the two most popular of these.

Hotel managers, recognizing the preference of their guests, even encouraged further segregation; William Miller noted that the Hotel des Iles Britanniques at Menton, which was well patronized by Britons, 'had one long table … set for the English and another long one for the foreigners'.[29] At the Hotel de France at Eaux Bonnes, according to the traveller Henry Blackburn, the table was divided into French and foreign sections, the latter evidently entirely populated by Britons:

> There were the grave *patres familiarum* who were there with their families, for the benefit of the waters, and who particularly disliked them; one or two members of the Alpine Club who had come down to Eaux Bonnes for a change; London physicians taking a brief but vigorous holiday; a

> few ordinary tourists; and the two English ladies that [one] met almost everywhere in Europe, travelling together.[30]

Social life at health resorts usually comprised dining, mutual visiting and excursions. Some invalids found even this limited range of activities taxing. Elizabeth Wynter, pleased to have escaped the burden of society at home in Devon, found its recreation in microcosm in Madeira tiresome: 'Far from lamenting the departure of visitors from this place', she wrote in July 1839, 'I am inclined to rejoice at every shipload that leaves the bay.'[31] She urged her brother to discourage the despatch of additional clothes: 'Tell Mamma that anything gay is quite useless to me ... for after what we have seen of the society here we are little inclined to enter into it again this winter.'[32] Elizabeth was no recluse however, but took pleasure in comforting the sick and bereaved, as befitted a clergyman's wife, taught German and music in invalid families, including to Emily Shore's sister, and held 'piano tea parties'.[33] Cecil Monro was equally uninterested in 'society' but when accompanied by his mother had necessarily to make some concession to the formalities of social life. He referred to the mutual exchange of visits as 'paying off old visiting scores'.[34] The sort of company that Cecil chiefly sought – intellectuals or attractive young women – was of little interest to his mother, who required 'ladies' to help her manage an extended period of exile from home.

Society in Madeira was famously soporific. Elizabeth Wynter dismissed it as 'a dull repetition of dinners' where conversation was characterized by 'little save the tittle tattle of the place or discussions about the various invalids and their status'.[35] For young people especially the lack of variety could be suffocating: 'This is the most *idle* place the mind can conceive', Cecil Monro noted soon after arrival in the island; 'the visitors concentrate their minds on billiards, whist, novels and riding at three miles an hour'.[36] 'Madeira is a bad place for unprotected males', he concluded during his third season – there simply was not enough to do.[37] Pau at first almost outdid Madeira in tedium, but it rapidly developed a peculiarly English social season. Dr Taylor confessed in 1856 that Pau was deficient in 'public amusements', but this was compensated for by the attraction of 'private soirées'; there was an English-style club, the *Cercle*, and plans for both theatre and library were afoot.[38] Frederick Johnson noted the whirl of evening activities: 'It may be some encouragement to fast, young people who anticipate a kind of exile in the Pyrenees', he advised, 'to know that in one evening of last season [1855–6], eight soireés and a fancy ball taxed the strength of the pleasure-seekers of Pau.'[39] By 1868 Fanny Blathwayt considered 'Pau had got to that pitch that people must have been made of money to even dress for it'.[40]

On the Riviera only Nice could match this. Cannes had a reputation for attracting religious types, with obvious implications for its attractiveness to the fast set, although it developed a more hedonistic character later in the century. Margaret Brewster found the society at Cannes 'very pleasant – so simple and kindly, without formality or overdressing'.[41] Menton was duller still. Dr Siordet admitted early in the 1860s that healthy people accompanying sick friends or relatives complained of the monotony.[42] The 1867–8 season was marked by balls, parties and picnics according to a witness, but William Chambers reported no such jollities in his account of the following two seasons: 'The English-speaking population are scattered about among the hotels and villas, and are generally unknown to each other', he explained; there were no social facilities worth the name – the *Cercle Philharmonique*, the club where the occasional ball and amateur theatricals were held, was so little advertised that 'so far as the general body of strangers were concerned the establishment might as well not exist'. The two Anglican and one Scottish church were the only institutions that provided any cohesion to the British expatriate community. 'It is a beauteous scene but you are alone in a strange land' was Chambers' summation.[43] In 1877 a group of British visitors, including invalids, put on several successful dramatic performances at the *Cercle*, leading the local paper to speculate that perhaps Menton was learning to enjoy itself.[44] But enjoyment was never really part of Menton's prospectus. Medical opinion assigned little therapeutic value to amusement.[45] In the words of J. R. Green, who died from tuberculosis at Menton in 1883, 'few places were more depressing in their social aspects as these picturesque little Britains; life was reduced to its lowest expression; people existed, rather than lived'.[46]

The company of compatriots in exile was important to most, but not all. William Chambers declared that living in pensions or boarding houses 'suited the gregariousness of the French character', but, he implied, not the British, or perhaps more precisely his own.[47] More commonly nationality was a necessary but not sufficient qualification for successful social relations. Victorian social relations among the 'higher' classes were highly regulated by convention and protocol so that the presence of numbers of compatriots with comparatively little to do did not necessarily promote a flourishing of uninhibited social intercourse. It was difficult to engage in easy interaction with those even of one's own class without a formal introduction. Consequently one of the first questions to exercise a new arrival at a health resort was whether anyone they knew was already in residence. The municipal authorities in many resorts published bulletins of arrivals, to allow guests to find their friends among other things. The German spa bulletins, so-called *Kurlisten*, giving details of newcomers, their status, companions and hotel or other residence, were especially detailed and regular. One of the first things writer G. H. Lewes (1817–1878), George Eliot's 'husband', did on arrival at Homburg in August 1873 was to consult the *Kurliste*, looking for acquaintances.[48] Non-German names were frequently garbled, but although corrections were invited they do not seem to have been made very often, so perhaps guests did not rely on these publications much.[49] In the absence of such bulletins new arrivals were expected to announce themselves to compatriots. Mary Eyre attended a ball at Bagnères-de-Bigorre in March 1863 to mark the marriage of the Prince of Wales but found herself a wallflower: 'The rule at Bagnères', she explained, 'is for the stranger to call upon the English residents, and I did not know this, and called on no-one.'[50]

If one was without friends or acquaintances, the company of strangers had to be embraced or endured. Revd Cecil Wynter and his wife Elizabeth contemplated sharing a large furnished house in Funchal with the Shore family, in order to economize, but the plan fell through as it became clear that Mr Shore, who like Cecil was a clergyman, held 'certain violent opinions in matters of politics and church government'.[51] Fanny Blathwayt avoided the table d'hôte at the Hotel de la Poste at Pau for most of her first season, as it meant sitting down to meals with as many as sixty other people, whom she dismissed as a 'gossiping, card-playing set'.[52] She only ventured into the hotel's dining room for breakfast for the first time five months after arriving.[53] Cecil Monro also baulked at eating in company at Miles's boarding house in Madeira, where the single sitting for dinner at six-thirty was for twenty-two guests. This arrangement was agreed by the majority of the other boarders, who wanted to be sociable. In consequence Cecil avoided dinner and merely took tea in his room until the owners turned over one of their private rooms for a common tea room. Cecil's reluctance to mix was partly owing to illness but probably also had something to do with his opinion of his fellow guests: 'The company at Miles's is not very choice this year', he informed his father; 'a good fraction of them are rather vulgar and one is a positive blackguard'.[54]

Cecil Monro had in general a low opinion of his fellow invalids wherever he went. After three seasons in the south he decided that 'this going abroad for people's health bred a childish sort of creature', implying presumably that the typical invalid was naïve, ill-prepared and dependent.[55] By the time he booked into the Pension Anglaise at Villa Garin, Cimiez, in 1868, the prospect of indifferent company was of no consequence, for he had 'done without society, especially of male persons … for some time'.[56] He kept mostly to his room, only venturing into the common sitting area in the evening. A modest infusion of interest was provided by the arrival of the consumptive humorist William Jeffery Prowse (1836–1870), who together with a young gentleman from Shropshire named Green were, Cecil was willing to concede by the new year, 'better than he should probably get elsewhere of that gender'. 'The other [gender] is certainly not well represented', he continued, 'and the whole lot are, Prowse excepted, (and possibly an old Indian I have not got to the bottom of) ignorant and insular beyond what I would have believed … possible'.[57] If Cecil Monro was an intellectual snob, his mother – a frequent companion in exile – looked for social equals of her own sex, who were apparently not always easy to find. Writing from Madeira in 1865 Cecil noted the lack of ladies as a potential drawback, should his mother decide to join him, for 'the *Quality*, as his mother called them … were said to have gone to the south of France'.[58] Perhaps they both eventually found their heart's desire at the Hotel des Ambassadeurs at Hyères in 1870, where fellow guests included the botanist Robert James Shuttleworth (1810–1874) – 'a great invalid, but very lively' – and two elderly spinster ladies related to the late bishop of Chichester and archbishop of York, respectively.[59]

## The church

One essential feature of colonization that did not spare the health resorts of continental Europe was the planting of Anglican – and to a lesser extent

Scottish Presbyterian – churches. They were not however established primarily for purposes of proselytism but to serve the needs of the expatriate community. Availability of a suitable place of worship was as important to most Victorian Britons overseas as any other staple of existence; for invalids perhaps more than most. Ann Vavasour, writing in the early 1840s, remarked on the proliferation of English clergy abroad: 'One of the greatest changes on the Continent in the last twenty years', she claimed, 'is that now there is an English clergyman in almost every town where a few English reside.'[60] At health resorts many of these clergy were themselves invalids, offering their services to fellow countrymen as they recovered their own health. Others were accompanying delicate wives or other relatives. Several were long-term residents on the Continent, moving from place to place as demand for their services dictated, in the same way as some expatriate doctors shuttled between resorts. Services were held in a variety of premises in the absence of a consecrated church – the British consul's house, as at Malaga, local Protestant chapels, hotel assembly rooms, even the ducal riding school at Wiesbaden, following the burning of the Lutheran church in the Revolution of 1848.[61]

It was obviously preferable to perform services in a dedicated building created for the purpose. Various obstacles might stand in the way. The first Anglican chapel at Nice, Holy Trinity, was built by private subscription in the Croix de Marbre district in 1822. The Sardinian authorities sanctioned construction only on condition that the building did not resemble a religious edifice and that its use was reserved exclusively to the British community. A perennial difficulty arose from the tendency of the chaplain, Revd Hubert McLaughlin, to disappear at regular intervals on health grounds, especially during the hot summer months, without making adequate arrangements for services in his absence. In 1836 the authorities were unimpressed to find the chapel's vacant pulpit occupied by non-Anglican dissenters, such as a Swiss pastor conducting services in French. The immediate risk of sanction was averted by regularizing the management of the chapel establishment, which became a consular chaplaincy, supported by a subvention from the Foreign Office.[62]

In 1857 a scheme for an additional Anglican church was launched; this was to be at Carabacel, half a mile or so inland from the shore, located for the greater convenience of invalids, with seating for about 200 to 250 worshippers.

Among sponsors of the scheme were expatriate doctors, such as Travis and Gurney.[63] Christ Church Carabacel opened for services in 1860. Holy Trinity in its turn was rebuilt soon afterwards, in fashionable Gothic style, 'a beautiful building', in the words of the British consul, 'far superior to any other Protestant church on the Continent'. It had accommodation for a congregation of 700, and the cost of £6,400 had been funded entirely by voluntary contributions.[64] However, the evident prosperity of the British colony at Nice that these developments seemed to demonstrate proved a mixed blessing to the church trustees. The Foreign Office had long bridled at the bother of supporting the English church at Nice, which had routinely annoyed officials in London by requests for money and irregular accounting. Government understandably expected a British colony overseas with the means to fund the building of two new churches to stand on its own feet: 'There is no church establishment under the [Consular] Act which has given so much trouble to the Foreign Office as this one at Nice', wailed an internal memorandum; there was apparently no good reason for any government subsidy – 'they are in difficulties because they insist on maintaining two churches and three chaplains'.[65] Consular status was finally withdrawn in 1874.

The Anglican Church on the Continent was something of a problem child for the ecclesiastical authorities at home. Superintendence was conventionally vested in the bishopric of London, but the bishop's authority was more notional than real, and the individual chaplaincies were largely left to their own devices unless and until a scandal or appeal for episcopal adjudication brought their affairs to wider notice. In the absence of close supervision and a lack of comprehensive and reliable information about membership of the Anglican ministry, errant clergy were sometimes able to continue to officiate on the Continent free from interference from superior authority. Revd W. G. Parminter spent several successive seasons at Bad Ems during the 1850s and 1860s, taking services and giving English lessons to supplement his income.[66] At other times of the year he lived in southern Germany, officiating at among other places Stuttgart and Freiburg.[67] This was despite the fact that he was widely known by fellow clergy to be incompetent. As the secretary of the Colonial and Continental Church Society informed the bishop of London in 1858, '[Parminter] was reported by other chaplains, of a respectable standing, to be not only useless but injurious to the cause of religion on the Continent, for he seemed to sanction by his presence every worldly amusement however unsuited to the position and profession of a clergyman of our Church'.[68] The quality of Anglican clergy in Europe at the time was not high – as the same correspondent added, 'it was probable that there were many even worse men and more glaring cases on the Continent than that of Ems' – and it may be that this was especially the case at spas, with their transitory and shifting British population, who would have been less able or indeed interested in monitoring standards than more permanently settled compatriots. Indeed Parminter's faults seem relatively minor compared with a chaplain at Spa, 'who had been censured by the Bishop as having kept race horses and been frequently seen in a state of intoxication even in church'.[69]

A few chaplaincies – so-called consular chaplaincies – had a higher profile because they attracted a government subvention on the basis of supporting the British community in places of commercial importance. Elsewhere the expenses of the chaplaincy, from the maintenance of buildings to the stipend of the chaplain, fell exclusively on the congregation. New church buildings were frequently financed by wealthy health-seekers. Christ Church Cannes was sponsored by the Lancashire industrialist Willam Garnett (1818–1873), who regularly wintered on the Riviera; the church opened in 1866 despite the loss of a specially commissioned stained glass window and church plate in transit by sea from England.[70] The Anglican church at Homburg was the project of Lady Janet Kay Shuttleworth (1817–1872), although it had other subscribers, including, it was rumoured, Messrs Blanc, the French proprietors of the *Kurhaus*.[71] The prime movers of the English church at Kissingen were two patients of Granville's, Sydney Herbert (1810–1861) and Charles Brindley MP, who visited the spa in 1855. All Saints Kissingen opened in 1862, with Granville as secretary of the trustees. Unfortunately he seems to have thought he enjoyed proprietary rights, falling into dispute with the bishop of London over the unlicensed appointment of a chaplain in 1865 and interfering in the arrangement of services.[72] Granville was a conspicuous presence in church during Louisa Campbell's time at the spa, singing loudly and tunelessly and taking the offertory.[73]

Most southern health resorts had, as we have seen, a settled expatriate population who typically provided the core of congregants, served as the church trustees and appointed the chaplain. But the variable influx of winter visitors often threatened the equilibrium of even the best-managed chaplaincy, partly because of the pressure of numbers that could not be easily accommodated in a building designed for far fewer congregants and also because of the tendency of winter visitors to contaminate sleepy ecclesiastical backwaters with the factional dissension of domestic church politics. Proposals for new churches to serve greater numbers were sometimes suspected of masking attempts to introduce modish metropolitan doctrines and liturgical innovations where they were not wanted. This was certainly the case at Pau, where St Andrew's, opened in 1866, and one of whose sponsors was Wynter Blathwayt, seemed to some to be an attempt by meddling invalids to introduce the Tractarian poison into a staunchly Protestant establishment.[74] The party feeling thus generated was evidently still alive and well as late as 1885.[75] At Menton, a new church, St John's, specially adapted for invalids, having a south-facing narthex at the west end, was opened in 1868 to serve residents of the west bay.[76] It quickly took on the High Church mantle and was by the later 1870s evidently better-attended than its sister church, Christ Church, attracting visitors with its music and more elaborate services.[77] In 1876 controversy arose at Nice over the services at Christ Church, leading to 'a most angry paper warfare', in the words of the vice-consul, stirred up by a recent arrival, Colonel Pughe, a former inspector of police in India.[78]

Nowhere was factional fighting more bitter than in Madeira. Even Madeira propagandists had to admit that the visitor community, in addition to being subject to the normal quotient of gossip and scandal associated with 'all little towns where three hundred people, without much to do, assemble for health's sake', was especially prone to religious dissension.[79] Soon after arriving on the island in 1838 Elizabeth Wynter remarked on the number of clergymen, who were regrettably 'divided into parties'.[80] The consular chaplain was Richard Thomas Lowe (1802–1874)[81], a noted naturalist who was appointed in early 1834. Lowe was a Tractarian who alienated the established Anglican congregation presided over by the British consul and the leading mercantile families to such an extent by his changes to services that in January 1846 a meeting of congregants voted to discontinue support for his salary. A minority of the congregation, largely comprising temporary visitors and invalids according to the consul, formed a body of Lowe partisans agitating for restoration of his income. In February 1846 the consul George Stoddart reported that twenty-two people had signed a 'protest' in Lowe's favour: 'Two or three visitors (here for purposes of health) of strong tractarian opinions are taking every means to create sympathy in Mr Lowe's favour chiefly with parties who are only here temporarily', he protested. The annual church meeting the following January saw an unsuccessful attempt to overturn the 1846 vote, despite efforts to pack the meeting with last-minute subscribers: 'No ladies ever attended our meetings before', complained Stoddart, 'and although I thought their presence did not shew a good feeling, still I did not think the Act gave me any right to object to their votes.' Nevertheless the vote was lost by thirty-six to twenty.

At the end of 1847 the British government terminated Lowe's official status as consular chaplain, but he did not go quietly, issuing a public protest on the arrival of his successor and announcing that he intended to continue holding services in a private room.[82] His ministrations bequeathed a legacy of bitterness: among his crimes, according to congregant Robert White, were his packing of the chaplaincy library with Tractarian publications in place of 'truly evangelical works', and his temerity in removing both the library and the communion plate on his dismissal, as if they were his own property; 'the great majority of the residents, however, were so pleased to obtain the removal of their ill-suited pastor … that they took no steps to recover the property belonging to their church'.[83]

Invalids were also heavily implicated in the more serious controversy surrounding the activities of Scottish medical missionary Robert Reid Kalley (1809–1888).[84] Kalley, who held an MD from the University of Glasgow, came to Madeira in 1838 for his wife's health but evidently found there a promising field for both his medical and missionary vocation. After returning briefly to England to be ordained into the ministry of the Congregational Church and obtaining a licence to practice medicine from the Portuguese authorities on his return, Kalley began to minister not only to British patients but also to poor Madeirans, for whom he additionally held religious services and encouraged in Bible study. This was unsurprisingly interpreted by the local authorities and the Catholic Church as Protestant proselytism. As with Lowe, the British consul detected the baleful influence of interfering invalids behind Kalley's work: 'I am given to understand that … Dr Kalley's supporters and advisers have been, and are, chiefly some invalids who have been only a short time in the island', he reported in May 1843, following complaints by Kalley of police intimidation. The consul forwarded a petition to London in favour of Kalley from his supporters, 'all I have no doubt exceedingly well-meaning persons but some of them certainly indiscreetly enthusiastic and injudicious – the greater number of the signatures are those of invalids, including many ladies, who are only here for a short time for the benefit of health'.

After Kalley was arrested later in 1843 and then released following diplomatic pressure, his claim for compensation elicited further invalid support: 'I write now to tell you that some of the invalids here and their friends are, as they did last year, getting up a memorial to Lord Aberdeen, in favour of Dr Kalley', Stoddart reported to London in February 1845. Things came to a head in August 1846 when a mob ransacked Kalley's house and those of some of his supporters, and he fled the island. One of the violated properties belonged to the Misses Rutherford, one an invalid: her 'life was endangered and she lay for hours in a state of insensibility'. Another supporter, a navy purser out in Madeira with an invalid mother and sister, was in the Rutherford house at the time and ascribed his mother's death some days later to the violence.[85] Madeira's religious dissensions, reported in detail by the consul to London, caused John Bidwell, superintendent of the consular department of the Foreign Office, to wish 'all the parsons at the bottom of the sea'.[86]

## Non-compatriots

British people visited continental health resorts to seek cure, to rest and recuperate, occasionally to play and be entertained. Although the advice literature was infused with the truism that a change was as good as a rest, there was no suggestion that immersion in a foreign culture was of any service in assisting recovery. On the contrary, every effort seems to have been made to render any cultural dislocation as imperceptible as possible. Some specialists railed against British health-seekers who overdosed on pharmaceutical remedies or insisted on luxuries that they were used to at home, but these were instances of folly betraying the patient's stubborn resistance to change the habits of a lifetime rather than criticism of his parochialism. Most British visitors had little desire to interact socially with foreigners. Their proverbial reserve went before them and the higher classes in the resorts they frequented, among whom they would in other circumstances have found their social equals, were in their turn viewed as standoffish and unwelcoming. Interaction with foreigners was largely confined to transactional relationships, usually with social inferiors. These conditions discouraged mutual sympathy. No tourists were more unpopular on the Continent than the British, thought Thomas Madden, for none were so reluctant to adapt to foreign habits and customs.[87] The British had not caught up with the societal change that had occurred in France since the Revolution, in the opinion of Adolphe Smith: 'In this democratic country, where caste has been abolished, the tradesman, the workman, the peasant, expect, and are generally treated with the same deference and civility as the lord or plutocrat', he warned. The peremptory manner in which British customers often barged into shops and barked out their demands without observing basic courtesies did not go down well.[88]

Such behaviour indicated not so much an antipathy to foreigners as a collision between the visitors' class-based expectations and the reality of continental life. Some commentators found the loosening of social restrictions liberating, but for most it seems to have been discombobulating. Spa life could be especially challenging. At continental watering places British visitors were unable to shelter within the warm embrace of an expatriate colony but were forced to enter a sometimes disconcerting world of social mixing. Most spas had a history of serving a primarily parochial clientele, and in the early Victorian period at least shopkeepers and artisans were as likely to feature among their adherents as lawyers, landowners and army officers. Many spas even had dedicated bathing facilities for paupers. British visitors consequently entered an unfamiliar world of blurred class boundaries, where, in the words of James Johnson, 'Mr Owen[89] might find his social system almost perfect … [for] we have our food in common, our physic in common and even our physician in common'.[90] For British women especially, according to a recent authority, 'eating in public in socially mixed company' was problematic.[91] At Rippoldsau in Baden, which few Britons visited, Ann Vavasour observed that 'the variety of ranks sitting down together would not be liked by the English, but in this country the countess and peasant sit side by side'.[92]

As the century advanced, social fragmentation set in as continental spas increasingly opened up to an international clientele, assisted by vigorous marketing, investment in new facilities and the growth of the railway network. Spas became at once more cosmopolitan but also more socially exclusive.[93] The Jewish shopkeepers who form such a conspicuous presence in the Carlsbad bath list for 1840, for example, are by no means so obvious twenty years later.[94] This may have encouraged more transnational mixing, even by British visitors, in the second part of the century, as social equals from across Europe found it easier to encounter each other at watering places. Lord Carnarvon found 'not a good deal' of 'society' at Wildbad in August 1869 but used the opportunity to become acquainted with several foreigners through the good offices of a fellow guest, Lady Olivia Cowley (d. 1885), wife of the former British ambassador in Paris, 'which as he was at a foreign watering place he looked upon as part of a day's work'. His wife Evelyn was at Bad Ems, where likewise there were 'apparently no English whom she cared to know' but like her husband could expect to fill the vacancy with 'a few foreigners whom she could know and who … would be some kind of society'.[95]

Mixing with foreigners who were fellow health-seekers was always more likely to occur than social interaction with the settled native population of the resorts that Britons visited, for they were not only usually social equals but also shared the common interests and identity of invalidity and exile. Cecil Monro often found the most congenial company in Madeira among the non-British guests – Americans, Germans and Scandinavians – including a Polish political refugee named Ritter, who had been wounded in a nationalist insurrection. Later, at Cimiez, the indifferent British company at the Villa Garin was mitigated by the opportunity to assist fellow guest Friedrich Schmidt in collecting botanical specimens.[96] Lone invalids may have been more inclined to mix with strangers – or at least compelled to find 'society' where they could. Louisa Campbell knew nobody at Kissingen when she arrived in June 1866, apart from a 'German gentleman and American lady' she had met on the Rhine steamer, who became her first friends. Subsequently she made several acquaintances, at the table d'hôte at the *Kurhaus*, through attending the English church or when music-making at the *Converzatione Saal*; these appear to have been mainly British though she also knew several Dutch guests. As an unaccompanied young woman she may have been particularly popular with gentlemen invalids, whose names pepper her journal, though there is no suggestion of impropriety.[97] If no suitable British company were available, foreigners might serve as substitutes. Even at Pau, the most Anglocentric social scene on the Continent was leavened somewhat by the participation of American and French visitors, who, according to an article in the *Times*, 'returned there season after season, [and were] notoriously hospitable'.[98]

Socializing with foreigners privileged some facility in foreign languages. Murray's sage advice that 'no-one should think of travelling before he had made some acquaintance with the language of the country he was about to visit' seems to have been largely neglected. English was of limited utility on the Continent beyond its use for basic practical transactions. Happily most educated Britons had some French, which for most of the nineteenth century operated as a European lingua franca in polite society; it was not only serviceable in the Francophone world but at many Rhineland watering places, which were heavily influenced by their proximity to and historical ties with France and existed in a sort of bilingual middle kingdom. Indeed many of the *kursaals* at the Rhineland spas were run by French entrepreneurs before 1870. At Baden Baden, Wiesbaden and Homburg French was the language of exchange, whether cultural, commercial or medical, and hotels had French names and bills of fare. Carlsbad also belonged to this bilingual world.

One did not have to move far from this zone of relative comfort to enter the world of Teutonic monolingualism, populated by impenetrable innkeepers and bewildered bath attendants. Ann Vavasour found French as useless as English at Rippoldsau. Mary Shelley's German interpreter at Kissingen was as incomprehensible as her interlocutor, while the servants at her lodgings tittered in bemusement at her attempts to order tea.[99] Mary at least made valiant if largely unsuccessful efforts to learn the language of Goethe and Schiller. For most Britons German remained beyond the pale, the object of derision and ridicule in equal measure. Returning to Spa in the Belgian Ardennes from his excursion up the Rhine, the author of *A Hot-Water Cure* was relieved to be free of the 'horrible ya boo language of Germany'.[100] Lord Carnarvon, taking the waters at Wildbad in 1869, had visited the opera, but 'it was unfortunately in German ... a detestably barbarous language'.[101] German was as comical as it was incomprehensible: 'it seems so odd not to hear "*Ja Ja, So So, Doch, Doch*"', a returning traveller reported to her friend on reaching Dover.[102] Many British invalids were however reluctant exiles, fundamentally home-sick, and used the intractable German language as a convenient whipping boy to assuage their misery. In France, the language could provide no such useful function for educated Britons, who were expected to have at least a working knowledge; here the main challenge was to reconcile the various local patois, especially in the Pyrenees and the Nice area, with the polite French the traveller brought with him from home, a language to which they seemed to bear distressingly little relation.

Class affinity could smooth the path of successful relations between British visitors and their continental counterparts in most circumstances, but there remained some continental habits which were shared, or at least tolerated, by foreigners of all classes that repelled British observers. By the early Victorian period the upper and middle classes in Britain had for the most part been bred to value privacy and decent segregation of the sexes. They were also used to a level of personal and public hygiene that often seemed woefully deficient across the Channel. In one area in particular – provision and use of toilets – these two concerns came together. Many British visitors were shocked by the apparent indifference of people on the Continent not only to provision of appropriate physical arrangements for hygienic evacuation of the bowels but also to observance of a fitting modesty in attending to what John Macpherson called 'the one daily recurring necesssity'; it would remain a struggle to persuade Britons to visit the smaller European spas, he asserted, until 'defective arrangements' were addressed.[103] The shock was worse, according to an experienced traveller who sought to warn his naïve countrymen what to expect, because returning tourists put the horrors they had encountered out of mind, so they never passed on appropriate warnings: in many a continental hotel, 'one glance, on the opening of the door [of the cabinet], was mostly sufficient to make any English gentlewoman run away, as from a chamber of horrors, to her room'.[104] Germans were dirty, the author of *A Hot-Water Cure* concluded on completion of his tour, as shown by 'the vehement filth of their most necessary apartments'.[105] Worse still was the brazen way in which two women had conducted a conversation with each other as each took turns in the dining room toilets at his hotel in Aachen, thus drawing attention to an activity that should have remained decently out of sight and mind.[106]

France if anything was worse. French provincial hostelries were notorious for inadequate toilets, providing no privacy. James Clark at the beginning of the century considered that women were especially vulnerable to the inconveniences of continental travel, such as the 'discomforts a lady must encounter in many of the smaller inns in [France]', so that misdirecting unsuitable female cases to spend winter in the south was doubly regrettable.[107] Four decades later the intrepid tourist Mary Eyre could still advise 'no lady traveller who could help it, to quarter herself at a French wayside inn'. 'What we consider the absolute necessities of life', she continued, 'is [*sic*] to the French mind superfluous luxury.'[108]

Privacy was a guiding watchword for the Victorian upper and middle classes. An anonymous contributor to *Blackwood's Magazine* in 1846 reckoned Vichy was no place for British families as life had to be lived in public, contradicting English notions of comfort, which 'implied both privacy and detachment'.[109] Yet at all continental spas life had to be lived to an extent in the public gaze. Dining was usually a communal activity that some British visitors could barely tolerate. The main meal at German spas took place in the middle of the day, and the sight of large groups of morning water drinkers descending on the hotel dining rooms at a time when most Britons would be diligently exercising their minds or bodies elicited amused comment, tinged with a dash of moral superiority: 'When most other people were actively pursuing their business', sniffed Madden, Germans 'sat themselves down to a meal, at which they consumed incredible quantities of watery soup, boiled beef with sour kreut [*sic*], roast veal, uncooked smoked ham, slices of raw herring, roast goose, *kartoffel salat*, stewed fruits and Dutch cheese, all mingled together in what appeared to one unused to German living most horrible confusion'. Besides, this dinner time was 'altogether too early and no invalid should dine at so absurd an hour'.[110] Sir Francis Head could stand the table d'hôte at Schwalbach for only two days before abandoning feeding in 'this gross manner'.[111]

If communal dining could be stressful, bathing in public was worse. By the opening of the Victorian period the use of mixed-sex baths was disappearing in Europe. Gastein in Austria was 'probably the only place where men and women bathed together', thought James Johnson, who visited in 1840.[112] John Macpherson, writing in the late 1860s, welcomed the abandonment of this 'most undesirable practice', which only persisted he believed at Leuk in Switzerland and one or two other minor spas in central Europe. At least the bathers were clothed, in contrast to Japan 'where men and women bathed promiscuously without any coverings'.[113] Indeed Johnson considered British objections to mixed bathing on the Continent illogical since 'the bathers were covered up from head to toe when bathing together – women showed more flesh on the dance floor'.[114] However, communal baths for each sex were still common, and this was objectionable enough to the sensibilities of many Britons, not through any hygienic fastidiousness but for reasons of privacy. Some form of clothing seems to have been generally used in these communal baths – Macpherson recommended 'a light shirt'– but the necessary level of undress was still a cause for concern.[115] At the Fürstenbad or Prince's bath at Wildbad, the most select of that resort's *piscinae*, Ann Vavasour was distressed at the lack of a 'screen to protect the modest stranger from the scrutinising glance of those already in the water below', which was 'most unpleasant to the English ladies, unaccustomed as they were to bathe in company'. Moreover there was only one dressing room, 'also without curtain or screen, so that the dressing was even more unpleasant than the bathing'. She looked forward to the opening of new facilities to enable 'English ladies to bathe in solitary dignity, as they did in other places'.[116]

It was not usually obligatory to bathe in public baths, but even individual baths were no guarantors of privacy: 'The Germans are decidedly gregarious, and no wise particular as to intruders', warned the author of *A Hot-Water Cure*, noting that the first cubicle locks he encountered were at Homburg.[117] Most single baths seem to have been housed in cubicles, open at the top like public lavatories, and British visitors were variously disturbed by chatting – German ladies had a fondness for sharing their baths according to the author of *A Hot-Water Cure* – whistling and the noise of douching in adjacent compartments. Anxieties about privacy diminished as the century progressed, presumably in line with the increasing privatization of space. French spas in the second half of the century offered 'individual bathrooms, private sedan chairs and personal changing rooms', according to a recent authority, reflecting 'the same conceptions of respectability, modesty and hygiene that the French bourgeoisie increasingly saw in itself'.[118]

Mixed-sex bathing was also the custom at French beach resorts. In Britain the sexes normally bathed apart, if only because men were used to bathing naked. The traveller Thomas Paris described the novel experience of donning a French bathing costume at Biarritz in 1842, which comprised a 'nether robe [scarcely] reaching the knees [and] jacket composed of the thinnest materials

… wholly guiltless of sleeves', and his nervous approach to the beach beneath the gaze of female onlookers.[119] Charles Weld some years later preferred to seek out a remote spot in the cliffs where he could strip off and bathe in private.[120] Bathing at Biarritz, as at other French seaside resorts, was a family affair, where the beach and the sea were merely extensions of social life on dry land. Henry Blackburn described a scene at the beach at Biarritz where, far from scuttling into the water as quickly as possible to hide their modesty, bathers paraded in their costumes, laughed and played, and both sexes spent hours in the water chatting and frolicking.[121] The difference between French and English attitudes to social life was never more obvious than at the beach, thought Charles Weld: 'In England we go generally to the seaside to enjoy repose and quiet', he concluded, 'whereas a visit to the coast is insufferably dull to our neighbours, unless gaiety and publicity are the order of the day.'[122]

## Politics and war

Victorian Britain was unusually peaceful. Warfare or insurrection were unknown. Even civil disturbance was muted by continental standards. Health-seekers contemplating a season abroad ran the risk of exchanging the comfort of home or the peace and repose of the English seaside for the volatility of a fractious Continent. Admittedly most established health resorts in Europe lay far from capital cities and other likely sites of violence, but they were not immune from the backwash of political strife, nor could they always be certain to remain off the path of armies. Edwin Lee considered the political events of 1848 only bore out the opinions he had expressed in *Continental Travel* regarding the deficiencies of the French character; he foresaw trouble in Italy through likely French intervention and ultimately war with Austria.[123]

Whether prospective visitors paid much attention to generalized warnings is doubtful. Many clearly avoided travelling at the height of or immediately after crises or bypassed more risky regions of Europe in favour of quieter ones. The British consul in Madeira expected an increase in visitor numbers for the 1848–9 season 'from a dread which invalids would have of the state of Italy and the south of Europe'.[124] British registrations at the spa at Homburg fell by about 40 per cent between 1847 and 1848, by almost two-thirds in 1866, the year of the Austro-Prussian war, and by about the same proportion in 1870; registrations at Bad Ems fell by roughly similar proportions over the same dates, although the decline was considerably less in 1870.[125] In 1856 the trustees of the English church at Malaga adduced civil disturbance as one of the reasons for the decline in visitor numbers that winter.[126] Outside these brief interludes prospective visitors do not seem to have ranked the threat of political conflict highly on their list of anxieties. As Britons they were doubtless confident in their passport to guarantee safe passage, their navy to intimidate foreigners and their government to protect their persons and property.

Even in times of peace British residents and visitors were likely to be regularly reminded that they had passed beyond the enlightened shores of their homeland. Long after the passport and customs restrictions that so exercised travellers in the early part of the century had largely eased, British newspapers remained liable to detention by the police in France. William Chambers blamed the French post office for the irregularity of delivery of papers from home: 'Frequently no paper arrives, and then perhaps two or three come together', he grumbled; 'such irregularities, often complained of, but never redressed, are the reproach of the French postal system'.[127] Since the normal mail generally suffered no such interruptions it is more likely the fault lay with the government censor.

Two new London titles, the *Pall Mall Gazette* (1865) and *Pall Mall Budget* (1868), were especially irregular at first, indicating that the authorities were exercising their habitual suspicion of unfamiliar publications. The Misses Smithers at Villa Garin in Cimiez considered cancelling their subscription to the former as its arrival was so uncertain.[128] When a promised copy of the latter failed to materialize with its covering letter from his brother, Cecil Monro was incandescent: '"Foreign circulation" seems humbug', he ranted, 'while France exists under this despicable regime'.[129] The following year, copies of two recently launched journals, *Nature* and the *Academy*, passed uncertainly under the gimlet eye of the censor; when one of two expected numbers of *Nature* failed to arrive at Hyères in late 1869 Cecil was perplexed – he suggested his brother complain to the secretary of the GPO, 'as it cannot possibly have been stopped on political grounds'.[130] The *Pall Mall Gazettes* now came without difficulty, having presumably passed their probation with the censor, even when on occasion they carried an article critical of government;

Cecil supposed that 'censorship could afford to let accidental strong language pass in articles not systematically directed against 'the head of state' or 'the constitution'.[131] Interruption of newspaper delivery was still a problem under the Third Republic, according to William Miller, who reported particular problems at the time of the political crisis of autumn 1877.[132]

The Franco-Prussian War and its aftermath was a period of heightened anxiety for British residents in France, for their country's neutrality was viewed by many French people as morally questionable. Alarm at the potential fall-off in business as a result of the war had led Dr Bennet to reassure his professional colleagues in September that the resorts of the Riviera 'would remain calm, peaceable and open to invalids' during the coming season, for 'their very existence depended on the winter influx of invalids and visitors'.[133] Although a disturbance by radicals had occurred at Nice on news of the proclamation of the republic in September, it was swiftly quashed by the authorities, who understood the importance of the tourist trade to the town's prosperity; 'The state of the town and the department is now such as to permit travellers, even invalids, to resort to it without fear', reported Adolphe Lacroix, British consul at Nice on 17 October.[134] 'On the whole a wonderful state of tranquillity had prevailed in the south of France', in the opinion of the consul at Marseilles, despite the defeat of the French army in the north of the country and the surrender of the Emperor.[135]

Nevertheless, anti-German feeling was predictably intense, and any suspicion of Britons favouring the enemy risked dire consequences. At the end of the year the vice-consul at Pau attempted to head off accusations of pro-German bias in the British colony in the pages of the *Indépendent* newspaper.[136] Already, Lacroix reported, an innocent Englishman had been assaulted in the street at Nice by a Frenchman as a supposed Prussian spy. Nice however was unlike the rest of France. Indeed it was hardly French at all, having been only recently incorporated into the French state. Here it was not the perfidious English who were unpopular but the French, and the assailant was almost lynched by onlookers. Nonetheless Lacroix was sufficiently alarmed by November to urge the immediate despatch of warships to defend British interests and reassure the colony, for 'a spirit of red republicanism had extended itself to Nice'.[137] The following February Lacroix was even more anxious, in view of recent disturbances, announcing that many winter visitors had left

Nice prematurely, although most of the Americans, reassured by the presence of four US warships at Villefranche, had stayed.[138] In the event no British ships were despatched, and it was rather the French navy that suppressed Nice's rebels. As for Pau, Dr Taylor assured his professional colleagues in late 1871 that 'there had never been any manifestation of excitement of a threatening character in the *département* of Basses Pyreneées' throughout the previous season; many Britons and Americans had kept away, but the 'residents of long standing', who knew better, had come as usual.[139]

The only continental health resort that saw a clash of regular armies during our period was Kissingen. In 1866, at the start of the Austro-Prussian war, it lay in the path of a Prussian army advancing into southern Germany, whose rulers were largely allied with Austria. Louisa Campbell was one of the unsuspecting British invalids whose placid summer was about to be rudely interrupted. Her journal betrays no suspicion of trouble ahead as she crosses Germany en route to the spa, apart from noticing 'crowds of soldiers' at Cologne. On 21 June she received a letter from her husband expressing concern about her staying in Germany any longer, but she appears to have taken little notice of the warning. On the contrary her routine continued without interruption despite evidence of troop movements and reports of military action elsewhere. On 9 July the tone of her journal changes quite suddenly as hurried preparations to defend the line of the Saale River at Kissingen are put in hand. Despite a warning from a Bavarian general that it was not safe to be outside, the following day Louisa accepted an invitation from a fellow guest to go and see the battle 'as the Prussians had commenced firing on the heights'. Bullets 'whiz overhead' as they move towards the battlefield and then hurriedly retreat from it to find Kissingen itself full of dead and wounded. Only now did Louisa appear to comprehend the gravity of events, as she and other spa guests were mobilized to care for the casualties. The battle of Kissingen disrupted spa life but did not annihilate it. Louisa continued to take regular baths and dine at the Hotel de Russie, but evidently she took an immediate decision to return home and left on 17 July by carriage for Würzburg, passing hurriedly through Bavarian forces moving up to the front.[140]

By early August an anonymous correspondent reported in the *Times* that Kissingen was now safe for visitors.[141] Baedeker's guide recorded that 'considerable damage had been done to several of the principal buildings ... to the no small consternation of the visitors'; traces of the battle could still be seen in 1868[142]. Louisa took a relatively minor role in caring for the wounded but seems to have been sorry to abandon them. Dr Granville's daughter, by contrast, was awarded a Prussian medal of honour in 1869 'in acknowledgement of her incessant care of the wounded Prussian soldiers after the battle of Kissingen'.[143]

## Conclusion

When Britons travelled south they packed their predilections and prejudices as well as their luggage. The prospect of freedom from social confinement and convention that expatriation offered was embraced by a few, deplored by more and ignored by most. Recreation of a familiar world of appropriate social relations, church services, foodstuffs and medicines, books and newspapers, games and pastimes was the overriding desire of all the British colonies in the sun. No one seems to have demurred from this ambition. Indeed the advice literature recognized that would-be travellers would be favourably impressed by accounts of resorts that had been thoroughly anglicized and repelled by descriptions of places that had resisted the tide. Murray might urge Britons to learn languages and behave with suitable humility as guests in a foreign land, but he really had no more interest than the most bone-headed of his readers in persuading tourists to engage with contemporary European culture and society. The British, in the words of John Pemble, 'regarded the countries of southern Europe, North Africa and the Levant primarily as museums, sanatoria and asylums, not as living societies'.[144]

Patients no doubt had more reason than most to welcome the comforting familiarity of the mature health resorts. There is no evidence however that anglicization was driven disproportionately by the demands of invalids. All British visitors demanded the same quality of accommodation, sanitation and services and craved the same foodstuffs and comforts. It may be the case that some invalids at least had more opportunity and inclination to break out of the insular straitjacket: with time of their hands they might have been more attuned to and appreciative of differences in landscape, flora and fauna; as more dependent on the help of others they might have formed more meaningful connections with foreign servants, hotel staff and others. One thinks of the young Charlie Marling nursed by his mother's Portuguese maid in Madeira, or as a young adult patient learning Portuguese and water-colouring, activities that one suspects would not have been top of his priority list if he had been in perfect health. In these circumstances, patients perhaps returned home – if they did – with their sympathies and imaginations widened, even if their bodies remained stubbornly resistant to reform.

# 6

# Outcomes

## Recovery and cure

'Many hundred patients migrate south every year, in search of health and a cure', observed the physician John Parkin in 1875, '[but] there are no statistical facts to show what the actual result of removal has been; we only know that a large proportion of them die, either before or after their return.'[1] Doubts about the efficacy of winter expatriation for consumptive patients especially were nothing new. Twenty-five years before, the Norwich physician Robert Hull questioned whether 'the expense, discomfort, wretchedness of travel and lodgings' were compensated by 'proportionate health and recovery'.[2] If the fate of consumptives was unclear, outcomes for other health-seekers were even more opaque. British people visited health resorts in every state of sickness and health imaginable. Contemporaries routinely distinguished between a minority of 'genuine' invalids and the rest, but the term was never defined, although it clearly implied a recognition that most health-seekers were not seriously ill. Indeed, those who were dangerously sick were invariably advised in the literature to remain at home.

Invalids were not segregated from the general visitor population in sanatoria, where their cases could be monitored systematically by their medical attendants, but distributed in hotels, pensions and villas, and seen by physicians irregularly, or perhaps not at all. They came and went as their wishes and circumstances dictated, sometimes, as we have seen, flitting between resorts in the hope of finding a better climate or more congenial living conditions. Only at watering places and to a limited extent in Madeira was there much prospect of compiling meaningful case histories by which treatment could be evaluated and progress – or lack of it – recorded. In the former, patients were typically undergoing a cure of predetermined duration under the supervision of a dedicated spa physician; this was not of course the case in Madeira, but the length of time invalids were obliged to spend on the island, as well perhaps as the more serious condition of the patients themselves, encouraged closer medical superintendence and generated the earliest published analyses of patient outcomes.

In 1826 Dr Renton was able to compute the medical outcomes of eighty-two cases of phthisis sent to Madeira for which he had notes, dating from the previous eight years. Of the forty-seven cases of 'confirmed' phthisis, thirty-two had died on the island within six months of arrival, six died on their return home, six more returned but had subsequently been reported deceased and the three others had returned but been lost sight of, though Renton concluded they were probably dead. In contrast to these grim figures, the thirty-five patients whose phthisis was only 'incipient' comprised twenty-six who left the island 'much improved in health, of which he had had good accounts', five who had also improved on the island but of whom no more was known and four who had since died.[3] Later, at the end of the 1839–40 season, Renton was able to provide James Clark with further details on the outcomes for recent cases of consumption sent to Madeira. Between 1 January 1838 and 31 May 1840, 182 invalids had arrived; of fifty-six 'with tuberculous lungs' thirty died on the island, twenty-two left and four still remained at the end of the season; meanwhile ninety-three of the 108 cases 'threatened with pulmonary disease' remained free from symptoms while thirteen had deteriorated and three had been lost sight of.[4]

Dr Lund subsequently supplied supporting evidence from a hundred cases of his own covering a period of about ten years up to 1853, divided into various stages of pulmonary disease: of forty-eight patients in the earliest stage, the disease was arrested in thirty-seven cases; of twenty-four in the second stage it was arrested in only five; and of twenty-eight in the last stage likewise in only five. Only one patient of the first group died on the island, five and a half months after landing; none of the second-stage patients died on the island but eleven were dead within four years; of the late-stage patients, eighteen died, almost all (fifteen) on the island during their first season. In all sixty-six of the one hundred were still living at the time of writing, thirty-four dead.[5]

Madeira was also the site of the only known climatological medical trial conducted with British patients at a foreign health resort during our period. In November 1865 twenty male patients from the Hospital for Consumption and Diseases of the Chest, Brompton, were despatched to the island, the only known occasion on which public charity cases were sent to Madeira. We do not know how they were selected, but some clue is provided by G. H. Brandt, the physician in Madeira responsible for their care. Writing in the *Lancet* early the next year he stressed the importance of selecting the right consumptive cases for treatment in the Madeira climate: 'From a climate like this the best results will be obtained in cases where disease is so far advanced as to have produced disintegration of tissue, where the constitution is so far impaired as not to be able to resist a cold atmosphere, and where living in the open air is the greatest desideratum.'[6] Early reports seemed hopeful. The *Times* reported on 27 June 1866:

> Of the twenty male patients sent out last year, eighteen have returned, one being still under treatment in the island. Of the whole twenty, twelve have improved considerably; six of them so much as to be restored to their several occupations; four others may be considered as stationary; three are not so well as they were six months ago; and one died suddenly, after a great improvement, from haemoptysis.[7]

In due course, however, the verdict was modified. Dr C. T. Williams, assistant physician to the hospital, later recalled that only three of the patients had returned improved; no medicines had been employed, so the climate alone offered perhaps some benefit but it was marginal at best.[8] The results were evidently sufficiently unconvincing to persuade the hospital not to repeat the experiment. Local expatriate physician Michael Grabham was unimpressed: in his view this decision amounted to effective strangulation at birth of an incipient Madeira sanatorium, for which generous funding had already been raised and which promised to provide the sort of clinical data that was sorely needed to support the therapeutic claims made for the island's climate.[9]

The published reports of medical outcomes relating to Madeira, limited and vague as they were, had no equivalent with respect to other European resorts. British physicians practising at continental spas published cases to advertise their success in treatment, but there was no systematic and objective analysis of outcomes and certainly no clinical trials. Elsewhere even this narrow and highly partisan evaluation was entirely absent. Patients and their medical advisers at home relied upon their own direct experience, individual word-of-mouth reports from others and the testimony of experts and authorities such as Clark and Granville.

In 1876, C. T. Williams's Lettsomian lectures attempted to shine a light into this mishmash of anecdotal evidence, hearsay and special pleading. Williams, now full physician to the Brompton Hospital in succession to his father, C. J. B. Williams, was able to collate results from 251 consumptive patients who had spent one or more winters at a foreign health resort. These were private patients whom Williams or his father had seen in London during the course of their careers. Williams analysed the development of their disease based on the winter locations the patients had visited. The majority of cases had been in the Riviera (82), Madeira (63), southern Europe generally, including Italy and Spain (52), and Pau (43); smaller numbers had visited Egypt and Syria (20), Rome (12), India (10), the Cape and Natal (9), Malaga (8) and Algiers (4); eighteen had been on sea voyages. The total amounted to 350 instances as obviously some patients had visited more than one resort. Patients wintering in the Riviera had clocked up the highest number of visits (135), followed by Madeira (102), Pau (74) and southern Europe (73). The percentage of patients whose condition improved ranged from 50 per cent for Pau and just under 54 per cent for Madeira to just above 58 per cent for the Riviera and 71 per cent for southern Europe. The patients who had taken sea voyages did even better. The more marked differential however was in the percentage of patients whose condition had worsened. Here the findings damned Pau with an egregious 45 per cent, with Madeira on 32 per cent; the figure for the Riviera was just under 21 per cent and for southern Europe 19 per cent.[10] The published findings caused predictable outrage at Pau, where Dr Alexander Taylor rushed into print to counter the challenge, but he had no statistical ammunition to deploy.[11] Dr Lund for his part tried to stand up for Madeira, though he no longer practised on the island, but again his case was essentially qualitative.[12]

Williams summed up the broad results of his survey thus: 'We see that in point of benefit received by the patients, sea-voyages occupy the first rank, the very dry climates the second, the south of Europe dry climates the third;

then follow the moist climates, viz. Rome fourth, Madeira and the Atlantic warm climates fifth, and at the bottom of the list comes Pau'. Williams himself acknowledged the limitations of his results – they took no account for example of the differential condition of the patients wintering in the several resorts. Separately however he provided tabulated data for the respective percentages of patients in various stages of phthisis, as well as the proportions with both lungs affected, which showed that although the patients wintering at Pau were more likely to be in the second or third stage of the disease than those at other resorts and that a relatively high proportion of them (38 per cent) had double affection of the lungs, this did not alter his conclusion that 'for the ordinary forms of consumption, a dry air, whether inland or marine, was better than a moist one, inland or marine, cold or hot'.[13] The survey in short seemed to provide inescapable proof that for the majority of consumptive patients the moist, sedative climates that had enjoyed widespread backing from specialists in the early Victorian period did more harm than good. A little later Edward Sparks was able to provide some further detail for consumptive patients on the Riviera. A survey of various published and unpublished results for patients of several nationalities, chiefly at Menton, Nice and Cannes, between 1868 and 1878, including Williams's cases, revealed that almost 63 per cent had been cured or improved, about 23 per cent were stationary and just under 15 per cent dead. While admitting the methodological limitations of the survey, Sparks considered the results broadly favourable and certainly something of a riposte to the advocates of winter expatriation in the Alps who were then emerging.[14]

For most interested members of the medical profession, Williams's survey of patient outcomes probably contained few surprises. The prevailing view of specialists on the etiology and consequent treatment of phthisis had changed since the days of James Clark. As John Thorowgood, physician to the City of London Hospital for Diseases of the Chest, observed in the late 1860s:

> Years ago consumption was regarded as an inflammatory disorder of the lungs, and was treated by depletion, by sedatives, and by a hot and humid climate; or else the unfortunate victim was smothered in a hot, close room into which no breath of air could enter … No wonder that under this method of treatment consumption was indeed a deadly and universally fatal disease.[15]

Such treatment had been 'founded on the most sublime ignorance of the nature and pathology of the disease'. Rather, Thorowgood continued, 'it was to the plan of tonic and invigorating constitutional treatment that we must look as the great method for the prevention and cure of phthisis in far the majority of cases'. The problem with sedative air was that it made the patient feel better without addressing the underlying organic conditions encouraging tuberculosis.[16] Nevertheless, the disease was mysterious. Many doubted whether it could be cured at all once established. The role of medicine was to try to reduce the patient's vulnerability to phthisis by salutary interventions in his domestic circumstances, his environment, his diet and occupations, even his mental health. Patients sometimes recovered from consumption; more often they were able to live with the disease for many years. The extent to which a change of climate assisted these happy outcomes remained unproven.

Even if they had been aware of them, patients would probably have been untroubled by Williams's findings. Invalids in the early Victorian period might have blundered onto the Continent on a wing and a prayer, but by the 1870s inexperienced patients contemplating a winter abroad rarely moved without medical advice, and the tide had already turned against the sedative resorts. Writing in 1867, Williams himself had noted the decline in Madeira's popularity, although he still regarded the climate as potentially useful in certain consumptive cases.[17] As we have seen, British visitor numbers do seem to have declined quite sharply after the 1850s, and although it is unclear how much of a role doubts about the efficacy of the climate played in this, it is unquestionably the case that fewer British patients were being directed to the island by their advisors after the mid-1850s. As for Pau, its climatic reputation always owed more to special pleading than objective analysis, and the number of patients directed there for climatic treatment per se was perhaps always relatively small. Most experienced health-seekers doubtless made up their minds according to their own personal experience. Looking back on his invalid career, Cecil Monro recorded its highs and lows – his worst season in Madeira in 1862–3, with 'a good deal of "strawberry-jam" expectoration', his best at Cimiez in 1868–9 – but there was no obvious pattern. Winter expatriation had not been entirely fruitless, as Cecil felt it had helped set him up for the summer, but he concluded that this meagre return for his health was not worth the outlay. After abandoning winters abroad in 1870 he found he 'usually got on very well at home till the late spring'. He then generally paid a price for missing the winter sun but this could be mitigated by a change of air within England in August or September.[18]

## Death and burial

Death was the imagined outcome for many who went abroad for the sake of health, especially confirmed consumptives. In the early nineteenth century, observers readily latched on to visible evidence that seemed to confirm the dread inevitability of expiring far from home in an unequal contest with chronic disease. Saunderson Walker, inspecting the inscriptions on the graves at Livorno's British cemetery in 1837, noticed the demise of their occupants 'at almost every town in Italy but transported thither to rest'.[19] The Irish lawyer James Whiteside 'could not comprehend the utility of despatching to distant countries patients for whom death and the doctor had long contended. The churchyards in the continental towns might teach, on this subject, a melancholy lesson', he concluded.[20] Italy was the archetypal hecatomb. William Bullar noticed the northbound Britons dressed in mourning black at dinner in his Milan hotel, 'some, likely enough, who had brought out relatives only to see them die away from home'.[21] But expatriation of consumptive patients to any warm, moist climate – the standard prescription of the early Victorian years – had been little more than a death sentence, according to Dr Bennet.[22]

The reality was more prosaic. Most British invalids who travelled for health survived, in the early nineteenth century as well as later. The practice of winter expatriation would obviously have quickly ceased if they had not. Many Britons found a grave on the Continent, but they were usually long-term residents rather than visitors, while those who returned home in a box were a small minority of winter expatriates. Even consumptive patients normally survived their winter exile. Nonetheless, death abroad was frequent enough to loom large in the correspondence and presumably conversations of patients and their families. It was an occurrence that commanded the attention of British consuls, church and burial ground trustees and hotel managers and for which suitable arrangements and procedures were required.

The one southern health resort that came closest to vindicating the imagined fate of the invalid in exile was Madeira. Death was an ever-present companion for patients on the island, whatever the outcome of their own personal medical journey. The first occasion that Emily Shore's spirits fell after arrival came with a visit to the stranger's graveyard.[23] This place evidently affected visitors, especially as so many graves belonged to the young. Analysis of burials between 1845 and 1856, when we have detailed statistics of visitor numbers, suggests that about 7 per cent of invalids found a grave on the island, assuming that roughly half the visitor population were patients.[24] If we allow for visitors who died but whose bodies were repatriated and those who died on the voyage home, we can perhaps posit a death rate of something approaching 10 per cent during the height of Madeira's popularity as a health resort. This was a rate far in excess of any other European invalid destination. As we have seen, Pau's record in assisting consumptive patients recover their health was even worse than Madeira's, according to Dr Williams's analysis, but this woeful outcome does not seem to have been reflected in mortality figures. It was easier for the sick to leave Pau so most fatalities were perhaps, as it were, deferred. We do not have statistics for the early Victorian period, but for the years 1865 to 1878 burials at Pau only exceeded single figures in one season (1867–8) and were usually nearer five than ten. Even allowing for the relative ease of returning the dead to England, deaths among British visitors to Pau by this date must have been comparatively rare.[25]

Did Madeira attract a disproportionate number of desperate cases, willing to submit to an unusually arduous journey because all else had failed? Perhaps the perception of the almost magical properties of the Madeira climate in the early Victorian period encouraged this last throw of the dice. Mrs Marling admired a memorial she saw to a young woman 'in delicate health' about to be married in England in February 1851, who was hurriedly despatched to the island when her condition worsened and who died there within three months of arrival.[26] 'People die very suddenly in Madeira', noted Cecil Monro; 'from one point of view at least it is a good thing, because it only means they go on living easily and comfortably enjoying the fresh air up to the last'.[27] It was a matter of some curiosity to learn who had expired between seasons: Cecil Monro reported to his father on his return for his second season that 'things are of course the same, except that people have been dying right and left'.[28]

When in 1863–4 he tried Algiers after three seasons in Madeira he discovered that his absence was treated as a sign of the worst – 'Kelly … has been giving out that I have been too ill to leave England', he noted.[29] Some deaths, like Emily Shore's, could be easily foretold; others appeared suddenly and from apparently unpredictable causes. A fellow house guest of Cecil Monro died in early 1862: 'He was consumptive', observed Cecil, 'but that is not what he died of; he died simply of his bowels being out of order … I suppose the weather was partly at fault; he was a German moreover and I think the climate disagrees with the German digestive system especially.'[30]

At the beginning of the nineteenth century the term 'graveyard of our consumptive invalids' was occasionally applied to Nice by British commentators, but at no stage did Nice take on the funereal mantle that hung about Madeira's visitor community during the height of the island's popularity as an invalid resort. For most visitors Madeira was journey's end – geographically if not metaphorically – whereas Nice was not merely a destination but a stage on the grand tour route to Italy, with all that implied for the profile of its visitor population. The newer resorts that developed later in the century also resisted the mark of mortality as best they could, at least as far as the British were concerned. Few English people died at Menton, according to Dr Bennet, because expatriation to the south lifted their spirits; by contrast no such consolation was available to French invalids, for whom a Mediterranean sojourn was but 'the last drop of bitterness in a cup of sorrow' – they were consequently more likely to die.[31] Bennet of course might be suspected of having a personal interest in making such a claim, but it was echoed by William Miller, who ascribed it to the good sense of the British, who unlike most continentals typically headed south in good time, before their affliction was well-entrenched. Figures for French patients given by Dr Farina, the town physician of Menton, appear to bear this out: almost 25 per cent of consumptive *hivernants* died, the majority as a result of delaying their visit till the disease was too far established to be assisted by medicine or climate.[32] Arthur Hill Hassall noted at about the same date the relative scarcity of English graves in the Protestant cemetery at San Remo, compared with German.[33]

There were certain obstacles to Protestant burial at almost all health resorts, which were generally in Catholic countries. Sharing a Catholic cemetery was out of the question so British expatriates and other non-Catholics were usually restricted to a small enclave of the town's graveyard. If fortunate enough to be allowed to create their own cemetery, it was normally confined to the edge of town and so constricted that it rapidly filled up. In the absence of any provision for decent burial the only alternative was to dispose of the body in some inconspicuous place and allow Nature to take its course. As the trustees of the English church at Malaga wrote in 1854, if no Protestant cemetery had been established there twenty-four years earlier, 'the remains of near one hundred of their countrymen [would have been] consigned ignominiously to the sands at the mercy of the waves'.[34] Frequently the relatives of the deceased preferred to repatriate the corpse. This does not seem to have been a problem for the most part, provided the distance was not prohibitive and the coffin could be accompanied. When the Youngs' youngest child Frank died from whooping cough during the family's excursion to the Rhineland spas in 1838, his body was returned for burial at home, accompanied presumably by one of the family servants, since his parents remained in Germany.[35] Occasionally repatriation was prevented by force majeure. The MP for Leicester, Joseph Noble (1799–1861), died from cholera at Malaga in January 1861, but his family was denied permission to repatriate his remains, as the local authorities insisted on immediate burial for fear of contagion.[36]

As for Madeira, it was just too far for the safe return of corpses unless they could be embalmed. On 24 May 1850 the *Times* reported the arrival at Plymouth of the remains of the late Lady Throckmorton aboard the *Dart*, together with her husband and children, after a passage of almost three weeks, so that the corpse must have been embalmed. The procedure was expensive, so no doubt confined to a minority, but there was evidently sufficient demand to support construction of a deposit vault at the stranger's graveyard at Funchal in about 1860, in which embalmed bodies could be held for up to six months.[37] One such corpse belonged to Thomas Wakley, editor of the *Lancet*, who died in 1862 after slipping on the beach.[38] The length of time was doubtless required to allow relatives to travel to Madeira to accompany a body home. If embalmed bodies were not removed after six months they were interred, but even this was not necessarily the end of proceedings, as from 1842 it was possible to obtain permission to disinter bodies for removal to Britain following a successful appeal to the Portuguese government for the repatriation of the remains of a Miss Caroline Emma Ellery.[39] A further peculiarity of Madeira was that invalids travelling to and from the island were disproportionately liable to die in transit. Some, possibly all, vessels kept coffins aboard against this eventuality. A Miss Macready died on the way home in 1869 aboard an unnamed ship, some nine days after departure from Madeira. Her funeral was recorded in a memorandum by her nurse: the ceremony was much like any other burial at sea, with the captain officiating and the coffin, draped in the Union flag, finally tipped into the sea off the coast of north-west Spain.[40]

Whether a body was to be returned home or buried locally, the death of an invalid abroad could entail plenty of trouble and expense for friends or relatives. The newly appointed British consul at Nice complained in May 1872 that hotel and lodging-house keepers at Menton had apparently purloined the effects of deceased British residents during the previous winter as there was no local representative to protect their property; he urged the appointment of a vice-consul at Menton accordingly.[41] An official presence was also highly desirable to satisfy insurance companies at home in the case of death on the Continent, according to Ughtred Kay-Shuttleworth, who petitioned the Foreign Office for appointment of Dr Frederick Rose as British vice-consul (unpaid) at San Remo.[42] Alexander Brown claimed that 'there was … an understood penalty attached to dying [at Menton], in some instances as high as twenty pounds sterling'.[43] This was the charge made by some hotels when a resident died, being rather tastelessly even advertised in the printed price list. This charge was justified to cover the costs of disposing of the bedclothes and leaving the room vacant for a short period.[44]

The death of a resident was bad news for hoteliers, who made every effort to keep it under wraps: 'When a death happens', reported Miller, 'the hotel people keep it as long quiet as possible [*sic*]; the authorities take charge of the burial, and the body, which must lie unburied twenty-four hours after death, is removed after dark in a coffin to the mortuary adjoining the cemetery, where the relations assemble usually on the following day, and it is buried.'[45] Local authorities were understandably anxious to ensure corpses were disposed of with despatch, but relatives, keen to arrange or attend a funeral or perhaps escort a coffin home, might be days away. At Cannes the British colony enjoyed the privilege of allowing bodies to be stored at the mortuary chapels of the three English churches for a number of days, pending local burial or transfer elsewhere. The practice was irregular under French law and when the privilege was briefly challenged in 1879 by the municipality a compromise was reached involving a defined time-limit before removal.[46]

## The limits of climate therapy

For as long as winter expatriation existed there had always been voices decrying the practice. Critics typically based their arguments on the failure of the Mediterranean or other invalid destinations to live up to expectations rather than on any serious questioning of therapeutic assumptions; the sun might shine, but it was countervailed by bitter winds, while the accommodations were ill-adapted to British standards of comfort. As early as the 1830s concern began to grow that Madeira's climate simply did not meet the strict desiderata for consumptive patients for a soft, equable and warm environment. Between the first (1830) and third (1841) editions of James Clark's standard work on climate for invalids, the submissions he received from fellow specialists about the suitability of the various climates he surveyed supported his own recommendations with the one exception of Madeira, which 'was almost the only place respecting which statements did not quite agree'.[47] Clark's own view that 'where the climate was likely to be useful in consumption, that of Madeira was preferable to any in the south of Europe' remained unchanged.[48] But the edifice was being undermined from below. In 1850 posthumous publication of J. A. Mason's *Treatise on the Climate and Meteorology of Madeira*, a moderate critique by a patient of Clark's who resided on the island in 1834–5 and made a minute analysis of the climate, indicated that, far from being a sort of subtropical greenhouse, there was in fact considerable year-round variability in both temperature and humidity.[49] This was taken up and exploited by medical opponents of the practice of winter expatriation, among them Thomas Burgess, who termed Madeira the 'Ultima Thule of hectic invalids', thus drawing attention to the perversity of journeying to as it were the edge of the known world for dubious health benefits.[50]

Pau's status was equally vulnerable. British visitors often felt short-changed when they encountered the rain and cold of Pau in winter, having made such a long journey. Louisa Costello arrived in early October 1842 to find the weather 'as cold as Christmas' and the rain incessant; 'The more experience I have of the climate of Pau', she continued, 'the more surprised I am at the crowds of English who resort to this town for the winter'; she supposed that most had been seduced by the 'mania of wintering at Pau', but once there were reluctant to leave before the weather improved in the spring.[51] In his review of Dr Taylor's book in the *Lancet*, George Lefevre observed that the author's description of the climate was very far from his own experience in 1819–20; it was not that Pau's climate was bad but that, as in almost all health resorts that British people frequented, it was unpredictable.[52] Thomas Madden, who visited Pau in the winter of 1861–2, concluded that the town's publicists had done a fine job in pulling the wool over the British invalid's eyes, the climate remaining 'what is was before the books were written – essentially cold, variable, damp and dreary during the winter'.[53] A correspondent in the *Times* pronounced the climate of Pau 'probably the worst in Europe', to be avoided by patients at all costs; only six weeks in the spring were tolerable.[54]

Ultimately neither Madeira nor Pau could sustain the extravagant therapeutic claims made on their behalf by propagandists. In face of the real-world experience of visitors, defenders of the resorts had recourse to a range of excuses: patients had left it too late in the course of their illness before coming; they had behaved carelessly while at the resort; the season had been in some way exceptionally wet, or hot, or cold, or windy. For those whose livelihoods depended on the invalid trade, questioning the value of the climate was inadmissible. It was 'hard to stand up for the Madeira climate so as to satisfy the Madeira people', so exacting were their demands, according to Cecil Monro.[55] Patients did not visit these resorts to undergo some dedicated pharmaceutical or dietary regime, dose themselves with mineral waters, take mud baths or bathe in the ocean. If the climate – the ultimate doctor – let them down, the resorts had little else to offer the patient. No wonder their defenders fought so doggedly to preserve their climatic reputation.

In addition to those who contested the climatic claims made for specific resorts there were others who questioned the entire therapeutic basis of the medical south. Thomas Burgess, physician to London's Blenheim Street Dispensary, was struck by the pathetic sight of his indigent consumptive patients lamenting that a cure was beyond reach since they lacked the means to travel to escape the British winter.[56] On the contrary, Burgess averred, 'Nature [had] adapted the constitution of man to the climate of his ancestors', so that 'change of air in his own climate or removal to one nearly approaching to it', was indicated for consumptives. Besides, the overland journey to the south was bad enough for the healthy traveller, wrote Burgess, 'but to the phthisical invalid absolute torture'.[57] Without indulging in such climatic nativism, Dr Cotton merely asserted that it was perfectly possible to find an appropriate change of air within the British Isles so that foreign travel for the purpose was so much wasted effort.[58] Some however even condemned the very concept of the health benefits of diversion and change of air: 'Fashion ruled everything', complained the London practitioner John Atkinson; 'nothing appeared to be more strikingly absurd than the almost daily removals of patients for the purposes of health, losing sight altogether of the importance of quietness, equable temperature and numerous other appliances of the medical art. Food properly selected and drink rightly ordered', he continued, 'would often do much more than "Change of Air."' The British were used to comfort and indoor life, so prescribing dislocation and outdoor living in a foreign land made no sense.[59]

Atkinson, who pointed out that scavengers and nightsoil men had better health than other workers, was at the extreme in contending that change of air was a delusion.[60] But as the century advanced, more and more questions were raised about exactly what sort of air benefitted respiratory cases and in particular about the role of warmth in promoting health. By the 1860s John Thorowgood could claim that the advantages of cool air over warmth for confirmed consumptives were widely agreed in the medical profession. He reckoned that plenty of advanced phthisitical cases had recovered on being removed from a warm to a cold climate and noted that the outpatients at his own London hospital tended to do better in winter than summer.[61]

Warm air relaxed the frame, diminished the appetite and depressed the spirits, according to William Ireland, who spent the winter of 1868–9 in Madeira, precisely the opposite of the intended results of winter expatriation. The most suitable consumptive cases were the advanced ones who were likely to die anyway but might escape the British winter and thus expire in relative comfort.[62] For John Parkin 'every degree of latitude, southwards, that a consumptive patient traversed was simply putting another nail in his coffin'.[63] 'It is evident', he continued, 'that an elevated temperature is injurious to all consumptive patients … and yet, with these facts before them … medical men in England were sending hundreds of patients from their country and their homes to seek an impossibility – health or a cure.'[64] Parkin's particular bugbear was Dr Bennet and his chosen resort of Menton – 'the favourite one at the present moment' – but the entire Mediterranean littoral was equally suspect. His conclusions were ostensibly based on the data available from British military and naval sources regarding the mortality from phthisis in overseas garrisons and from disease statistics among continental populations, but his diatribe is better viewed as a late example of the nativist critiques of invalid expatriation more familiar from earlier in the century. More careful investigators, like C. T. Williams, were able to demonstrate that there was no clear correlation between latitude and the incidence of the disease and that cold certainly did not confer immunity, as some had suggested.[65] Few specialists would be prepared to echo William Thomson's prediction that 'climate per se would be found to have no sort of influence whatever, causative or curative, over phthisis'.[66] But quite what that influence was, and how significant a part it played, was no clearer at the end of our period than at the beginning.

## Paradigm shift

The key to successful treatment of consumption appeared to C. T. Williams to be attention to humidity rather than temperature.[67] None of his patients had wintered in the Alps although he noted that the Alpine resorts were already attracting many German and Swiss invalids. The Alps and indeed the Pyrenees had long provided a summer retreat for British patients unable or unwilling to return home from Italy, the Riviera or Pau between winter seasons. Bennet had recommended 'some of the high mountain sanatoria to which medical men of Switzerland sent their patients'.[68] The suggestion that high altitude per se could be helpful in combating pulmonary disease struggled to gain wide acceptance, even though it had been remarked by several practitioners since the 1830s.[69] To recommend life in thinner, colder air to a patient threatened with or suffering from diseased lungs quite naturally made little sense. Although Thorowgood noted that cases of phthisis decreased with elevation, he considered that the cold air at altitude would simply be too irritating to the lungs of confirmed consumptives.[70]

Hermann Weber, physician to the German Hospital in London and one of the first British practitioners to direct consumptive patients to the Alps, noted that 'in almost every case of incipient consumption in which he had advised a prolonged residence in St Moritz or Davos, or any other elevated region, it had happened that either one or other of the relatives, or a medical man connected with the family, strongly objected to the plan'.[71] Weber admitted in 1869 that the processes by which high altitude favoured consumptives were as yet matters for debate, for 'the agents under which the invalid was placed were very unclear'. His own directions to patients were based largely on empirical evidence: few did worse in the mountains, and the majority reported considerable benefit. It was not a question of finding a new 'wonder-working' climate but of being open to alternatives to the standard prescription of the warm south for consumptives, for, as Weber's colleague William Gull explained to a patient, 'his experience with regard to the warmer health resorts was great but it was unfortunately not favourable'.[72]

The Alpine valleys that were to become the chief sites of invalid expatriation to high elevations, the Upper Engadin and Davos valleys in the Graubünden canton of Switzerland, were already well known to British summer visitors by the 1860s. They had not been deemed suitable places for the sick however: Weber recalled in 1870 that about a decade or so earlier a recommendation to a patient to 'spend a prolonged stay in the Engadin and other high places during summer' would be met with 'every kind of good-natured abuse from medical men and invalids'; now the Engadin in summer was 'regarded as good for everybody and every ailment'.[73] Winter expatriation was a considerably harder sell. The first documented consumptive patients at Davos were two Germans who arrived in February 1865, one of whom was a doctor who stayed to practise for twenty years; the other, a former bookseller, took over management of the hotel where they had lodged. The first-known British case was the wife of a Dutch banker, Mrs Holsboer, who was directed to Davos by Weber in May 1867 only to die there within a short time. Holsboer however stayed on, providing finance for the first Davos *Kurhaus* or invalid hotel.[74] The earliest known British consumptive patient to overwinter at high altitude in Switzerland was a young man whose case was described by Weber, who was directed to the Upper Engadin by Gull in May 1866 and whose 'cough, expectoration and breathlessness disappeared' during the winter of 1866–7 under the supervision of a British expatriate physician Dr Berry, at St Moritz.[75] But although St Moritz was already welcoming more winter than summer visitors by 1873, the resort resisted conversion into an invalid asylum; its hotels turned away consumptive patients in favour of winter sports enthusiasts.[76]

Weber confessed to having suffered 'great anxiety' in directing patients who were 'not progressing in England to high elevations in autumn and early winter' but had discovered that 'almost all the invalids in the Engaddin [*sic*] and Davos felt during the winter better than during the summer, and that the fear of the so-called winter climate in these valleys was to a great degree groundless'.[77] Far from being inimical to health, a cold atmosphere it seemed desiccated the ground, purified the air and maximized the healing power of the sun, providing just the sort of dry, bright and bracing climate that specialists by the 1860s agreed was best suited to most pulmonary cases. Weber's publications were instrumental in shifting medical opinion in favour of the benefits of high altitude for treating consumption.[78] His advocacy was based on the practical outcomes for patients, informed by his knowledge of German experiments in Bavaria and the Harz mountains, which long antedated British trials, and exposure to German and Swiss patients through his hospital practice. Theoretical underpinning for the virtues of winter cold for the consumptive patient was eventually provided for the profession in Britain by the Leeds physician Clifford Allbutt, who had experimented with open-air treatment of typhus patients in Yorkshire in 1865–6.[79] In a series of contributions in the *Lancet* Allbutt explained that the high Alps provided an aseptic environment that prevented putrefaction of tissue, just as meat hung out to dry by the locals did not rot. The majority of patients who died from consumption, Allbutt held, were poisoned by septicaemia. Once the patient was stabilized, natural healing could be left to take its course, safe in the knowledge that the poison formerly issuing from the body's internal sores had been staunched.[80]

Discovery of the tuberculosis bacillus in 1882 did nothing to undermine the putrefaction theory; on the contrary it merely identified the causative microbe that specialists had suspected from the work of Pasteur and others inhabited the atmosphere along with thousands of other bacteria.[81] Neither did this knowledge do much to assist therapy, which continued to be based largely on empirical foundations. Many patients seemed to prosper in the high Alpine winter but by no means all did, and there remained a variety of opinions on exactly which aspects of the high altitude environment were implicated in assisting cure. Was it low temperature or humidity, low barometric pressure, lack of wind, an air devoid of impurities, strong winter sunshine or a combination of several or all of these? Perhaps these features were largely enabling conditions that allowed patients to regain appetite and tone, both physical and psychological. For Alfred Tucker Wise, physician to the Infirmary for Consumption, Margaret Street, who visited Davos in 1879 and 1880 for research purposes, the natural environment of the high Alpine winter was clearly conducive to health, but he already foresaw a time when the popularity of Davos would lead to overcrowding and 'the benefits of living among a sparse population in scattered dwellings would be modified'.[82] Here was implicit recognition that perhaps the chief attraction of the high Alps for patients was escape, not merely from a gloomy northern winter but increasingly from the oversubscribed invalid asylums of the Mediterranean. Medical validation of the high Alps in winter as a sanatorium from the 1870s did not so much transform the approach to treatment as provide another venue to the suite of alternatives available to wealthy invalids in search of relief and cure for phthisis above all, but eventually for a range of other complaints.

Patient numbers at Davos rose from two hundred in 1872–3 to five hundred in 1875–6 and seven hundred in 1878–9.[83] British invalids began to winter at Davos in numbers from the mid-1870s onwards. Allbutt reckoned between twenty and thirty of his compatriots wintered there in 1877, heavily outnumbered by Germans and Swiss, rising to more than 250 by 1879.[84] There were about a thousand by 1883.[85] Most were directed there by consultants at home, but as with Madeira and Pau earlier in the century patient publications also played a significant part in promotion. The earliest seems to have been the anonymous *Davos-Platz: A New Alpine Resort for Sick and Sound* (1878), by a female invalid who apparently stumbled on Davos by accident, and the writer John Addington Symonds's contribution to the *Fortnightly Review* in the same year, 'Davos in Winter', a work that a later lay commentator thought 'probably had more to do with bringing English people to Davos than all the other publications put together'.[86] Both emphasized the primacy of the Davos air in assisting cure of lung disease but also painted a picture of a life unencumbered by the artificiality and sophistry of the established invalid resorts. 'Davos was refreshingly free from all the meaningless paraphernalia of a modern watering place', declared the lady invalid, an observation echoed by Allbutt, who noted his surprise at the absence of 'pretentious cure systems, and of all the machinery of quackery'; there were 'no mud-baths, no pine-baths, no elaborate regulation of food, or habits of life'.[87] Once more it was the natural environment that was the key to cure, rather than the ministrations of medicine, just as the unique qualities of the climate had formerly been held supreme at Madeira and Pau.

No one could claim that winter in the Alps was suitable for patients in an advanced state of pulmonary disease without the fundamental bodily means for recovery. Rather it was those patients with the capacity and inclination to lead a wholesome outdoor life to the full who were most likely to benefit. 'It was of the greatest importance that invalids who went to Davos should have a fair reserve of physical vigour to enable them to resist the intense cold', thought R. A. Otter, who spent two winters there between 1878 and 1880.[88] Many, possibly most, patients were refugees from the Riviera or at least individuals disappointed by the results of winter expatriation in the warm south. For some of these patients the very severity of winter weather was to be embraced: 'I never found that my health suffered from bad weather', recorded Symonds; 'on the contrary I had the exhilarating consciousness that I could bear it, harden myself against it, and advance steadily in conditions that in England would have been hopeless'.[89] Let the feeble languish in the warm south or be coddled in some fussy continental spa – the high-altitude cure offered British patients the opportunity to escape from established health resorts that had become ever more accessible, comfortable and tame. In the words of John Pemble, 'When the Victorian doctor sent his patients into the wilderness he became identified – if only subconsciously – with the Old Testament deity, summoning his votaries from the fleshpots to a new life.'[90]

Flight to the Alps appealed because it offered not only a new therapeutic paradigm but also the prospect of escape from the increasingly flaccid Mediterranean littoral. As soon as Davos itself seemed threatened by overdevelopment, as Tucker Wise had envisaged, Symonds took fright. After four winters he called time on a resort that risked becoming 'an ill-drained, over-crowded, gas-lighted centre of cosmopolitan disease and second-rate gaiety'.[91] Whether the appeal of Davos had much to do with 'middle class values of discipline and duty', as has been claimed, seems more questionable.[92]

Choosing Davos represented a decision to put oneself under continual medical supervision without significant distraction. It was undoubtedly an exercise in self-denial but hardly self-discipline since life was reduced to a matter of following the rules. In this as in other respects there was little echo of the experience of the invalid abroad of fifty years before, apart perhaps from the last stage of his journey to Davos by *diligence*. There was no lottery in securing suitable accommodation, no trouble with couriers or servants, no desperate search for cod liver oil or familiar patent medicines. On the contrary invalidity had become regulated, monitored and predictable in its contours, if not its outcome.

## Conclusion

For as long as invalids had fled the British winter for the south, medical voices had been raised against the tendency of patients to ignore professional advice but conduct themselves according to their own lights and consequently jeopardize their chances of recovery. The fact that, as we have seen, surviving documentary evidence appears to suggest precisely the opposite may help to elucidate the context from which such accusations of patient perversity arose. For John Pemble, sending patients to winter in the south burdened with a long list of dietary and behavioural injunctions provided doctors with a useful means of escaping blame for failure: they were implicitly admitting that the chances of recovery were slight but placing the onus for cure on the self-discipline of the patient rather than the skill of the physician, enabling them to 'assume the aggrieved attitude that had been the patient's prerogative' in the past. He even suggests that sending consumptives to the Mediterranean may only have persisted for so long because it provided this handy benefit to their medical advisers.[93] However persuasive this speculation might be for the later Victorian and Edwardian periods, it does not really work for earlier decades. Although the suspicion that the warm south provided a handy means for doctors at home to get rid of troublesome patients had a long ancestry,[94] the speculation surely places too much weight on the role of medical professionals in initiating and sustaining winter expatriation, or spa-visiting for that matter, in the period before 1880. The notion of being 'ordered' south obscures the reality that travelling for health for most of the nineteenth century was at bottom a patient-driven enterprise, however much medical professionals attempted to steer, mould and capitalize on it.

It is perhaps more profitable to interpret the tension between medical injunction and patient obedience as part of the struggle by doctors to gain and keep control of the therapeutic programme. After all, in an environment where climate was king, the traditional role of the medical practitioner in prescribing medicines was marginalized, so it was only too easy for a patient to avoid routine medical supervision, with all that implied not only for his health but also for his doctor's purse. Just as the Continent seemed to be full of rogue Anglican clergy, so was it replete with British invalids, unmoored from the familiar ties and certainties of their homeland, sorely in need of medical direction or superintendence. Moreover, as any lingering belief in the therapeutic benefits of climate per se, which had never been very strong in medical circles anyway, dissipated, it was ever more imperative for patients to follow professional directions.

Various attempts were made from the 1860s to provide bespoke accommodation and services for invalids so that their diet and regimen could be organized and treatment supervised. This development had been anticipated to some extent at certain German spas, where accommodation was often available at the government-owned *Kurhaus* or provided by physicians at their own residences, in both cases offering obvious advantages in terms of ready access to medical and therapeutic resources. At Kissingen, for example, Adam Hailmann's guest house seems to have regularly received about one in ten of all British spa guests over the three and a half decades from 1844, when Dr Travis made it his base for the season.[95] As we have seen, several individual practitioners on the Riviera took boarders into their own homes. British nursing institutes were set up at Cannes and planned at least for San Remo in the early 1870s.[96] The move to the Alps offered doctors the chance to gain complete control of patient care, free from the distraction of sightseeing and social activities. Patients were usually directed to Davos by specialists at home, but even if they were not there was really no escape from medical supervision as there were only two or three hotels available at first.

The concentration of consumptive patients that necessarily ensued brought its own problems, especially as the hotel 'improvements', such as double windows and indoor stoves, that discriminating British visitors demanded hampered the free circulation of air. What was the point of wintering in the high Alps if the patient spent most of his time in badly ventilated hotel rooms where, in Tucker Wise's words, he breathed 'sewer-gas, kitchen and basement air, exhalations from the lungs and skin of organic matter, scales of epithelium, fibres of cotton, wool, wood, etc., the products of combustion from gas, lamps and candles, bacteria and fungi and … the bacillus tuberculosis floating about in the air'.[97] For Wise, consumptives required specialized sanatoria so that they were not condemned to live cheek by jowl in unsuitable hotels. He planned to open his own sanatorium by converting two hotels at Wiesen, in the Davos valley.[98] By 1884 he was consulting on the design of the first purpose-built sanatorium in the Alps at Maloja, near St Moritz, now the luxury Majola Palace Hotel.[99]

Creation of specialized sanatoria held out the prospect of being able to evaluate the role of climate in health based on robust clinical evidence. For clinicians and others at the end of our period were no more able to disentangle the contribution, if any, of climate per se in the recovery from illness or stabilization of patients at health resorts than their colleagues had been in 1830. As the Irish physician James Lindsay pointed out, 'rates of mortality, proportions of cures etc., tell us little, unless such information be accompanied by full medical details, supplied on competent authority, and unless the many sources of fallacy be rigidly excluded'.[100] These conditions were still entirely absent as far as British patients wintering in the south were concerned. The medical truism that little help could be expected from climate alone, which was founded on long experience of disappointing patient outcomes, was as firmly held at the end of our period as it had been by James Clark at the beginning. The difference over fifty years was that by 1880 doctors were beginning to envision the prospect of ensuring that patients finally observe the injunctions concerning diet, exercise, rest, clothing and so on that were deemed essential adjuncts to successful climatic treatment. Debate about the merits of particular climates for consumption and a range of other illnesses continued, but the notion long held by a few that climate therapy as such was a sham remained very much a minority view.

Climate therapy was still alive and well in 1880. But a half-century of experience had shown that no climate suited every case, and certainly none held miraculous powers. The exaggerated claims of promoters and expectations of patients had given way to an appreciation of the complexity and unpredictability of the interactions between environment and health. Nevertheless the British winter remained grim and the lure of the south undiminished. An editorial in 1880 in the *British Medical Journal* might have read like a throwback to the nativist critiques of old if not for the allowance that in winter there were indeed pleasanter places to reside, not only for the genuinely sick but also for those 'who, without being absolutely ill, were tired and wearied by the excitement and by labours of active life':

> There is probably no better climate in the world for the Anglo-Saxon race than that of England in the summer of an ordinary year. If a better climate be sought for in winter, probably the one that approaches the nearest to it, in the majority of cases, is best for our race. More and more generally we are learning to work in England while the weather is fine and the environs of our cities full of rural attraction, and to take our foreign travel when climatic conditions are least favourable here, and may be most profitably exchanged for the happier influences of sunnier lands.[101]

The 'diseases of modern life' that physicians of the later nineteenth century began to associate with the increased speed, urgency and competitiveness of contemporary civilization do not sound so different from those identified at the beginning, before some of the supposed culprits, such as railways and the electric telegraph, had been invented.[102] Benjamin Ward Richardson's category of 'disease from worry or mental strain', with its tendency to afflict scientists, artists, writers, politicians, businessmen, students and scholars, seems uncannily like James Johnson's 'wear and tear' of almost fifty years before.[103] Richardson did not prescribe foreign travel as an antidote to mental strain, but he did insist that 'occupations of every kind … required to be alternated … with rest and recreation'.[104] By the time he was writing the British had discovered a region that seemed tailor-made for both, a region that could be reached and left with ease, where British preferences and habits were generously accommodated, above all where expatriation in a benign climate could be enjoyed without the necessity of relinquishing the comforts of home.

The Riviera remained the foremost foreign destination for British health-seekers after 1880; indeed it consolidated and increased its dominance as alternative venues declined. It did not lose its invalids, but its consumptive cases, who were drawn off to the Alps or increasingly attracted to sanatoria in Germany and later at home, became less visible. Whether such cases vanished because of disillusion with climate therapy, as has been claimed, is moot.[105] As we have seen, few doctors had ever invested much confidence in climate per se as therapy for consumption. Before the 1880s medicine had little to offer the consumptive patient so that 'change of air' was, rather like cod liver oil, a prescription dispensed more in hope than expectation. After 1880 confidence in the capacity of medicine to prevent or cure the disease grew, leading to increased interest in the active management of patients. Clearly this could best be achieved in a closed, aseptic environment where diet, regimen and exercise could be supervised.[106]

As 'genuine' invalids disappeared the health-seekers who remained on the Riviera were refugees from the northern winter, a species whose avoidance of 'what God had put to harden it, the English winter and English winter pursuits' filled visiting clergyman Laughton Alison with contempt: 'Shooting and hunting are not the last aims in life', he declared, 'but they are at least more manly and more elevating than lounging (in stays) under a parasol and dawdling over to Monte Carlo.'[107] Here was confirmation of the region's destiny as Europe's premier pleasure resort, a destiny that had been long foretold. The change did not represent a rupture so much as a foregrounding of an important element of the Riviera's appeal from its earliest discovery by British expatriates. Health and recreation had always been intimately entwined in winter expatriation. Through all the changing currents in society, medicine and disease, and culture in nineteenth-century Britain, one constant of relevance to our study is clearly discernible, a restless but relentless search for a place where one could feel whole, in body and mind.

# Notes

## Preface

1 George Weisz, 'Historical Reflections on Medical Travel', *Anthropology & Medicine*, vol. 18, no. 1 (2011), 137–8.
2 See Ralph Jackson, 'Waters and Spas in the Classical World', in *The Medical History of Waters and Spas*, ed. Roy Porter, *Medical History* Supplement no. 10 (London: Wellcome Institute for the History of Medicine, 1990), 1–13.
3 Marjorie Morgan, *National Identities and Travel in Victorian Britain* (Basingstoke: Palgrave, 2001).
4 This is not to say that Pau's only importance for British visitors was as an invalid station. On the contrary it served as a gateway to the Pyrenees, a major attraction for British visitors from early in the century; see Martyn Lyons, *The Pyrenees in the Modern Era: Reinventions of a Landscape, 1775–2012* (London: Bloomsbury, 2018).

## Introduction

1 Peter Bailey, *Leisure and Class in Victorian England: Rational Recreation and the Contest for Control, 1830–1885* (London: Routledge, 1978), 56.
2 For a discussion of doctor–patient relations in the eighteenth century, see Roy Porter, 'The Patient in England, c. 1660–c. 1800', in *Medicine in Society: Historical Essays*, ed. Andrew Wear (Cambridge: Cambridge University Press, 1992), 91–118.
3 Vladimir Janković, *Confronting the Climate: British Airs and the Making of Environmental Medicine* (New York: Palgrave Macmillan, 2010), 121.
4 Sheila M. Rothman, *Living in the Shadow of Death: Tuberculosis and the Social Experience of Illness in America* (New York: Basic Books, 1994), 5.
5 Janković, *Confronting the Climate*, 125.
6 See especially Jane M. Adams, *Healing with Water: English Spas and the Water Cure, 1840–1960* (Manchester: Manchester University Press, 2015); Phyllis Hembry, *The English Spa 1560–1815, a Social History* (London: Athlone Press, 1990); Phyllis Hembry and *British Spas from 1815 to the Present*, ed.

and completed by W. Cowie and Evelyn E. Cowie (London: Athlone Press, 1997); John K. Walton, *The English Seaside Resort, a Social History 1750–1914* (Leicester: Leicester University Press, 1983); John Hassan, *The Seaside, Health and Environment in England and Wales since 1800* (Aldershot: Ashgate, 2003).

7 Examples include Jill R. Steward, 'Moral Economies and Commercial Imperatives: Food, Diet and Spas in Central Europe, 1800–1914', in *Mineral Springs Resorts in Global Perspective*, ed. John K. Walton (London: Routledge, 2014), 109–31 and Jill R. Steward, 'The Role of Inland Spas as Sites of Transnational Cultural Exchange in the Production of European Leisure Culture (1750–1870)', in *Leisure Cultures in Urban Europe, c. 1700–1870*, ed. Peter Borsay and Jan Hein Fumée (Manchester: Manchester University Press, 2016), 234–59, both of which include the experience of British curists among others at the continental spas; Hermann Sommer's *Zur Kur nach Ems: ein Beitrag zur Geschichte der Badereise von 1830 bis 1914* (Stuttgart: Franz Steiner, 1999) includes a section on British curists at Bad Ems. Notable contributions to the history of British presence at individual resorts include Pierre Tucoo-Chala, *Pau, Ville Anglaise: Promenades Historiques* (Pau: Société Nouvelle d'Editions Régionales et de Diffusion, 1979) and Desmond Gregory, *The Beneficent Usurpers: a History of the British in Madeira* (Rutherford, NJ: Farleigh Dickinson University Press; London: Associated University Presses, *c.* 1988).

8 John Pemble, *The Mediterranean Passion: Victorians and Edwardians in the South* (Oxford: Clarendon, 1987).

9 Rothman, *Living in the Shadow of Death*, 1.

10 The chief protagonists of Thomas Hood's *Up the Rhine* comprise a nephew, 'yearning to the abounding river', and his hypochondriacal uncle, who, despite challenging his doctor to 'name a single instance of a man who had lived the longer for wandering over the world', is nonetheless persuaded to accompany his nephew, *Up the Rhine*, 2nd edn (London: A. H. Baily, 1840), 1–5.

11 Rothman, *Living in the Shadow of Death*, 7.

## 1 Travel, climate and health

1 James Buzzard, *The Beaten Track: European Tourism, Literature and the Ways to 'Culture', 1800–1918* (Oxford: Clarendon, 1993), 159.

2 Hood, *Up the Rhine*, vi.

3 Letters from Germany and Belgium by an Autumn Tourist (London: Simpkin, Marshall, 1839), 167.

4 Jonathan Andrews, 'Letting Madness Range: Travel and Mental Disorder, c. 1700–1900', in *Pathologies of Travel*, ed. Richard Wrigley and George Revill

(Amsterdam: Rodopi, 2000), 25–88; Vladimir Janković, 'The Last Resort: A British Perspective on the Medical South', *Journal of Intercultural Studies* 27, no. 3 (2006): 273.

5 Bailey, *Leisure and Class in Victorian England*, 64–6.

6 Janet Oppenheim, *Shattered Nerves: Doctors, Patients and Depression in Victorian England* (New York: Oxford University Press, 1990), 131.

7 Thomas More Madden, *The Spas of Belgium, Germany, Switzerland, France and Italy* (London: T. C. Newby, 1867), 72.

8 The poet Samuel Rogers characterized travel as 'medicine for the troubled mind'; Buzard, *The Beaten Track*, 102. The physician-traveller James Johnson even advocated an appropriately organized continental tour to 'prevent many a hypochondriac and dyspeptic from lifting his hand against his own existence'; James Johnson, *Change of Air, or the Pursuit of Health and Recreation (through France, Switzerland, Italy, etc)*, 3rd edn (London: S. Highley, 1832), 19.

9 Memoranda of an excursion by Saunderson Walker, Society of Friends Library (SF), MSS 84–5.

10 'With respect to modes of travelling from Great Britain to Italy, that considered as the least fatiguing, and best calculated to benefit consumptive persons, is to go by sea, in a vessel bound for Leghorn'; Mariana Starke, *Travels in Europe, for the Use of Travellers on the Continent*, 9th edn (Paris: Galignani, 1839), 3.

11 For discussion of the literary genre, see Pemble, *The Mediterranean Passion* and Maria H. Frawley, *Invalidism and Identity in Nineteenth-Century Britain* (Chicago: University of Chicago Press, 2004).

12 Henry Matthews, *The Diary of an Invalid Being the Journal of a Tour in Pursuit of Health in Portugal, Italy, Switzerland and France in the Years 1817, 1818 and 1819*, 2nd edn (London: John Murray, 1820); the author's consumption is introduced on page 58.

13 Johnson, *Change of Air*, 247.

14 W. F. Cumming, *Notes of a Wanderer in Search of Health, through Italy, Egypt, Greece, Turkey, Up the Danube, and down the Rhine* (London: Sanders & Otley, 1839).

15 Letters of William Money-Kyrle to his parents, 1843–6 Money-Kyrle papers, Wiltshire and Swindon History Centre (WS) 1720/843.

16 [Albert Denison, Lord Londesborough], *Wanderings in Search of Health* (London: printed for private circulation, 1849).

17 Andrew Scull, Charlotte MacKenzie and Nicholas Hervey, *Masters of Bedlam; the Transformation of the Mad-Doctoring Trade* (Princeton, NJ: Princeton University Press, 1996), 134–5.

18 [Ann, Lady Vavasour], *My Last Tour and First Work; Or, a Visit to the Baths of Wildbad and Rippoldsau* (London: H. Cunningham, 1842).

19 Janković, *Confronting the Climate*, 122–6; Oppenheim, *Shattered Nerves*, 124–8.

20 Johnson, *Change of Air*, 2–19.

21 Ibid., 7–8.

22 Edwin Lee, *Bradshaw's Companion to the Continent; A Descriptive Hand-Book to the Chief Places of Resort, Their Characteristic Features, Climates, Scenery and Remedial Resources, with Observations on the Influences of Climates and Travelling* (London: W. J. Adams, 1851), 371–2.

23 D. J. T. Francis, *Change of Climate Considered as a Remedy in Dyspeptic, Pulmonary, and Other Chronic Affections* (London: Churchill, 1853), 56.

24 Johnson, *Change of Air*, 264.

25 Janković, *Confronting the Climate*, 128.

26 Janković, 'The Last Resort', 274, quoting the anonymous *Best and Easiest Method of Preserving Uninterrupted Health to Extreme Old Age* (1748).

27 Janković, *Confronting the Climate*, 122.

28 Ibid., 120–2.

29 Richard E. Morris, 'The Victorian Change of Air as Medical and Social Construction', *Journal of Tourism History* 10, no. 1 (2018): 52–3.

30 J. C. Atkinson, *Change of Air: Fallacies Regarding It* (London: John Ollivier, 1848), v.

31 Johnson, *Change of Air*, 7–8.

32 Morris, 'The Victorian Change of Air', 58

33 Lee, *Bradshaw's Companion to the Continent*, 334.

34 Janković, *Confronting the Climate*, 134.

35 Edwin Lee, *Notes on Italy and Rhenish Germany; With Professional Notices of Climates of Nice, Pisa, Florence, Rome, and Naples* (Edinburgh: Laing & Forbes, 1835), 17–19.

36 Ibid., 50.

37 Lee, *Bradshaw's Companion to the Continent*, 342.

38 Joseph Cox, *Hints for Invalids About to Visit Naples* (London: Longman, 1841), 36–7.

39 Mrs Carleton, *Brief Advice to Travellers in Italy* (Paris: Galignani, 1847), 6, 69–70.

40 Lee, *Bradshaw's Companion to the Continent*, 150.

41 Pemble, *The Mediterranean Passion*, 168.

42 Report of the trustees of the Anglican church at Nice, 4 January 1864 The National Archives, Kew (TNA) FO27/1545.

43 'I do like Rome, I must say … Have you been in Rome, Mrs Proudie?' Mrs Proudie sighed as she replied in the negative and declared her belief that danger

was to be apprehended from such visits. 'Oh! – ah! – the malaria – of course – yes; if you go at the wrong time; but nobody is such a fool as that now.' 'I was thinking of the soul, Miss Dunstable', said the lady-bishop;, Anthony Trollope, *Dr Thorne* (London: Penguin, [1858] 1991), 187–8.

44 Richard Wrigley, 'Pathological Topography and Cultural Itineraries: Mapping "Mal'aria" in 18th and 19th Century Rome', in *Pathologies of Travel*, ed. Richard Wrigley and George Revill (Amsterdam: Rodopi, 2000), 212–13.

45 Stefania Arcara, 'Constructing the South: Sicily, Southern Italy and the Mediterranean in British Culture, 1773–1926' (PhD diss., University of Warwick, 1998).

46 Johnson, *Change of Air*, 269–79.

47 Lee, *Bradshaw's Companion to the Continent*, 371–2.

48 Thomas King Chambers, *Some Effects of the Climate of Italy* (London: Churchill, 1865), 71–2.

49 Vavasour, *My Last Tour and First Work*, 51, 85.

50 Janković, *Confronting the Climate*, 124.

51 James Clark, *The Influence of Climate in the Prevention and Cure of Chronic Diseases* (London: John Murray, 1830), 197. He did however rely extensively on the experience of two local expatriate physicians, Drs Heineken and Renton, to support his claims.

52 Ibid., 103–6.

53 Alexander Taylor, *On the Curative Influence of the Climate of Pau, and the Mineral Waters of the Pyrenees, on Disease* (London: John W. Parker, 1842).

54 Alexander Taylor, *A Comparative Enquiry as to the Preventive and Curative Influence of the Climate of Pau* (London: J. W. Parker, 1856), 30.

55 Drewry Ottley, 'Observations on the Climate of Pau', *Medical Times and Gazette* 17 (1858): 294–5.

56 Francis, *Change of Climate*, 67.

57 Frederick H. Johnson, *A Winter's Sketches in the South of France and the Pyrenees* (London: Chapman & Hall, 1857), 156–60.

58 Thomas Dormandy, *The White Death: A History of Tuberculosis* (London: Hambledon Press, 1999), 22–3.

59 The proposition advanced by William Budd in 1867 that consumption was analogous to typhoid fever and other contagious diseases received little support; Michael Warboys, *Spreading Germs: Disease Theories and Medical Practice in Britain, 1865–1900* (Cambridge: Cambridge University Press, 2000), 198–9.

60 James Clark, *Medical Notes on Climate, Disease, Hospitals, and Medical Schools in France, Italy and Switzerland* (London: printed for T. and G. Underwood, 1820), 41.

61 Janković, *Confronting the Climate*, 134–6.

62 For the eighteenth and early nineteenth century medical foundations of the consensus, see Roy Porter, 'Consumption: Disease of the Consumer Society?', in *Consumption and the World of Goods*, ed. John Brewer and Roy Porter (London: Routledge, 1993), 58–81; and Clark Lawlor and Akihito Suzuki, 'The Disease of the Self: Representing Consumption, 1700–1830', *Bulletin of the History of Medicine* 74, no. 3 (2000): 458–94.

63 Janković, *Confronting the Climate*, 134.

64 Ibid., 136.

65 Julius Jeffreys, *A Few Remarks on Climate and the Rational Treatment of Affections of the Throat and Lungs by Means of Atmospheres of Soothing Properties: With an Explanation of the Action and Use of Respirators* (London: Longman, 1849).

66 James Edward Pollock, 'Considerations on the Climate of Italy, with Reference to the Treatment of Chronic Disease', *London Medical Gazette* xi (ns) (1850): 1018.

67 Johnson, *A Winter's Sketches in the South of France and the Pyrenees*, 313–14.

68 Thomas More Madden, *On Change of Climate: A Guide for Travellers in Pursuit of Health* (London: T. C. Newby, 1864), 35–6.

69 John C. Thorowgood, *The Climatic Treatment of Consumption and Chronic Lung Diseases*, 3rd edn (London: H. K. Lewis, 1868), 3.

70 Pollock, 'Considerations on the Climate of Italy', 1017.

71 Madden, *On Change of Climate*, iii.

72 F. B. Smith, *The Retreat of Tuberculosis, 1850–1950* (London: Croom Helm, 1988), 4–5.

73 Edwin Lee, *Memoranda on France, Italy and Germany, with Remarks on Climates, Medical Practice, Mineral Waters etc.* (London: Saunders and Otley, 1841), 300.

74 Thorowgood, *The Climatic Treatment of Consumption*, 41.

75 Madden, *On Change of Climate*, 34.

76 Henry M'Cormac, *On the Nature, Treatment and Prevention of Pulmonary Consumption* (London: Longman, 1855), 80.

77 Thorowgood, *The Climatic Treatment of Consumption*, 34.

78 George Bodington, 'An Essay on the Treatment and Cure of Pulmonary Consumption' (1840), reprint ed. A. E. Bodington (Lichfield: Lomas Successors, 1906).

79 Thomas H. Burgess, *Climate of Italy in Relation to Pulmonary Consumption: With Remarks on the Influence of Foreign Climates upon Invalids* (London: Longman, Brown, Green, and Longmans, 1852), 168.

80 Francis, *Change of Climate*, 25.

81 Ibid., 77–8; Richard Payne Cotton, *The Nature, Symptoms, and Treatment of Consumption* (London: Churchill, 1852), 69.

82 For the history of tuberculosis in Victorian Britain, see Smith, *The Retreat of Tuberculosis*; Dormandy, *The White Death*; Helen Bynum, *Spitting Blood: The History of Tuberculosis* (Oxford: Oxford University Press, 2012).

83 Lawlor and Suzuki, 'The Disease of the Self', 470–5.

84 The longevity of the association is explored by Clark Lawlor in *Consumption and Literature: The Making of the Romantic Disease* (London: Palgrave Macmillan, 2006).

85 Clark, *The Influence of Climate*, 8.

86 Christopher Hoolihan, 'Health and Travel in Nineteenth-Century Rome', *Journal of the History of Medicine* 44, no. 4 (1989): 468, citing *The Italian Journal of Samuel Rogers*, ed. J. R. Hale (1956). Henry Matthews likewise put the number of Britons in Rome at Easter 1818 at 2000, *The Diary of an Invalid*, 162. Precise statistics are unavailable before the advent of hotel registration in the 1880s.

87 Clark, *Medical Notes on Climate*, 74–5.

88 Pollock, 'Considerations on the Climate of Italy', 1016.

89 Clark, *The Influence of Climate*, 137.

90 Starke, *Travels in Europe*, 499–500.

91 Clark, *Medical Notes on Climate*, 68.

92 Clark, *The Influence of Climate*, 135; Lee, *Notes on Italy and Rhenish Germany*, 43.

93 Ibid., 57.

94 Clark, *Medical Notes on Climate*, 86.

95 Pemble, *The Mediterranean Passion*, 87.

96 When J. H. Bennet used the term in *Mentone and the Riviera as a Winter Climate* (1861) he seems to have been restricting it to its original Italian meaning of the Ligurian coastline. Two decades later it had been appropriated by the British for the entire French coast as far as Hyères – see for example Adolphe Smith, *The Garden of Hyères: A Description of the Most Southerly Point on the French Riviera* (London: J. Evans, 1880) – a rare example of reverse acculturation following the incorporation of the county of Nice into the French state. The term was not used by the French themselves however, who only began to designate the entire coast of the Var and Alpes-Maritimes departments *la Côte d'Azur* towards the end of the nineteenth century; until that time it was merely the coast of Provence.

97 Edward I. Sparks, *The Riviera: Sketches of the Health Resorts of the North Mediterranean Coast of France and Italy from Hyères to Spezia* (London: Churchill, 1879), 27.

98 Clark, *Medical Notes on Climate*, 37–46. Montpellier had been a favoured resort for British patients before the Victorian period.

99 Clark, *The Influence of Climate*, 122–6.

100 Return by HM consul at Nice to the Royal College of Physicians' questionnaire on local health conditions, 1829 Royal College of Physicians, London (RCP) MS 3082.

101 William Farr, *A Medical Guide to Nice … with Separate Remarks on All Those Diseases to Which Its Climate Is Proved to Be Injurious or Beneficial, Especially Consumption and Scrofula* (London: Churchill, 1841), 3–4.

102 Sparks, *The Riviera*, 96.

103 Farr, *A Medical Guide to Nice*, 56–7.

104 *Hand-Book for Travellers in Northern Italy*, 1st edn (London: John Murray, 1842), 73. The *bise* is in fact a north-east wind.

105 Francis, *Change of Climate*, 55–6.

106 Carleton, *Brief Advice to Travellers*, 61–5.

107 Margaret Maria Brewster, *Letters from Cannes and Nice* (Edinburgh: Thomas Constable, 1857), 109.

108 Francis, *Change of Climate*, 80.

109 Charles Theodore Williams, *The Climate of the South of France, and Its Varieties Most Suitable for Invalids; With Remarks on Italian and Other Winter Stations* (London: Churchill, 1867), 53, 66.

110 J. Henry Bennet, *Mentone, the Riviera, Corsica and Biarritz as Winter Climates* (London: Churchill, 1862), 113; James Lewis Siordet, *Mentone in Its Medical Aspect* (London: Churchill, 1863), 62.

111 William Chambers, *Wintering at Mentone* (London: W. & R. Chambers, 1870), 50.

112 M'Cormac, *On the Nature, Treatment and Prevention of Pulmonary Consumption*, 78–9.

113 Chambers, *Wintering at Mentone*, 49.

114 Brewster, *Letters from Cannes and Nice*, 157.

115 Chambers, *Wintering at Mentone*, 54.

116 Madden, *The Spas of Belgium*, ii–iv.

117 Lambeth Palace Library, London (LPL) Fulham Papers, Jackson 29, ff. 151–2.

118 For British spa development and statistics during the Regency period, see Phyllis Hembury, *The English Spa 1560–1815, a Social History* (London: Athlone Press, 1990), esp. 105–12 and the same author's *British Spas from 1815 to the Present*, ed. and completed by W. Cowie and Evelyn E. Cowie (London: Athlone Press, 1997).

119 A. B. Granville, *The Spas of Germany*, 2nd edn with a supplement (London: Henry Colburn, 1843), xiv.

120 Vavasour, *My Last Tour and First Work*, 69.

121 James Johnson, *Pilgrimages to the Spas in Pursuit of Health and Recreation; With an Inquiry into the Comparative Merits of Different Mineral Waters* (London: S. Highley, 1841), 216.

122 Sir Alexander Mackenzie Downie, *The Spas of Homburg, Considered with Reference to Their Efficacy in the Treatment of Chronic Disease* (London: Churchill, 1842), 46–8.

123 Hood, *Up the Rhine*, 254–7.

124 Johnson, *Pilgrimages to the Spas*, 225–6. Blue pill was a mercury-based preparation normally used for digestive complaints.

125 F. H. Prytherch, *The Mineral Waters of Homburg and Kissingen Compared, with a Medical Topography of the Environs, etc.* (Frankfurt: Charles Jugel, 1844), 92–3.

126 *Liste der Kur-und Badgäste in Karlsbad* (Carlsbad: Franieck, 1840).

127 Phillip A. Nicholls, *Homeopathy and the Medical Profession* (London: Croom Helm, 1988), 111.

128 Phillip Nicholls, 'Class, Status and Gender: Toward a Sociology of the Homeopathic Patient in Nineteenth-Century Britain', in *Patients in the History of Homeopathy*, ed. Martin Dinges (Sheffield: European Association for the History of Medicine and Health Publications, 2002), 149.

129 The role of chemical analysis in the validation of the efficacy of mineral waters is explored by Christopher Hamlin, 'Chemistry, Medicine, and the Legitimization of English Spas, 1740–1840', *Medical History of Waters and Spas*, ed. Roy Porter, Medical History Supplement no. 10 (London: Wellcome Institute for the History of Medicine, 1990), 67–81.

130 Anon., *A Hot-Water Cure, Sought Out in Germany in the Summer of 1844. The Journal of a Patient* (London: Saunders and Otley, 1845).

131 Vavasour, *My Last Tour and First Work*, 133.

132 It was widely recognized by the early nineteenth century that water was not merely a vehicle for conducting chemical ingredients to the body, but a medium within which chemical substances could be rearranged; Hamlin, 'Chemistry, Medicine, and the Legitimization of English Spas', 76.

133 Jane M. Adams, *Healing with Water: English Spas and the Water Cure, 1840–1960* (Manchester: Manchester University Press, 2015), 40–5.

134 Johnson, *Pilgrimages to the Spas*, 164.

135 A. B. Granville, *Kissingen, Its Sources and Resources* (London: G.W. Nickisson, 1846), 224–5.

136 Granville, *The Spas of Germany*, 524.

137 Letter to his mother, 2 June 1863, Wilkie Collins, *The Letters of Wilkie Collins*, ed. W. Baker and W. M. Clark (London: Palgrave Macmillan, 1999), vol. 1, 224–6.

138 Johnson, *Pilgrimages to the Spas*, 108.

139 Madden, *The Spas of Belgium*, 141–2.

140 Johnson, *A Winter's Sketches in the South of France and the Pyrenees*, 325.

141 Mary Eyre, *A Lady's Walks in the South of France in 1863* (London: Richard Bentley, 1865), 69.

142 Edwin Lee, *Practical Observations on Mineral Waters and Baths; With Notices of Some Continental Climates* (London: Churchill, 1846), 33.

143 Janković, *Confronting the Climate*, 123.

## 2 Destinations

1 Letter from HM consul Mark to Lord Clarendon, 14 July 1855 TNA FO72/874.

2 E. W. L. Davies, *Algiers in 1857, Its Accessibility, Climate and Resources Described with Especial Reference to English Invalids* (London: Longman, Brown, Green, Longmans, and Roberts, 1858), 1.

3 Francis, *Change of Climate*, 87.

4 Mariana Starke, *Letters from Italy, Between the Years 1792 and 1798 … With Instructions for the Use of Invalids and Families Who May Not Choose to Incur the Expence of Travelling with a Courier* (London: R. Phillips: 1800), vol. 2, 257–68. The appendix to this work eventually evolved into a fully-fledged guidebook to Europe, *Travels on the Continent*, which went through several editions from 1820 onwards, while never losing its primary focus on Italy.

5 James Clark published revised editions of this work until 1846, by which date it had acquired the title *The Sanative Influence of Climate: With an Account of the Best Places for Resort for Invalids in England, the South of Europe, Etc.* (London: J. Murray, 1846).

6 Edwin Lee, *Bradshaw's Companion to the Continent*, iii–iv. The second edition of this work made this intention more explicit in the title, *Bradshaw's Invalid's Companion to the Continent: Comprising General and Medical Notices of the Principal Places of Resort* (London: W. J. Adams, 1861).

7 On the publication history of Murray's handbooks, see W. B. C. Lister, *A Bibliography of Murray's Handbooks for Travellers* (Dereham: Dereham Books, 1993).

8 *Cook's Handbook to the Health Resorts of the South of France and the Riviera, with descriptions of Marseilles, Hyères, Cannes, Nice, Monaco,Mentone, Bordighera, San Remo, Oneglia, Genoa, Spezzia, and Pisa* (London: Thomas Cook, 1878); in 1893 Cook added the resorts of south-west France.

9 'In *Medical Climatology* I recognise much of the matter, both respecting baths and climates, which I have communicated for several years past', Edwin Lee, *The Principal Baths of Germany, France, and Switzerland, Considered with Reference to Their Remedial Efficacy in Chronic Disease* (London: Churchill, 1863), viii.

10 R. E. Scoresby-Jackson, *Medical Climatology: Or, a Topographical and Meteorological Description of the Localities Resorted to in Winter and Summer by Invalids of Various Classes, both at Home and Abroad* (London: Churchill, 1862), x.

11 Madden however later revised and expanded the work as *The Principal Health-Resorts of Europe and Africa for the Treatment of Chronic Diseases* (London: Churchill, 1876), by which date he was able to include continental spas, based on visits in the intervening period. He never visited Madeira.

12 Francis, *Change of Climate*, vi. The author used this justification for privileging coverage of the Iberian Peninsula in the book, at the expense of Italy and the south of France, regions that he claimed would in other circumstances have been well within his orbit.

13 For both Granville and Lee see *ODNB*.

14 [Sir Francis Bond Head], *Bubbles from the Brunnens of Nassau by an Old Man* (London: John Murray, 1834). The relevant *Kurlisten* for Schwalbach and Schlangenbad show that Head and his wife made a brief visit to Schwalbach in July 1832 and a longer one to Schlangenbad the following year. These separate visits are conflated in the published account, a minor deception in keeping with Head's assumed literary persona as an elderly curist; he was after all barely forty.

15 *Verzeichnis der Kurfremden und Durchreisenden zu Bad Ems, Langenschwalbach, Schlangenbad und Weilbach in Jahre 1833* (Wiesbaden: Ludwig Riedel, 1833); identical title and imprint for 1835.

16 *A Handbook for Travellers on the Continent* (London: John Murray, 1836), 391.

17 Granville, *The Spas of Germany*, 2nd edn (London: Henry Colburn, 1839), xvii, 460. Head had been appointed assistant poor law commissioner for East Kent in 1834, deputy-governor of Upper Canada the following year, and made a baronet in 1837, *ODNB*.

18 Sir Alexander McKenzie Downie, *A Practical Treatise on the Efficiency of Mineral Waters in the Cure of Chronic Diseases* (Frankfurt am Main: Charles Jugel, 1841), 3.

19 Granville, *The Spas of Germany*, 62–3.

20 Ibid., 72.

21 Johnson, *Pilgrimages to the Spas*, 105. This represented just over 10 per cent of all visitors and the largest non-German-speaking contribution to numbers, *A Handbook for Travellers in Southern Germany* (London: John Murray, 1843), 20.

22 Letter from Allan Young to his aunt, 21 May [1838] Young of Orlingbury papers, Northamptonshire Archives (NA) YO/710 (iv).

23 Letter from J. H. Rowland to his parents, 2 June 1838 Wellcome Library, London (WL) Western MS 8439.

24 Sparks, *The Riviera*; the work was based on a series of articles published by in the *Medical Times and Gazette* in 1876–7.

25 Scoresby-Jackson, *Medical Climatology*, ix.

26 Madden, *On Change of Climate*, ii.

27 Chambers, *Some Effects of the Climate of Italy*, 4–5.

28 Letter to his mother 18 [Feb.], 1844 WS 1720/843.

29 Johnson, *Change of Air*, 28.

30 That the vast and featureless interior of eastern France held few attractions for nineteenth-century tourists was not exclusive to Britons: in 1827 Stendhal, en route for Rome, wrote that 'from Paris, travelling the ugliest country in the world which simpletons call "France the beautiful", we came to Basel', *A Roman Journal by Stendhal*, ed. and trans. Haakon Chevalier (London: Orion Press, 1959), 7.

31 Pemble, *The Mediterranean Passion*, 8.

32 Bennet, *Mentone, the Riviera, Corsica and Biarritz*, 107.

33 Chambers, *Some Effects of the Climate of Italy*, 95.

34 Ibid., 66.

35 Bennet, *Mentone, the Riviera, Corsica and Biarritz*, 177.

36 *Bradshaw's Invalid's Companion to the Continent*, 365.

37 William Bullar, *Letters from Abroad from a Physician in Search of Health* (London: John Van Voorst, 1861), 215–17.

38 Thomas Burgess termed Pisa 'the great central depot for foreign consumptive invalids', *Climate of Italy*, 148.

39 Johnson, *Change of Air*, 240.

40 Farr, *A Medical Guide to Nice*, 9.

41 Ibid., 140.

42 Notable examples include the draughtsman and lithographer Andrew Picken (1815–1845), whose *Madeira Illustrated* (1840) was based on work undertaken during two years of convalescence on the island, and the surgeon William Wilde (1815–1876), whose *Narrative of a Voyage to Madeira, Teneriffe and Along the Shores of the Mediterranean* (1840) arose from his role as medical attendant to a consumptive invalid. See *ODNB* Picken, Andrew, and Wilde, Sir William Robert Wills.

43 Sarah Ellis, *Summer and Winter in the Pyrenees* (London: Fisher, 1841), 33.

44 Taylor, *On the Curative Influence of the Climate of Pau*, 22.

45 Louisa Stuart Costello, *Béarn and the Pyrenees: A Legendary Tour to the Country of Henri Quatre* (London: Richard Bentley, 1844), vol. 2, 16–17.

46 Johnson, *Change of Air*, 64.
47 Clark, *Medical Notes on Climate*, 19–26.
48 Clark, *The Influence of Climate*, 114–15.
49 *Hand-book for Travellers in France* (London: John Murray, 1843), 485.
50 Lee, *Memoranda on France, Italy and Germany*, 91.
51 *The Taylor Papers, Being a Record of Certain Reminiscences, Letters, and Journals in the Life of Lieut.-Gen. Sir Herbert Taylor* (London: Longmans, Green, 1913), 480.
52 *Hand-Book for Travellers in France* (London: John Murray, 1843), 490.
53 Lee, *Bradshaw's Companion to the Continent*, 23
54 Brewster, *Letters from Cannes and Nice*, 163, 193.
55 Francis, *Change of Climate*, 168–92.
56 Edwin Lee, *Notes on Spain: With a Special Account of Malaga and Its Climate* (London: Hope, 1854).
57 Ibid., iv.
58 Ibid., 50–95.
59 Despatch from HM consul Mark, 14 July 1855 TNA FO 72/874.
60 Reports by the trustees, TNA FO72/1068, 1085, 1106, 1150, 1191.
61 Mrs Ramsay, *A Summer in Spain* (London: Tinsley Brothers, 1874), 376–7.
62 Francis, *Change of Climate*, 263.
63 Letter from HM consul Bell to the Foreign Office, 13 September 1851 TNA FO27/911.
64 Letter from HM consul Bell to the Foreign Office, 5 April 1862 TNA FO27/1455.
65 Letter from HM consul Playfair to the Foreign Office, 24 January 1868 TNA FO 27/1725.
66 Letter from Cecil Monro to his mother, 7 March 1869 Monro papers, London Metropolitan Archives (LMA) ACC/1063/1573. William Douglas-Hamilton (1845–1895), 12th Duke of Hamilton, described by an infatuated Russian admirer as 'a man who lives only for racing, horses, shooting, hunting, and who adores good wine and bad women', Patrick Howarth, *When the Riviera Was Ours* (London: Routledge, 1977), 105.
67 Diary of Dr Robert J. Lee, WL Western MS 3222.
68 Bennet, *Mentone, the Riviera, Corsica, and Biarritz*, 182–3; [W. B. Aspinall], *San Remo as a Winter Residence, by an Invalid, 1863–65* (London: William Hunt, 1869), 19.
69 Lee, *Bradshaw's Companion to the Continent*, 73; Edwin Lee, *The Effect of Climate on Tuberculous Disease … with an Appendix of Corroborative Observations and Notices of Several Places of Winter Resort* (London: Churchill, 1858), 188.

70 Augustus J. C. Hare, *A Winter at Mentone* (London: Wertheim, Macintosh, & Hunt, 1862), 14–16.
71 Bennet, *Mentone, the Riviera, Corsica, and Biarritz*, 137.
72 Hare, *A Winter at Mentone*, 163.
73 J. Henry Bennet, *Mentone and the Riviera as a Winter Climate* (London: Churchill, 1861), v–vi. The Italian spelling of the place name remained common in English-language publications for at least two decades after unification with France.
74 Bennet, *Mentone, the Riviera, Corsica, and Biarritz*, 180.
75 Hare, *A Winter at Mentone*, xiii.
76 Bennet, *Mentone, the Riviera, Corsica, and Biarritz*, 181.
77 Letter from 'A Pioneer', *Times*, 13 October 1858.
78 [Aspinall] *San Remo as a Winter Residence*, 32.
79 Ibid., 127–42.
80 Chambers, *Wintering at Mentone*, 6.
81 Sparks, *The Riviera*, 327–33.
82 Ibid., 334–9.
83 Johnson, *A Winter's Sketches in the South of France and the Pyrenees*, 65–6.
84 *Times*, 18, 22 September 1858.
85 John Altrayd Wittitterly [alias Elizabeth Carne], *Three Months' Rest at Pau, in the Winter and Spring of 1859* (London: Bell and Daldy, 1860), 27.
86 Pierre Tucoo-Chala, *Pau, Ville Anglaise*, 78.
87 *Times*, 4 June, 15 September 1868.
88 Alfred Drysdale, *Wintering Abroad: Mentone and the Riviera* (London: printed by J. S. Virtue, 1884), 28–30.
89 *Times*, 18 December 1883.
90 Letter from Revd Rolfe to William Garnett, 9 June 1868, Garnett papers, Lancashire Archives (LA) DDQ/7/4/29.
91 William Miller, *Wintering in the Riviera with Notes of Travel in Italy and France and Practical Hints to Travellers* (London: Longmans, Green, 1879), 152–3.
92 *Cook's Handbook to the Health Resorts of the South of France and the Northern Coast of the Mediterranean* (London: Thomas Cook, 1881–2), 36.
93 See *ODNB*.
94 Douglas Galton, *Report on the Works of Sewerage and Drainage Proposed for the Town of Cannes* (London: Wyman, 1883), 6–7.
95 Ibid., 21.
96 *Cook's Handbook to the Health Resorts of the South of France and the Riviera* (London: Thomas Cook, 1893), 45.
97 Madden, *On Change of Climate*, 32.
98 Pemble, *The Mediterranean Passion*, 40.

99 Reports of the trustees of the Anglican church at Nice, 1837–61 TNA FO 97/256.

100 Sparks, *The Riviera*, 197, 217–18.

101 Ibid., 306. Caution is needed in interpreting Sparks's definition of 'foreign', which includes both French and Italian families.

102 Ibid., 307.

103 Letter from Ughtred Kay Shuttleworth to Arthur Otway, 18 January 1869 TNA FO45/150. These were doubtless chiefly winter visitors rather than permanent residents.

104 Miller, *Wintering in the Riviera*, 245. As the author makes clear, official statistics relied on visitor self-identification so almost certainly undercounted numbers.

105 J. Henry Bennet, *Winter and Spring on the Shores of the Mediterranean; Or the Riviera, Mentone, Italy, Corsica, Sicily, Algeria, Spain, and Biarritz as Winter Climates* (New York: D. Appleton, 1870), 190.

106 William White Cooper, *The Invalid's Guide to Madeira* (London: Smith, Elder, 1840), 24; Robert White and James Y. Johnson, *Madeira, Its Climate and Scenery, a Handbook for Visitors* (Edinburgh: Adam and Charles Black, 1860), 322. These statistics were compiled by the British consul.

107 The figure for 1856 is given in a return of numbers sent by the Anglican chaplain to the bishop of London, LPL Tait 423, 181. The cholera outbreak of 1856 killed almost 10 per cent of Madeira's population, including the prominent expatriate doctor Archibald Ross, and a daughter of the British consul, TNA FO 63/807; burial register of the British cemetery, Funchal, Holy Trinity Church archives, Archivo e Biblioteca da Madeira (ABM), HTC /13.

108 James Clark, *The Sanative Influence of Climate: With an Account of the Best Places of Resort for Invalids in England, the South of Europe, etc.* (London: John Murray, 1841), 271.

109 Anon., *Madeira: A Brief Letter of Advice to an Invalid by an Ex-Invalid* (London: Bell and Daldy, 1859), 8.

110 The visiting physician W. W. Ireland, who had access to visitor statistics kept by the British consul, quotes four-year averages of 227 for 1861–4 and 155 for 1865–8, *The Climate of Madeira* (Edinburgh: Oliver and Boyd, 1869), 5.

111 Tucoo-Chala, *Pau, Ville Anglaise*, 12. Note that 'foreigners' comprised all visitors from outside the Pau region.

112 Despatch from HM vice-consul Church, 25 June 1869 TNA FO27/1770.

113 LPL, Tait papers 413, 189. This total seems broadly consistent with the figure of 365 British families given in *Liste des Etrangers Fixés ou Résident à Pau et aux Environs – Station Hivernale 1867–68*, published by the Syndicat de la ville de Pau at the end of 1867 (see the copy in the Blathwayt papers, Gloucestershire Archives (GA) D1799/Z20).

114 Thorowgood, *The Climatic Treatment of Consumption*, 38.

115 Tucoo-Chala, *Pau, Ville Anglaise*, 150.

116 Lady Emmeline Stuart-Wortley, *The Sweet South* (London: printed for private circulation, 1856), vol. 2, 340.

117 Letter from HM consul Mark to Lord Clarendon, 14 July 1855 TNA FO72/874.

118 Mrs H. Lloyd Evans, *Last Winter in Algeria* (London: Chapman & Hall, 1868), 335.

119 John Richard Green, *Stray Studies from England and Italy* (London: Macmillan, 1876), vol. 1, 77.

120 Scoresby-Jackson, *Medical Climatology*, viii–ix.

121 Tucoo-Chala, *Pau, Ville Anglaise*, 13.

122 See note 112.

123 Henry Blackburn, *The Pyrenees: A Description of Summer Life at French Watering Places* (London: Sampson Low, Son, and Marston, 1867), 29.

124 Ibid., 29–30.

125 Green, *Stray Studies*, vol. 1, 77.

126 Brewster, *Letters from Cannes and Nice*, 194. It is noteworthy that clergy were also prominent supporters of homeopathy, suggestive perhaps of the general appeal of 'natural' cures to clerical types; see Nicholls, 'Class, Status and Gender', 149.

127 Pemble, *The Mediterranean Passion*, 46.

128 Sparks, *The Riviera*, 333–4.

129 Clark, *Medical Notes on Climate*, 118.

130 Ann Vavasour recalled seeing the names of two unmarried English ladies who were travelling from Athens to Paris – 'a long step for lone ladies' – inscribed in the visitors book of a Swiss inn, *My Last Tour and First Work*, 232.

131 Katherine Byrne, *Tuberculosis and the Victorian Literary Imagination* (Cambridge: Cambridge University Press, 2011), 30–5. Official mortality statistics provide no support for this perception, see Smith, *The Retreat of Tuberculosis*, 5–7.

132 Davies, *Algiers in 1857*, 32.

133 Sparks, *The Riviera*, 104.

134 Lee, *Memoranda on France, Italy and Germany*, 308–9; see also his *Treatise on Some Nervous Disorders*, 2nd edn (London: Churchill, 1838), 13–39.

135 Sparks, *The Riviera*, 141.

136 Chambers, *Some Effects of the Climate of Italy*, 85.

137 Taylor, *On the Curative Influence of the Climate of Pau*, 82–4; John Macpherson, *The Baths and Wells of Europe; Their Action and Uses* (London: Macmillan, 1869), 160.

138 Letter to Charlotte Blathwayt, 2 January 1865 GA D1799/C63.

139 See the Marling papers in the Gloucestershire Archives (GA) D873.

140 Dr Siordet of Menton, for example, informed Dr Sparks that 'judging from his experience there were many more phthisitical girls from the age of sixteen to twenty years than boys', Sparks, *The Riviera*, 104.

141 Brewster, *Letters from Cannes and Nice*, 118.

142 Head, *Bubbles from the Brunnens of Nassau*, 20.

143 Pierre Lafagne, *Spa and the English, or, English Influence in the History of Spa* (Spa: Association for the Promotion and Encouragement of Tourism in Spa, 1948), 22.

144 Edwin Lee noted that Spa was 'out of favour with the English', *An Account of the Most Frequented Watering Places on the Continent, and of the Medicinal Application of their Mineral Springs* (London: Longman, 1836), 86.

145 Collins, *The Letters*, vol. 2, 216–23.

146 Hermann Weber claimed towards the end of the century that 70 per cent of patients at Aachen were syphilitic, Hermann Weber and F. Parkes Weber, *The Spas and Mineral Waters of Europe* (London: Smith, Elder, 1896), 212.

147 Macpherson, *The Baths and Wells of Europe*, 246.

148 Hermann Sommer, *Zur Kur nach Ems* (Stuttgart: Franz Steiner Verlag, 1999), 714–19.

149 *Emser Kurliste vom Jahr 1846* (Bad-Ems: Druck und Verlag von H. Chr. Sommer, 1846).

150 Sommer, *Zur Kur nach Ems*, 724–5.

151 Macpherson, *The Baths and Wells of Europe*, 114–15.

152 The *Kurlisten* provide details of registrations, indicating among other things the sex of visitors. However it is not clear how many visitors took the cure, or were merely, as it were, non-playing members of the team. Hermann Sommer's statistics by contrast are based on active curists under medical supervision.

153 Granville, *Kissingen, Its Sources and Resources*, 3–13. The total number of incidences of different ailments tabulated by Granville amounts to 893, presumably because several cases presented more than one ailment.

154 The published *Kurlisten* for 1858, 1869 and 1878 give an official figure of 430, 503 and 483, respectively, *Liste der im Jahre 1858 angekommenen und abgereisten Kur-und Badgäste von Bad Kissingen und Bocklet* (n.p., n.d.) and subsequent editions.

155 A. B. Granville, *Autobiography of A. B. Granville*, ed. Paulina B. Granville (London: Henry S. King, 1874), vol. 2, 351. Granville presumably used registrations as a proxy for patients, an inexact tool, but he would have had nothing better.

156 The proportion of British female registrations rose from about 15 per cent in 1844 to 32 per cent in 1878. These were either single women or women accompanied by female companions or mixed-sex family groups. Comparison

with Hermann Sommer's figures for female curists under medical supervision at Ems suggests that the statistics of female registrations typically undercount the total number of female curists by the equivalent of several percentage points.

157 Granville, *The Spas of Germany* (1843), 420, 569–70.

158 Erasmus Wilson, *A Three Weeks' Scamper through the Spas of Germany and Belgium* (London: Churchill, 1858), 201.

159 Anon., *A Hot-Water Cure*, 223.

160 John Macpherson provides a figure of 12,000 annual visitors to Homburg at the end of the decade, putting it third behind Baden Baden (50,000) and Wiesbaden (30,000), *The Baths and Wells of Europe*, 21.

161 Ibid., 222.

162 Vavasour, *My Last Tour and First Work*, 133.

163 Lee, *Memoranda on France, Italy and Germany*, 259.

164 *Handbook for Travellers in Southern Germany*, 10th edn, revised (London: John Murray, 1867), 38.

165 Macpherson, *The Baths and Wells of Europe*, 113.

166 Collins, *Letters*, vol. 2, 223–8.

167 Edwin Lee, *The Baths of Germany, Considered with Reference to Their Remedial Efficacy in Chronic Diseases*, 2nd edn (London: Whittaker, 1843), 218.

168 Lyons, *The Pyrenees in the Modern Era*, 7.

169 Taylor, *On the Curative Influence of the Climate of Pau*, 181.

170 Ibid., 339.

171 Ibid., 208–32.

172 Ibid., 335.

173 Statistics quoted in Peter Thorold, *The British in France* (London: Continuum, 2008), 76. By the end of the 1860s Eaux Bonnes had almost 10,000 annual visitors according to Macpherson, *The Baths and Wells of Europe*, 21.

174 Jérôme Penez, *Histoire du Thermalisme en France au XIXe Siècle: Eau, Médicine et Loisirs* (Paris: Econimica, 2005), 47.

175 Lee, *Memoranda on France, Italy and Germany*, 59.

176 Charles Richard Weld, *The Pyrenees, West and East* (London: Longman, Brown, Green, Longmans & Roberts, 1859), 209. 'Hells' was a common term of disapproval for gambling establishments.

177 Blackburn, *The Pyrenees*, 213.

178 Taylor, *On the Curative Influence of the Climate of Pau*, 316–22.

179 Douglas Peter Mackaman, *Leisure Settings: Bourgeois Culture, Medicine and the Spa in Modern France* (Chicago: University of Chicago Press, 1998), 48.

180 F. Gros, *Vichy and Environs* (Vichy, 1884), 100; Macpherson, *The Baths and Wells of Europe*, 20–1. Comparative statistics need to be treated with care

in view of the different approaches adopted by the various spa authorities in keeping and presenting them, but the broad outlines are clear.

181 'Vichyana', *Blackwood's Magazine* 59 (1846), 309.

182 *A Handbook for Travellers in France* (London: John Murray, 1854), 360.

183 Letter from Hilary Bonham-Carter to her mother, 25 July 1850 Bonham-Carter papers, Hampshire Archives (HA) 94M72/F532.

184 Penez, *Histoire du Thermalisme*, 73–4.

185 *A Handbook for Travellers in France* (London: John Murray: 1870), 388.

186 Penez, *Histoire du Thermalisme*, 74.

187 *A Handbook for Travellers in France* (London: John Murray, 1878), vol. 2, 34.

188 This development is discussed by Mackaman, especially in relation to Vichy and Aix-les-Bains, in *Leisure Settings*.

189 Bertram M. Gordon, 'Reinvention of a Spa Town: The Unique Case of Vichy', *Journal of Tourism History* 4, no. 1 (2012), 45.

190 Macpherson, *The Baths and Wells of Europe*, 116.

191 Letter to Mr Blackwood, 24 August 1863, George Eliot, *The George Eliot Letters*, ed. G. H. Haight (New Haven: Yale University Press, 1954–78), vol. 5, 429–30.

## 3 Travelling

1 Margaret Brewster on the other hand remarked in 1856 on the number of private villas at Cannes that had been booked by electric telegraph, *Letters from Cannes and Nice*, 33. Communication by telegraph between Britain and the Riviera was achieved by about 1853, see report from HM consul Turnbull, Marseilles, 1 May 1852 TNA FO27/944.

2 Mariana Starke, *Travels on the Continent: Written for the Use and Particular Information of Travellers* (London: John Murray, 1820), appendix, 5.

3 Lee, *Memoranda on France, Italy and Germany*, 341. A personal supply of tea (and portable apparatus for boiling water) remained a constant recommendation for British invalids abroad throughout the following half century: see for example T. Lauder Brunton, *Winter Health Resorts* (London: printed by Adlard, 1884), 16.

4 The respirator was patented in 1836. Henry M'Cormac was not a fan: 'This so-named respirator never saved anyone from consumption, or any one in consumption', he complained; 'in fact the respirator impedes respiration', *On the Nature, Treatment and Prevention of Pulmonary Consumption*, 102–3.

5 Letter from Margaret Marling to her husband, 29 January 1853 GA D873/C10.

6 Lee, *Memoranda on France, Italy and Germany*, 340–2.

7 LMA ACC/2668. The catalogue suggests a date of *c.* 1860, but the contract is certainly much earlier, probably *c.* 1800.
8 Selina Bunbury, *Rides in the Pyrenees* (London: Newby, 1844), vol. 1, 16.
9 Letter to his mother, 19 March 1863, Collins, *Letters*, vol. 1, 216–17.
10 Letter from Cecil Monro to his father, 6 December 1866 LMA ACC/1063/1493.
11 Travel journal of Dr Charles Brodie Sewell, 1882 WL Western MS 4507.
12 Starke, *Travels in Europe*, 503–4. Obadiah Elliott patented a method of mounting coach bodies on elliptical iron springs rather than the traditional wooden perch or frame, giving a more stable ride.
13 Lee, *Memoranda on France, Germany and Italy*, 340–1.
14 Johnson, *Change of Air*, 253.
15 Letter to her mother, 25 July 1850, HA 94M72/F532.
16 Vavasour, *My Last Tour and First Work*, 125.
17 Clark, *The Sanative Influence of Climate*, 113–14.
18 Letter from Charles Baring to his brother, 29 October 1839 Baring papers, HA 92M95/NP7/1.
19 Letters from Alice and Hilary Bonham-Carter, 31 October, 7, 13 November 1843 HA 94M72/F532.
20 Letter from Rosamund Fox Talbot to her brother, 8 October 1867 Talbot of Lacock papers, WS 2664/3/1B/22.
21 Bennet, *Mentone, the Riviera, Corsica, and Biarritz*, 276, 281–2.
22 Taylor, *On the Curative Influence of the Climate of Pau*, 16–18.
23 Elizabeth Grant, *A Highland Lady in France 1843–1845*, ed. Patricia Pelly and Andrew Tod (East Linton: Tuckwell Press, 1996), 3.
24 Wittitterly, *Three Months' Rest at Pau*, 14–15.
25 Letter to his brother, 7 September 1868 LMA ACC/1063/1540. Walshe was presumably Dr Walter Hayle Walshe (1812–1892), an authority on phthisis. Clark had been made a KCB in 1866.
26 Taylor, *A Comparative Enquiry*, 5.
27 Ibid., 29.
28 Starke, *Travels in Europe* (1839), 3–4. This edition of Starke's guidebook notes in addition that the St Gothard Pass had recently been made accessible to carriages.
29 Ibid., 103.
30 Johnson, *Change of Air*, 238–9. Although the coast road was made accessible to wheeled transport in 1827 there were still some 'fifty or sixty torrents' to cross in the 1850s according to Murray, *Handbook for Travellers in Northern Italy* (London: John Murray, 1853), 64.
31 Vavasour, *My Last Tour and First Work*, 309.
32 Starke, *Travels in Europe*, 530.
33 Clark, *Medical Notes on Climate*, 58–9.

34 Edwin Lee, *Continental Travel; With an Appendix on the Influence of Climate, the Remedial Advantages of Travelling, etc.* (London: W. J. Adams, 1848), 22, and *Bradshaw's Companion to the Continent*, 18.
35 Pemble, *The Mediterranean Passion*, 26.
36 Brewster, *Letters from Cannes and Nice*, 14–15.
37 Lee, *Bradshaw's Companion to the Continent*, 19.
38 *A Hand-book for Travellers in France* (1858), 482.
39 Miller, *Wintering in the Riviera*, 38. Murray noted in 1875 that 'Mentone [could be] reached in little more than 24 hours by the express train from Paris', but this comment seems to be based on railway timetables rather than real-world experience, *A Handbook for Travellers in France* (London: John Murray, 1875), part 2, 185.
40 *Times*, 3 February 1872.
41 'Railway Accident at Antibes, Near Cannes, Dragging for the Dead', *Illustrated London News*, 10 February 1872. By the 1890s some 100,000 annual visitors, a substantial minority of whom were British, arrived at Nice alone, Pemble, *The Victorian Passion*, 41.
42 Sparks, *The Riviera*, 150–1.
43 Taylor, *On the Curative Influence of the Climate of Pau*, 15–16.
44 Murray noted that the *malle-poste* from Paris to Bordeaux took thirty-six hours in the early 1840s, *A Hand-book for Travellers in France* (London: John Murray, 1844), xxv. This would equate to an average speed of ten mph.
45 Johnson, *A Winter's Sketches in the South of France*, 23.
46 Taylor, *A Comparative Enquiry*, 26.
47 Letters from Fanny Blathwayt to Charlotte Baker, 8 December 1865, 29 July 1868 GA D1799/C63.
48 Blackburn, *The Pyrenees*, 15.
49 Head, *Bubbles from the Brunnens of Nassau*, 10. Travellers heading for Ems typically disembarked at Koblenz, those for Wiesbaden and Homburg at Biebrich.
50 Letter from Anne Bourne to Miss Dyson, n. d. [1856] HA 9M55/F29.
51 Lee, *Bradshaw's Companion to the Continent*, 325.
52 Letter from E. H. Bradby to his mother, Namur, 2 September 1849 Bradby of Hamble papers, HA 46A06/A4/6.
53 Madden, *The Spas of Belgium*, 85–6. 'Forty minutes' for crossing the Channel is clearly an exaggeration; the fastest crossing seems to have been about ninety minutes, *A Handbook for Travellers on the Continent* (London: John Murray, 1868), 103.
54 *A Handbook for Travellers on the Continent* (1843), 206.
55 *A Handbook for Travellers on the Continent* (1863), 201; ibid. (1868), 92.
56 Madden, *The Spas of Belgium*, 204.

57 Lee, *Memoranda on France, Italy and Germany*, 341–2.

58 Clark, *The Sanative Influence of Climate*, 108–14.

59 Francis, *Change of Climate*, 91. By contrast Mrs Starke claimed the Italian post roads were so good that the chief danger for travellers was speeding by enthusiastic postillions, *Travels in Europe*, 3.

60 Letters from Cecil Monro to his father and brother, 12, 15 May 1860 LMA ACC/1063/1375-6.

61 Revd W Phelps, *A Mirror of the Duchy of Nassau* (Wiesbaden: printed for the author by A. Scholz, 1842), 280–1.

62 Granville, *Kissingen*, 59–61.

63 'Daily journal of Mrs Louisa Wilmot Campbell (née Cave-Brown-Cave) 16th September 1865 to 17th September 1866', ts copy Stoke-on-Trent City Archives (STA) SD 1705/MS 38.

64 Journal of Dr R. J. Lee, WL MS 3222.

65 Letter to his father, 2 November 1866 LMA ACC/1063/1490. The misery of long hours in a first-class railway carriage between Marseilles and Paris in 1867 is captured by Mark Twain: 'If you are worn out and must sleep, you must sit up and do it in naps, with cramped legs and in a torturing misery that leaves you withered and lifeless the next day', *The Innocents Abroad* (London: Penguin, [1869] 2002), 74.

66 He seems to have taken the overnight train from Paris again in November 1869, bound for Hyères, LMA ACC/1063/1597. It is not known how he travelled to Nice in 1868.

67 Journal of Dr R. J. Lee, WL MS 3222.

68 Bennet, *Winter and Spring on the Shores of the Mediterranean*, 608.

69 Ibid., 602.

70 Chambers, *Wintering in Mentone*, 8.

71 W. B. Aspinall, *San Remo as a Winter Residence by an Invalid, 1863–65*, 3rd edn, edited by his widow (London: William Hunt, 1869), 149.

72 Sparks, *The Riviera*, 144–6.

73 Ibid., 147–52.

74 James Livesey to the editor, Mentone 31 December 1875, *Times*, 7 January 1876. Livesey's complaints focused on lack of adequate sleeping accommodation, noise and vibration, want of ventilation, and of course expense.

75 The Reckitt family's first visit to Menton, 1861–2, is described in Major Desmond Chapman-Huston, *Sir James Reckitt: a Memoir* (London: Faber & Gwyer, 1927), 131–41.

76 Wittitterly, *Three Months' Rest at Pau*, 13–14.

77 Diaries of Fanny Blathwayt, 1864–68 GA D1799/F255-59.

78 Lee, *Memoranda on France, Germany and Italy*, 308.

79 Ibid., 295.
80 Letters of William Money-Kyrle, 1844–6 WS 1720/843.
81 Letter from Rosamund to Charles Fox Talbot, 27 August [1867] WS 2664/3/1B/22.
82 The story of the Fox Talbot tour of 1867–8 is reconstructed from letters written home to Charles Fox Talbot WS 2664/3/1B/22
83 Mary Shelley, *Rambles in Germany and Italy in 1840, 1842, and 1843* (London: Edward Moxon, 1844), vol. 1, 155–278.
84 Young papers, NA YO/710.
85 Lee, *A Treatise on Some Nervous Disorders*, 39.
86 Johnson, *Pilgrimages to the Spas*, 86.
87 Bonham-Carter papers, HA 94M72/F532.
88 Letters from Lady Naesmyth to Richard Long, 1856–7 Lord Long Papers, WS 947/1904.
89 Rothman, *Living in the Shadow of Death*, 24.
90 Correspondence and papers of Cecil Monro, LMA ACC/1063.
91 Letter from Fanny Blathwayt to Charlotte Baker, 3 February 1865 GA D1799/C63.
92 Letter to his mother, 14 November 1869 LMA ACC/1063/1602.
93 Letter to his father, 3 January 1861 LMA ACC/1063/1381.
94 Letters from Revd A. H. and Mrs Hosmer to Cecil Monro, 1869–70 LMA ACC/1063/2255-2258, 2327–2328, 2343.
95 Letter from Cecil Monro to his father, 23 February [1864] LMA ACC/1063/1404. The letter is dated 1862 and has consequently been misfiled, but this is clearly a scribal error.
96 Letter to his brother 16 January [1869] LMA ACC/1063/1567. The letter is misdated 1868. Lady Dunbar published *A Family Tour Round the Coasts of Spain and Portugal During the Winter of 1860–1861* (Edinburgh: Blackwood, 1862), which gives some background on the Dunbars' earlier travels.
97 W. H. Kittoe, *The Pocket Book of Practical Medicine, or Manual for Emergencies* (London: Sherwood, Gilbert and Piper, 1844), 217.
98 Ebenezer Gilchrist, *The Use of Sea Voyages in Medicine* (London: printed for A. Millar, and D. Wilson, and T. Durham, 1757), vii.
99 Katherine Foxhall, *Health, Medicine and the Sea: Australian Voyages, c. 1815–1860* (Manchester: Manchester University Press, 2012), 17–19.
100 William S. Wilson, *The Ocean as a Health-Resort: A Handbook of Practical Information as to Sea Voyages for the Use of Tourists and Invalids* (London: Churchill, 1880), 2–3.

101 The cruise was written up by William Wilde, Meiklam's medical companion, in *Narrative of a Voyage to Madeira, Teneriffe and along the Shores of the Mediterranean*, 2 vols (Dublin: William Curry, Jun., 1840).

102 Memoranda of an excursion, SF MS 84. Walker himself later took a more ambitious therapeutic sea voyage to the East Indies, Journal, 1840–1 SF MS 76.

103 Taylor, *The Curative Influence of the Climate of Pau*, 16; see for comparison the same author's *Comparative Enquiry*, 26.

104 C. B. Faber, *On the Influence of Sea-Voyages on the Human Body, and Their Value in the Treatment of Consumption* (reprints from *The Practitioner*, 1876–7), 1–2.

105 Granville, *Kissingen*, 58.

106 Francis, *Change of Climate*, 90.

107 Wilson, *A Three Weeks' Scamper*, 12.

108 Kittoe, *The Pocket Book of Practical Medicine*, 216, 220–2.

109 Emily Shore, *Journal of Emily Shore*, ed. Barbara Timms Gates (Charlottesville: University Press of Virginia, 1991), 290–6. See also *ODNB*.

110 Cooper, *The Invalid's Guide to Madeira*, 2.

111 Robert White, *Madeira, Its Climate and Scenery, Containing Medical and General Information for Invalids and Visitors* (London: Cradock, 1851), 101–3. Confusingly there were two sailing brigs named *Dart*; the first of 180 tons was wrecked in October 1842 but was replaced by a slightly larger namesake within a year, *Times*, 22 November 1842 and 25 October 1844; report by HM consul Stoddart, 14 November 1842 TNA FO 63/553.

112 Letters to her brother, 24 September 1839, 13 February 1840, Elizabeth Wynter letters, Surrey History Centre (SHC) 2185/79/53, 55.

113 White, *Madeira*, 103–4. From 1850 the Royal Mail packets continued on to Brazil from the West Indies, leading to their popular nickname, 'Brazilians'.

114 Shore, *Journal*, 290.

115 Letters from Margaret Marling to her husband, 7–14 February 1853 GA D/873 C10.

116 White, *Madeira*, 135.

117 Michael C. Grabham, *The Climate and Resources of Madeira, as Regarding Chiefly the Necessities of Consumption and the Welfare of Invalids* (London: Churchill, 1870), 198–9. Grabham does not mention reaching Madeira by sail so perhaps the practice had largely fallen out of use by this date.

118 Letter from Cecil Monro to his brother, 20 November 1860 LMA ACC/1963/1378.

119 Letter to the editor dated 24 October, *Times*, 22 November 1842.

120 Lady Emmeline Stuart-Wortley, *A Visit to Portugal and Madeira* (London: Chapman and Hall, 1854), 221.

121 This would appear to be the implication of White and Johnson's statement that 'their times of sailing are made to accommodate the greatest number of persons who secure berths in them', White and Johnson, *Madeira, Its Climate and Scenery: A Handbook for Visitors*, 47.

122 Ibid.

123 Letters from Cecil Monro to his brother, 15 May, 12 June 1861 LMA ACC/1083/1392, 1395; letter from Charles Marling to his father, 1 June 1862 GA D873/ C22.

124 Pemble, *The Mediterranean Passion*, 22.

125 Report by HM consul Turnbull, Marseilles, 12 December 1842 TNA FO 27/657A.

126 Letter from William Money-Kyrle to his mother, 21 December 1843 WS 1720/843.

127 'List of all the steamers which frequent the port of Marseilles for the conveyance of goods and passengers', 30 May 1853 TNA FO 27/984.

128 Letters from Cecil Monro to his family, 2 November 1864–1, January 1865 LMA ACC/1083/1463-1470.

129 Charles Dickens, *Little Dorrit* (London: Penguin, [1857] 2003), 30.

130 Despatch from HM consul Turnbull, 19 October 1853 TNA FO27/984.

131 Despatch dated 24 December 1857 TNA FO 63/822.

132 Copy letter from John Kennedy, 18 November 1857 TNA FO 63/822.

133 Letter from John Kent to Gwendoline Herbert, October [1873] Carnarvon of Highclere papers, HA 75M91/X2.

134 Jackson, *Medical Climatology*, 410.

## 4 Living and spending

1 Lady Chatterton, *The Pyrenees and Excursions into Spain* (London: Saunders and Otley, 1843), vol. 1, 2.

2 *Hand-Book for Travellers in Northern Italy* (1842), 72; ibid. (1847), 69.

3 Brewster, *Letters from Cannes and Nice*, 144; *Handbook for Visitors to Northern Italy* (1858), 69.

4 *Handbook for Travellers in France* (1864), 502. A correspondent in the *Times* had made similar complaints the previous year, extending the calumnies to the hotel-keepers of Cannes and Menton as well, *Times*, 1 April 1863.

5 Taylor, *The Taylor Papers*, 467.

6 *Hand-Book for Travellers in France* (1844), 492, 497.

7 Ibid. (1852), 475, 480.

8 *Handbook for Travellers in Northern Italy* (1854), 71.
9 Ibid. (1858), 83.
10 Sparks, *The Riviera*, 83–4.
11 *Handbook for Travellers in France* (1864), 502.
12 Chapman-Huston, *Sir James Reckitt*, 133. Ann described Miss Stafford as 'an agreeable lady about thirty who had suffered from ill health, and had found Mentone to suit her so well, she had chosen it as her residence'. This Miss Stafford was reported by Murray as running a second pension at Nice by 1864 ('generally full') and another at the Villa Christiana at Cannes in 1870, *Handbook for Travellers in France* (1864), 503; ibid. (1870), 539.
13 *Handbook for Travellers in France* (1864), 499–516. The designation *Pension Anglaise* does not seem to have been invariably applied to British-run pensions, and in at least one case, Clerici's Pension Anglaise at Menton, was used for an establishment run by a local.
14 Letter to his mother, 22 November 1868 LMA ACC/1063/1554.
15 Letter to his father, 5 May 1870 LMA ACC/1063/1633. M. and Mme Suzanne were the proprietors.
16 Sparks, *The Riviera*, 286.
17 *Handbook for Travellers in France* (1875), part ii, 185. This was probably the same establishment as William Miller identified in 1877: 'An institution maintained by subscription and called *Helvetia*, [providing] at a small rate of board (about £1 per week) a home for … fifteen invalid ladies, who are not in circumstances to incur the much heavier expense of boarding at a hotel', *Wintering in the Riviera*, 176.
18 See advertisements in the *Times*, 14 July 1883, 2 February 1884.
19 The Reckitt family found no vacancies when they arrived in October 1861, Chapman-Huston, *Sir James Reckitt*, 133.
20 Letter to his mother, 9 November 1866 LMA ACC/1063/1491. Quite what the 'Bennet clique system' was is unclear, but it seems from Cecil's letter that it had ceased by the time of writing. William Chambers reported in 1870 that Bennet was still in residence at the (renamed) Hotel des Anglais during the season, together with a resident English dentist, Dr J. Martin, *Wintering in Mentone*, 41.
21 Letters to his parents, 2–24 November 1866, LMA ACC1/063/1490-1492. Augustus Hare likewise found the meals from the Pension Anglaise inadequate, *A Winter at Mentone*, 16.
22 Letter to his father, 24 April 1867 LMA ACC/1063/1499.
23 Letter to his father, 23 February [1864] LMA ACC/1063/1404.
24 Letter to his brother, 1 March 1864 LMA ACC/1063/1454.
25 Letter to his mother, 8 February 1869 LMA ACC/1063/1568.
26 Aspinall, *San Remo as a Winter Residence*, 138.

27 *Handbook for Travellers in France* (1864), 503.

28 Alexander M. Brown, *Wintering at Menton on the Riviera: A Compagnon de Voyage with Hints to Invalids* (London: Churchill, 1872), 165–7.

29 See the advertisement for the Smithers' pensions anglaises in the notices section of *A Handbook for Travellers in France* (1864), 33. This advertisement shows that the Smithers had also recently opened a summer *Pension Anglaise* in a chateau at Nyons on Lake Geneva. The proprietors of these establishments are named in 1864 as 'Mr and Mrs Smithers'. The identity of Mr Smithers is a little obscure; as is evident from Cecil Monro's letters, one of the sisters was married to a Frenchman, M. Debrassine, but he makes no reference to any British husband.

30 Letter from Cecil Monro to his father, 17 November 1868 LMA ACC/1063/1553.

31 Letter to his mother, 28 October 1868 LMA ACC/1063/1545.

32 Wilde, *Narrative of a Voyage to Madeira*, 76.

33 Grabham, *The Climate and Resources of Madeira*, 64.

34 Johnson, *A Winter's Sketches in the South of France*, 66.

35 Tucoo-Chala, *Pau, Ville Anglaise*, 135, 162; Miller, *Wintering in the Riviera*, 440.

36 Granville, *Kissingen*, 91. There appears to be no evidence this was ever established.

37 Ibid., 128–32.

38 Anon., *A Hot-Water Cure*, 202. Granville quoted £7 16s. 0d. per person for a four-week cure at a second-level hotel, *Kissingen*, 128.

39 Macpherson, *The Baths and Wells of Europe*, 26.

40 Letter to his mother, 21 May 1863, Collins, *Letters*, vol. 1, 223.

41 Letter to her mother, 25 July 1850 GA 94M72/F532; *A Handbook for Travellers in France* (1854), 360.

42 Gordon, 'Reinvention of a Spa Town', 37.

43 Lee, *Vichy and Its Mineral Springs*, 4.

44 *A Handbook for Travellers in France* (1864), 357.

45 Madden, *The Spas of Belgium*, 299.

46 Weld, *The Pyrennees*, 203; Eyre, *A Lady's Walks*, 40.

47 *A Handbook for Travellers in France* (1877), part i, 333–4, 359, 364.

48 See for example ibid., 264.

49 Ibid. (1875), part ii, 33.

50 Clark, *Medical Notes on Climate*, 35.

51 Clark, *The Sanative Influence of Climate*, 116.

52 Jackson, *Medical Climatology*, 33.

53 Clark, *The Sanative Influence of Climate*, 112; Farr, *A Medical Guide to Nice*, 137.

54 Jackson, *Medical Climatology*, 33.

55 Francis, *Change of Climate*, 92.

56 Letter from Charles Baring to his brother, 29 October 1839 HA 92M95/NP7/1.

57 Wittitterly, *Three Months' Rest at Pau*, 38–9.
58 Wilde, *Narrative of a Voyage to Madeira*, 76. A broadly similar price range is quoted by Dr Grabham in 1870, *The Climate and Resources of Madeira*, 61.
59 Letter from Margaret Marling to her husband, 14 February 1853 GA D873 C10.
60 Letter to his aunt, Nice 22 November 1838 NA YO/710 (vi).
61 Brewster, *Letters from Cannes and Nice*, 113–14.
62 *Handbook for Travellers to Northern Italy* (1858), 70.
63 Hare, *A Winter at Mentone*, x, 3. Hare does not specify the rent he paid but quotes sixty to seventy pounds as the going rate for apartments at Menton for the season. It is not clear if the Hares paid by the month or for the entire season.
64 Letter from Hilary Bonham-Carter to her mother, 7 November 1843 HA 94M72/F532; Grant, *A Highland Lady in France*, 33.
65 *Handbook for Travellers in Northern Italy* (1858), 70; *Handbook for Travellers in France* (1864), 503.
66 Chambers, *Wintering at Mentone*, 41–3.
67 Miller, *Wintering in the Riviera*, 78. Four thousand francs accords with J. R. Green's notional £150 for seasonal rent of a villa at Menton, *Stray Studies*, vol. 1, 77.
68 Tucoo-Chala, *Pau, Ville Anglaise*, 162.
69 Letter to her aunt, 10 September 1838 NA YO/710 (i).
70 Shelley, *Rambles in Germany and Italy*, 196.
71 'To obviate as much as possible any quarrels with the proprietors of the furnished appartements – generally arrising [*sic*] from some misunderstanding – the strangers are earnestly requested to put down their engagements in writing', *Emser Fremden-Liste für das Jahr 1856* and subsequent editions.
72 Journal of W. F. Wrottesley, Wrottesley papers HA 109M94/FW4/2.
73 *A Handbook for Travellers on the Continent* (1842), 195–6.
74 Eyre, *A Lady's Walks*, 8.
75 Ibid., 72.
76 Letter from Allen Young to his aunt, Nice 22 November 1838 NA YO/710(vi).
77 Brewster, *Letters from Cannes and Nice*, 119–20.
78 Hare, *A Winter at Mentone*, 16.
79 AlisonCunningham, *Cummy's Diary: A Diary Kept by R. L. Stevenson's Nurse, Alison Cunningham, while Travelling with Him on the Continent during 1863* (London: Chatto & Windus, 1926), 47, 84.
80 *Handbook for Travellers in France* (1864), 504.
81 Wittitterly, *Three Months' Rest at Pau*, 21.
82 Letter to his brother, 17 September 1867 LMA ACC/1063/1505.
83 Costello, *Béarn and the Pyrenees*, vol. 2, 26–7.
84 Farr, *A Medical Guide to Nice*, 143.

85 Wittitterly, *Three Months' Rest at Pau*, 20.
86 Johnson, *A Winter's Sketches in the South of France*, 113.
87 'The manners of Portuguese servants … are such as would be pronounced very free-and-easy in England', Shore, *Journal*, 322.
88 Brewster, *Letters from Cannes and Nice*, 83.
89 Ellis, *Summer and Winter in the Pyrenees*, 55–6.
90 Costello, *Béarn and the Pyrenees*, vol. 2, 29.
91 Farr, *A Medical Guide to Nice*, 143.
92 Brewster, *Letters from Cannes and Nice*, 33–7, 104.
93 Arthur Hill Hassall, *San Remo and the Western Riviera* (London: Longman, Green, 1879), 26.
94 Anon., *Madeira, a Brief Letter of Advice to an Invalid*, 4.
95 Letter from Margaret Marling to her husband, 7 February 1853 GA D873 C10.
96 *Liste der in Jahre 1844 Angekommenen und Abgereisten Kur-und Badegueste von Kissingen & Bocklet* [1844].
97 At Carlsbad the average size of a British party was about 2.5 individuals in 1840, 2.1 in 1850 and 1.9 in 1860; these figures are between 0.8 and 0.45 higher than the average for all parties, irrespective of geographical origin, during these years. This pattern is broadly similar in the ratios for Kissingen in 1844, 1858, 1869 and 1878 (2.9 to 1.75, 2.4 to 1.6, 2.06 to 1.66 and 2.0 to 1.56, respectively).
98 Copy despatch from HM consul Lacroix at Nice to Lord Lyons, ambassador in Paris, 26 April 1869 TNA FO27/ 1770.
99 Williams, *The Climate of the South of France*, 7, 128.
100 Clark, *Medical Notes on Climate*, 31, 35.
101 RCP MS 3082.
102 Letter to his aunt, 22 November 1838 NA YO/710 (vi).
103 Farr, *A Medical Guide to Nice*, 82.
104 Clark, *The Sanative Influence of Climate*, 112. The warning about vegetables clearly appears to contradict Farr's advice, but the injunctions of specialists were often misaligned.
105 The Stevenson family at Menton were exceptional in enjoying olives, Cunningham, *Cummy's Diary*, 83.
106 Jackson, *Medical Climatology*, 37.
107 Williams, *The Climate of the South of France*, 77.
108 Hare, *A Winter at Mentone*, x–xi, 16.
109 Siordet, *Mentone in Its Medical Aspect*, 78–9.
110 Brewster, *Letters from Cannes and Nice*, 37.
111 Bennet, *Mentone, the Riviera, Corsica and Biarritz*, 181.
112 Adolphe Smith, *The Garden of Hyères. A Description of the Most Southern Point on the French Riviera* (London: J. Evans, 1880), 122–3.

113 Grabham, *The Climate and Resources of Madeira*, 65, 165–6.
114 Grant, *A Highland Lady in France*, 33.
115 Letter to Mrs Barton, 10 July 1838 NA YO/710 (vii).
116 Granville, *The Spas of Germany*, viii, xiv.
117 Wilson, *A Three-Weeks' Scamper*, 136.
118 Granville, *The Spas of Germany*, xxxiv.
119 Granville, *Kissingen*, 308.
120 Granville, *The Spas of Germany*, 264.
121 *A Handbook for Travellers in Southern Germany* (1843), 372.
122 *A Hand-Book for Travellers on the Continent* (1836), 398. This encomium survived in all editions until 1860.
123 *Emser Kurliste vom Jahr 1846*, 186. Original in French.
124 F. H. Prytherch, *Observations on the Mineral Waters of Homburg* (London: Churchill, 1853), 46–50.
125 Hoeber, Dr, *Bad Homburg and Its Resources: For the Use of English Visitors Especially* (Bad Homburg: printed at Louis Schick's office, 1875), 55–7.
126 Anon., *A Hot-Water Cure*, 284.
127 Letter to Charles Collins, 22 April 1863, Collins, *Letters*, vol. 1, 220–2.
128 Madden, *The Spas of Belgium*, 35–6.
129 Letter to her brother, 17 December 1838 SHC 2185/79/49.
130 Letter to his father, 25 December 1869 LMA ACC/1063/1613.
131 Letter to his father, 26 December 1863 LMA ACC/1063/1445.
132 Postscript by his father to Cecil Monro's letter to his mother, 24 October 1868 LMA ACC/1063/1545.
133 *Handbook for Travellers in France* (1875), part ii, 168.
134 Lee, *The Effect of Climate on Tuberculous Disease*, 48.
135 Williams, *The Climate of the South of France*, 84–6.
136 Hare, *A Winter at Mentone*, 147.
137 Williams, *The Climate of the South of France*, 80.
138 Ibid., 61.
139 J. Henry Bennet, *On the Treatment of Pulmonary Consumption by Hygiene, Climate, and Medicine* (London: Churchill, 1866), 17.
140 Diary of Dr R. J. Lee, WL MS 3222. The horses arrived eight days after their owner.
141 Brewster, *Letters from Cannes and Nice*, 196; Hare, *A Winter at Mentone*, 11–12; Chambers, *Wintering at Mentone*, 94. Augustus Hare quotes a rate of 3 francs a day at Nice in 1861, *A Winter at Mentone*, 164.
142 Brewster, *Letters from Cannes and Nice*, 176–7, 196.
143 Letters to his father, 24 November 1866, 3 April 1870 LMA ACC/1063/1492, 1629.

144 Letter to her brother, 7 December 1838 SHC 2185/79/49.

145 See for example Stuart-Wortley, *A Visit to Portugal and Madeira*, 244–5 and Marianne North, *Recollections of a Happy Life, Being an Autobiography of Marianne North*, ed. Janet Catherine Symonds (New York: Macmillan, 1894), 192.

146 Letter from William Marling to his sister, 19 January 1853 GA D873/C10.

147 Letters to his family, 20 November, 2, 19 December 1860 LMA ACC1063/1378-1380.

148 Letter to his father, 12 April 1864 LMA ACC/1063/1459.

149 Diary of Fanny Blathwayt, 1868 (entry for 22 June) GA D1799/F259.

150 Lord Harrington's personal physician Robert Lee pronounced the water at Cannes in December 'as warm as it is at Brighton in the middle of June', Diary, WL MS 3222.

151 Alain Corbin, *The Lure of the Sea: The Discovery of the Seaside in the Western World, 1750–1840* (Cambridge: Polity, 1994), 82–4.

152 Macpherson, *The Baths and Wells of Europe*, 160.

153 Letter from G. B. Whiteley MD to the *Times*, 18 October 1865.

154 *Handbook for Travellers in Northern Italy* (1858), 75; *Handbook for Travellers in France* (1864), 500; ibid. (1870), 542; WL MS 3222.

155 Aspinall, *San Remo as a Winter Residence*, 25.

156 Miller, *Wintering in the Riviera*, 152.

157 Bullar, *Letters from Abroad*, 106–7.

158 Brewster, *Letters from Cannes and Nice*, 87–8.

159 Carleton, *Brief Advice to Travellers*, 73.

160 Letter to his aunt, 22 November 1838 NA YO/710 (vi).

161 Lee, *Bradshaw's Companion to the Continent*, 11–12.

162 Brewster, *Letters from Cannes and Nice*, 105, 163.

163 See his obituary in the *British Medical Journal* (*BMJ*) 1602 (1891), ii: 620–1. 1887 was the date of his retirement from practice.

164 On Daubeny, see the photograph of his memorial tablet at San Remo in LMA ACC/1096/114.

165 List of church subscribers, 1865 TNA FO27/1635.

166 Letter from Revd Rolfe to William Garnett, 17 November 1868 LA DDQ/7/4/30.

167 Chambers, *Wintering at Mentone*, 69; *Handbook for Travellers in France* (1870), 548.

168 Brown, *Wintering at Menton*, 166.

169 *Handbook for Travellers in France* (1870), 564.

170 Chapman-Huston, *Sir James Reckitt*, 140.

171 Chambers, *Wintering at Mentone*, 104.

172 Letter to his mother, 20 December 1869 LMA ACC/1063/1612.

173 Letters to his parents, 1 December 1868, 7 December 1869 LMA ACC/1063/1557, 1610.

174 Mrs Ellis may have been thinking of Hazelwood when she refers to 'an English doctor … who with his amiable family has for several years been resident at Pau and … has the happy art of blending all the kindness of friendship with the solicitude of a medical advisor', *Summer and Winter in the Pyrenees*, 221–2.

175 Correspondence of Lord Cowley, including an address by British residents of Pau in favour of Hazlewood, 7, 27 May 1844 TNA FO 27/690, 696.

176 Grant, *A Highland Lady in France*, 96.

177 Ibid., 110.

178 Tucoo-Chala, *Pau, Ville Anglaise*, 86–7.

179 Letter to Charlotte Baker, 2 January 1865 GA D1799/C63.

180 Letter from HM consul Graham to the Foreign Office, 5 March 1864 TNA FO 27/1539.

181 *Liste des Etrangers Fixés ou Résident* [*sic*] *à Pau et aux Environs – Station Hivernale 1867–68* GA D1799/Z20.

182 Arthur Hill Hassall, *The Narrative of a Busy Life. An Autobiography* (London: Longmans, Green, 1893), 117–18.

183 Papers on the Gurney affair, 1850–1 TNA FO 67/180.

184 Lee, *The Baths of Germany*, x–xvii. According to James Johnson this occurred in the summer of 1839, when Lee and a colleague 'Dr Downie' were peremptorily ordered to leave the duchy within forty-eight hours, an act that he humorously termed the 'Order off the Bath', *Pilgrimages to the Spas*, 76 note. Dr Downie was of course Sir Alexander Downie, who merely refers to an unnamed local physician at Wiesbaden 'who was so occupied … in endeavouring to prevent English medical men from affording advice to their own countrymen at the baths' that he neglected a young English patient he was treating, whose care had to be taken in hand by Downie, *A Practical Treatise*, 160.

185 Shelley, *Rambles in Germany and Italy*, vol. 1, 192–3.

186 Prytherch, *The Mineral Waters of Homburg and Kissingen Compared*, 34–5.

187 Granville, *Kissingen*, 355–9.

188 Ibid., 361–5.

189 'I have passed the last five summers practising in the duchy of Nassau', *The Baths of Germany*, 1. The Schwalbach *Kurlisten* for 1840–5 show Lee residing at the *Hotel des Postes* from July or August to the end of the season for six consecutive years, *Liste der Kurgäste und Durchreisenden zu Ems, Schwalbach, Schlangenbad und Weilbach*.

190 Granville, *The Spas of Germany*, 470; Lee, *The Baths of Germany*, 1.

191 *Handbook for Travellers in southern Germany* (1843), 78. In 1869 between 3 and 4 per cent of registered British visitors (eighteen individuals) lodged with

Welsch and another three individuals with another local physician, Balling, *Liste der im Jahre 1869 Angekommenen und Abgereisten Kur-und-Bad-Gäste in Bad Kissingen, Bocklet und Brückenau.*

192 'Daily journal', 1865–6 STA SD/1705 MS 38.

193 Collins, *Letters*, vol. 1, 216–28.

194 Letter from Revd L. P. Acland to William Garnett, 27 September 1869 LA DDQ/7/15/1.

195 Cooper, *The Invalid's Guide to Madeira*, 23.

196 Correspondence relating to the dispute, 1847 ABM HTC/21; *Correspondence between Dr Gillham and Other Medical Men in Madeira* (Funchal: at A.L. da Cunha's P. Office: [1847]). The upshot of the case is unknown.

197 *Times*, 27 September 1856.

198 G. H. Brown, *Lives of the Fellows of the Royal College of Physicians of London* (London: published by the College, 1955), 129, 248.

199 Letter from Hilary Bonham-Carter to her mother, 19 March 1844 HA 94M72/F532.

200 Letter to his brother, 22 March 1864 LMA ACC/1063/1456.

201 Davies, *Algiers in 1857*, 35.

202 Diary of Helen Mason, 1859 Wickham papers HA 38M49/16.

203 Carleton, *Brief Advice to Travellers*, 73.

204 Lee, *The Effects of Climate on Tuberculous Disease*, 102–3.

205 Revd Edward Davies pronounced the cod liver oil of Algiers 'undrinkable', *Algiers in 1857*, 18.

206 Green, *Stray studies*, vol. 1, 77–8.

207 Letter from Dr Ross to Samuel Marling, 1 June [1853] GA D873/C12.

208 Letter from [Hilary Bonham-Carter] to an unidentified correspondent [February 1844] HA 94M72/F532.

209 Letters to his family, 5 March 1861, 31 March, 2 May 1862 GA D873/C21-2.

210 Letter to his brother, 1 May 1863 LMA ACC/1063/1425.

211 Letter to his father, 2 May 1866 LMA ACC/1063/1487.

212 Letter to his father, 7 November 1867 LMA ACC/1063/1507.

213 Sparks, *The Riviera*, 121.

214 Macpherson, *The Baths and Wells of Europe*, 53n.

215 Clark, *The Sanative Influence of Climate*, 108–13.

216 Bennet, *Treatment of Pulmonary Consumption*, 18.

217 Letter to her brother, 17 December 1838 SHC 2185/79/49.

218 Shore, *Journal*, 296–351.

219 Letter to her brother, 9 July 1839 SHC 2185/79/51.

220 See Pat Jalland, *Death in the Victorian Family* (Oxford: Oxford University Press, 1996), 40–1.

221 Nan Marie McMurry, '"Am I? I Am in a Consumption": The Tuberculosis Patient, 1780–1930', PhD diss., Duke University, 1985, 147–8.
222 Rothman, *Living in the Shadow of Death*, 8.
223 Letter to her brother, 11 November 1839 SHC 2185/79/54.
224 Letter to her brother, 13 February 1840 SHC 2185/79/55.
225 Letter from William Marling to his father, 21 January 1853 GA D873/C10.
226 Letter to her husband, 29 January–1 February 1853 GA D873/C10.
227 Letters to his mother, 29 November 1860, 27 January 1861 GA D873/C21.
228 Letter from Ann Miles to Margaret Marling, 18 February 1861 GA D873/C21.
229 Letter to his father, 5 March 1861 GA D873/C21.
230 Letter from Henry Gedge to [Samuel Marling], 1 January 1862 GA D873/D22.
231 Letters to his brother, 15–31 January 1840 HA 92M95/NP7/1.
232 Letter to his mother, 2 April 1840 HA 92M95/NP7/1.
233 Grant, *A Highland Lady in France*, 18–157.
234 Letter to Charlotte Baker, 7 February 1868 GA D1799/C63.
235 Diaries of Fanny Blathwayt, 1867–8 GA D1799/F258-9.
236 Telegram announcing her death, 22 February 1869 GA D1799/C63.
237 Letter to his father, 2 February 1870 LMA ACC/1063/1619.
238 Letters to his parents, 1–10 November 1868 LMA ACC/1063/1548, 1550–1.
239 R. L. Stevenson, 'Ordered South', *Macmillan's Magazine*, 30 (May–October 1874): 69.
240 Miller, *Wintering in the Riviera*, 230.
241 Grant, *A Highland Lady in France*, 123.
242 Morris, 'The Victorian Change of Air', 60–1.
243 *Pall Mall Gazette*, 18 May 1872.

## 5 Meeting and mixing

1 Letter from HM consul Lacroix, 6 May 1861 TNA FO 27/1404.
2 Letter from HM consul Veitch to the Foreign Office, 1 November 1835 TNA FO 63/441.
3 Letter from John Bidwell to HM consul Stobbart, 18 November 1841 TNA FO 63/532.
4 White and Johnson, *Madeira, Its Climate and Scenery*, 203; W. W. Ireland, *The Climate of Madeira* (Edinburgh: Oliver and Boyd, 1869), 5. Charlie Marling remarked on the number of German passengers aboard his ship, the *Derwent*, on his final passage to Madeira, letter to his mother, 24 September 1861 GA D873/C22.

5 About forty German and fifteen other north European burials are recorded in the British cemetery register between 1860 and 1880, out of a total of 303 burials for that date-span, the large majority in the 1870s, a decade during which barely fifty British burials can be plausibly assigned to invalid visitors ABM PT/ABM/HTC /13.

6 Costello, *Béarn and the Pyrenees*, vol. 2, 18.

7 Tucoo-Chala, *Pau, Ville Anglaise*, 150–3.

8 Ibid., 153–4 and unpaginated tables. The British made up almost half the total of habitual visitors in both seasons, 164 out of 350 in 1877–8 and 157 out of 340 the following year.

9 Bills for goods purchased at Pau by the Blathwayt family, 1866–9 GA D1799/A424.

10 Tucoo-Chala, *Pau, Ville Anglaise*, 170–4. The attraction of hunting was no doubt one reason why Major Grantly, threatened with being disinherited by his father for an unsuitable marriage, contemplated decamping to Pau in Trollope's *Last Chronicle of Barset*; Anthony Trollope, *The Last Chronicle of Barset* (London: Penguin, [1867] 1979), 229.

11 *La Vie hors de Chez Soi (Comédie de Notre Temps … par Bertall)* (Paris: E. Plon et Cie, 1876), 214–59.

12 Green, *Stray Studies*, vol. 1, 32.

13 Francis, *Change of Climate*, 65.

14 *Cook's Handbook to the Health Resorts of the South of France and the Riviera* (1878), 20–2.

15 C. J. B. Williams, *Memoirs of Life and Work* (London: Smith, Elder, 1884), 468.

16 Despatch from HM consul Lacroix, 18 February 1871 TNA FO27/1894.

17 Letter from Frances Garnett to her son, 7 February 18[72] LA DDQ/7/19/3.

18 Report on Menton, dated 20 July 1864 TNA FO27/1545. The total number of visitor families for this year is not provided by Sparks, but if we assume it was a little less than his figure for 1865–6 (439) we can tentatively compute a British proportion of something in the region of 40 per cent.

19 Chambers, *Wintering at Mentone*, 45; Sparks, *The Riviera*, 306.

20 Miller, *Wintering in the Riviera*, 245–6.

21 Wilkie Collins, *Armadale* (London: Penguin, [1866] 1995), 12.

22 Sommer, *Zur Kur nach Ems*, 714–19.

23 *Verzeichnis der Kurfremden und Durchreisenden zu Bad Ems, Langenschwalbach, Schlangenbad und Weilbach im Jahre 1835* (Wiesbaden: Ludwig Riedel, 1835) and subsequent issues till 1839. From 1840 onwards the bulletins lack a title page.

24 Breakdowns of numbers by nationality are given at the end of the *Emser Fremden-Listen* from 1857 onwards. The printed *Kurlisten* for Ems from 1818 to 1869 are available online via the *Dilibri* portal of Rheinland-Pfalz libraries, with

the exception of the year 1848, presumably missing owing to political turmoil in Germany in that year. After 1869 coverage on the site is patchy, with the only continuous run covering the period 1883–9, although it is largely complete from 1896 to 1930.

25 The published *Kurlisten* for Homburg from 1834 to 1918 are available online at the *Homburger Kur-und Bade-Listen* project site https://www.lagis-hessen.de/de/klhg/. Although the originals do not give a breakdown by nationality the site provides a geographical year-by-year view, based on analysis by the project team, as well as other search functions.

26 *Liste der im Jahre 1858 Angekommenen und Abgereisten Kur-und Badgäste in Bad Kissingen und Bocklet* and subsequent editions for 1859, 1869 and 1878. Unfortunately it has not been possible to locate complete *Kurlisten* for the period before 1857. Granville however had access to them, and his figures for the British contribution to overall visitor numbers for the period up to 1845 indicate a ratio of something over 10 per cent for the early 1840s, *Kissingen*, 13. An incomplete series for 1844 implies a British proportion of about 13 per cent in that year. It must be remembered however that these lists record all visitors, not just patients.

27 A complete series of printed *Kurlisten* for the spa from 1795 to 1949 is available at https://www.portafontium.eu/contents/kurliste.

28 William Marcet, *The Principal Southern and Swiss Health Resorts* (London: Churchill, 1883), 1–2.

29 Miller, *Wintering in the Riviera*, 174 footnote 19.

30 Blackburn, *The Pyrenees*, 87–8.

31 Letter to her brother, 9 July 1839 SHC 2185/79/51.

32 Letter to her brother, 26 July 1839 SHC 2185/79/52.

33 Letters to her brother, 1839–40 SHC 2185/79/50-55; Shore, *Journal of Emily Shore*, 347.

34 Letter to his father, 19 December 1867 LMA ACC/1063/1515.

35 Letter to her brother, 26 July 1839 SHC 2185/79/52.

36 Letter to his brother, 20 November 1860 LMA ACC/1063/1378.

37 Letter to his brother, 18 December 1862 LMA ACC/1063/1416.

38 Taylor, *A Comparative Enquiry*, 49–54.

39 Johnson, *A Winter's Sketches*, 128.

40 Letter to Ellen Philips, 22 January 1868 GA D1799/C103.

41 Brewster, *Letters from Cannes and Nice*, 97.

42 Siordet, *Mentone in Its Medical Aspect*, 83.

43 Chambers, *Wintering at Mentone*, 68–74.

44 Miller, *Wintering in the Riviera*, 75–6.

45 Morris, 'The Victorian Change of Air', 59.

46 Green, *Stray studies*, vol. 1, 74–5.

47 Chambers, *Wintering at Mentone*, 46.

48 Letter to his brother, 8 August 1873; Eliot, *Letters*, vol. 5, 424–5.

49 For example the Bad Ems list for 1846 includes the following notice: 'People who find errors in their names, titles or place of origin are requested to provide a correction in writing, in a legible hand', *Emser Kurliste vom Jahr 1846* (Bad Ems: Sommer, 1846), 223. Original in French.

50 Eyre, *A Lady's Walks*, 206.

51 Letter from Elizabeth Wynter to her brother, 24 July 1839 SHC 2185/79/53.

52 Letter to Sophy, 7 December 1864 GA D1799/C59.

53 Diary of Fanny Blathwayt, 1865 GA D1799/F256.

54 Letters to his family, 4 November 1861–29 January 1862 LMA ACC/1063/1400-03.

55 Letter to his father, 26 December 1863 LMA ACC/1063/1445.

56 Letter to his mother, 24 October 1868 LMA ACC/1063/1545.

57 Letters to his parents, 28 October–12 January 1869 LMA ACC/1063/1548, 1550, 1556, 1566 .

58 Letter dated 27 November 1865 LMA ACC/1063/1474. This letter has been misfiled and occurs out of chronological sequence.

59 Letter to his father, 23 February 1870 LMA ACC/1063/1623.

60 Vavasour, *My Last Tour and First Work*, 53.

61 Letter from the trustees of the English church at Wiesbaden, 23 August 1858 LPL Tait 422, 178–9.

62 Correspondence between the British consul at Nice and the Foreign Office, 1836–7 TNA FO 67/98, 102.

63 Letters from the chaplain on the English church at Nice, 1857–8 LPL Tait 418, 161–6.

64 Report by HM consul Lacroix, 29 December 1862 TNA FO 27/1452.

65 Internal memorandum dated 24 March 1864 TNA FO 27/1545. The three chaplains comprised the consular chaplain, Revd Childers and two curates, one to serve Christ Church, Carabacel, and one to assist with services at Holy Trinity.

66 See his advertisement in *Emser Kurliste vom Jahr 1852*, 62.

67 Letters from Revd W. G. Parminter to the bishop of London, 15 February 1858, and 1867 LPL Tait 147, 383–4 and 413, 296–7.

68 Letter to the bishop of London, 1 March 1858 LPL Tait 418, 373–4.

69 Letter from Revd J. W. Birch to the Bishop of London, 21 July 1858 LPL Tait 419, 324–8.

70 Letters from Revd Rolfe to William Garnett, 18 May 1865–25 November 1866 LA DDQ/7/4/3-21. The window was later salvaged and installed in St Peter's Quernmore, Garnett's local parish church near Lancaster, see https://www.youtube.com/watch?v=E-bfLfkGNtA.

71 Letter to the bishop of London, 9 July 1863 LPL Tait 132, 389–92; *A Handbook for Travellers on the Continent* (1867), 534.
72 Correspondence on the Anglican chaplaincy at Kissingen, 1863–6 LPL Tait 132, 335–6 and 415, 21–70.
73 'Daily journal' STA SD 1705/MS 38.
74 Papers on building a new Anglican church at Pau, 1866 GA D1799/Z19.
75 Correspondence on the Anglican chaplaincy at Pau, 1885 LPL Benson 32, 9–41.
76 Letter to the editor by 'a Wanderer', *Times*, 4 June 1868. The architecture of St John's did not impress Cecil Monro, letter to his brother, 28 November 1868 LMA ACC/1063/1555.
77 Miller, *Wintering in the Riviera*, 177.
78 Correspondence on the Anglican chaplaincy at Nice, 1876–7 TNA FO 27/2180 (filed under Marseilles); LPL Tait 234, 134–62.
79 Anon., *Madeira, a Brief Letter of Advice to Invalids*, 7.
80 Letter to her brother, 17 December 1838 SHC 2185/79/49.
81 See *ODNB*.
82 Correspondence of HM consul Stoddart with the Foreign Office, 1846–8 TNA FO 63/628, 666, 692.
83 White, *Madeira, Its Climate and Scenery*, 124.
84 See *ODNB*.
85 Correspondence of HM consul Stoddart with the Foreign Office, 1843–6 TNA FO 63/570, 608, 628; William B. Forsyth, *The Wolf from Scotland; The Story of Robert Reid Kalley – Pioneer Missionary* (Darlington: Evangelical Press, 1988), 27–83.
86 Letter from HM consul Stoddart to John Bidwell, 5 February 1847 TNA FO 63/666. Bidwells's wish was partially fulfilled years later when Lowe tempted the gods of the Western Approaches once too often and drowned with his wife off the Scillies in April 1874, on his thirty-eighth passage to Madeira.
87 Madden, *The Principal Health-Resorts*, xvii–xviii.
88 Smith, *The Garden of Hyères*, 134.
89 Robert Owen (1771–1858), socialist and philanthropist.
90 Johnson, *Pilgrimages to the Spas*, 209.
91 Jill R. Steward, 'Moral Economies and Commercial Imperatives: Food, Diet and Spas in Central Europe, 1800–1914', in *Mineral Springs Resorts in Global Perspective*, ed. John K. Walton (London: Routledge, 2014), 116.
92 Vavasour, *My Last Tour and First Work*, 446.
93 Steward, 'Moral Economies and Commercial Imperatives', 118; see also the same author's 'The Role of Inland Spas as Sites of Transnational Cultural Exchange in the Production of European Leisure Culture (1750–1870)', in *Leisure*

*Cultures in Urban Europe, c. 1700–1870*, ed. Peter Borsay and Jan Hein Fumée (Manchester: Manchester University Press, 2016), 252–4.

94 See *Liste der im Jahre 1840 Angekommenen und Abgereisten Kur-und Badegäste in Karlsbad* (Carlsbad: Franieck, 1840) and *Liste der Angekommenen und Abgereisten P.T. Curgäste in Carlsbad* (1860).

95 Letter to his mother, 5 August 1869 HA 75M91/L21.

96 Letters to his family, 31 March–18 April 1869 LMA Acc. 1063/1578, 1581, 1584. Friedrich or Fedor Schmidt (1838–1908), Livonian geologist and botanist, was like Cecil an invalid but evidently continued to pursue his scientific interests on the Riviera with vigour. He published a catalogue of local flora in which he credited the contribution of '*la colonie anglaise qui habite Menton*', especially John Traherne Moggridge (1842–1874), a consumptive patient.

97 'Daily journal', SD 1705/MS 38.

98 *Times*, 4 January 1875.

99 Shelley, *Rambles in Germany and Italy*, vol. 1, 180–1.

100 Anon., *A Hot-Water Cure*, 267.

101 Letter to his mother, 5 August 1869 HA 75M91/L21/27.

102 Letter from Anne Bourne to Miss Dyson, n. d. [1856] HA 9M55/F29/25.

103 Macpherson, *The Baths and Wells of Europe* (1869), 19n. In the second edition of this work the author noted that in 1872 he had 'observed a great improvement in this respect in France', *The Baths and Wells of Europe* (1873), 19n. 'Such arrangements were very much better in all European countries' by the date of the third edition (1888), 20n.

104 Viator Verax, *Cautions for the First Tour on the Annoyances, Short Comings, Indecencies and Impositions Incidental to Foreign Travel*, 4th edn (London: W. Ridgway, 1863), 36.

105 Anon., *A Hot-water Cure*, 280.

106 Ibid., 57.

107 Clark, *Medical Notes on Climate*, 118–19.

108 Eyre, *A Lady's Walks*, 112.

109 'Vichyana', *Blackwood's Magazine*, vol. 59 (1846), 309.

110 Madden, *The Spas of Belgium*, 56, 59.

111 Head, *Bubbles from the Brunnens of Nassau*, 71.

112 Johnson, *Pilgrimages to the Spas*, 228.

113 Macpherson, *The Baths and Wells of Europe*, 99. The bathers at Leuk wore long bathing gowns, ibid., 122.

114 Johnson, *Pilgrimages to the Spas*, 108.

115 As with mixed-sex bathing, attitudes to dress may have been more relaxed in the Austrian lands: Johnson records being invited to observe the women's bath at Teplitz in 1840 by a local physician, where the bathers were all naked,

*Pilgrimages to the Spas*, 234; Granville had been granted the same privilege in 1836, *The Spas of Germany*, 325.

116 Vavasour, *My Last Tour and First Work*, 82, 152.

117 Anon., *A Hot-Water Cure*, 222.

118 Mackaman, *Leisure Settings*, 84.

119 T. Clifton Paris, *Letters from the Pyrenees during Three Months' Pedestrian Wanderings* (London: Murray, 1843), 35.

120 Weld, *The Pyrenees*, 58.

121 Blackburn, *The Pyrenees*, 14–17.

122 Weld, *The Pyrenees*, 53.

123 Lee, *Continental Travel*, postscript.

124 Letter to John Bidwell, 29 September 1848 TNA FO 63/692.

125 Sixty and forty per cent, respectively in 1866 and 1870, Sommer, *Zur Kur nach Ems*, 714–15; there is no separate figure available for foreign curists at Ems in 1848, but the decline in total numbers was of the order of 50 per cent, ibid., 711–13.

126 Report of the trustees to the Foreign Office, 28 February 1856 TNA FO72/900.

127 Chambers, *Wintering at Mentone*, 72.

128 Letter from Cecil Monro to his mother, 10 November 1868 LMA ACC1063/1551.

129 Letter to his brother, 12 December 1868 LMA ACC/1063/1559.

130 Letter to his brother, 27 November 1869 LMA ACC/1063/1606.

131 Letter to his father, 25 December 1869 LMA ACC/1063/1613.

132 Miller, *Wintering in the Riviera*, 100–1.

133 Letter to the editor, *Lancet* (7 September 1870), ii: 419.

134 Despatch from HM consul Lacroix, 17 October 1870 TNA FO27/1829.

135 Despatch from HM consul Mark, 7 November 1870 TNA FO27/1829.

136 Tucoo-Chala, *Pau, Ville Anglaise*, 88.

137 Despatch from HM consul Lacroix, 3 November 1870 TNA FO27/1829.

138 Despatch from HM consul Lacroix, 18 February 1871 TNA FO27/1894.

139 'The Climate of Pau', *Lancet* (1871), ii: 535–7.

140 'Daily journal' STA SD 1705/MS 38.

141 *Times*, 9 August 1866.

142 K. Baedeker, *Southern Germany and the Austrian Empire: Handbook for Travellers* (Coblenz: Karl Baedeker, 1868), 123.

143 *Times*, 13 March 1869.

144 Pemble, *The Victorian Passion*, 266.

## 6 Outcomes

1 John Parkin, *Climate and Phthisis* (London: Longman, Green, 1875), 3.
2 Robert Hull, *A Few Suggestions on Consumption* (London: Churchill, 1849), 114.
3 A. H. Renton, 'Observations on the Inexpediency of Sending Consumptive Patients to Madeira', *Edinburgh Medical and Surgical Journal* 27 no. 91 (1827): 305–7.
4 Clark, *The Sanative Influence of Climate*, 271.
5 George Lund, 'Examination of Different Opinions as to the Value of the Climate of Madeira in Chest Disease', *Association Medical Journal*, s3–1, no. 35 (1853): 767–73.
6 Letter to the editor, *Lancet* (January 1866), i: 133.
7 *Times*, 27 June 1866.
8 Williams, *The Climate of the South of France*, 62–3.
9 Grabham, *The Climate and Resources of Madeira*, 3–4.
10 Charles Theodore Williams, *The Influence of Climate in the Prevention and Treatment of Pulmonary Consumption* (London: Smith, Elder, 1877), 78–83.
11 Tucoo-Chala, *Pau, Ville Anglaise*, 92–4.
12 George Lund, 'Remarks on the Climate of Madeira', *BMJ* 796 (1876), i: 408–9.
13 Williams, *The Influence of Climate*, 113–15.
14 Sparks, *The Riviera*, 112–16.
15 Thorowgood, *The Climatic Treatment of Consumption*, 93.
16 Ibid., 25, 41, 98.
17 Williams, *The Climate of the South of France*, 61–2.
18 Memorandum by Cecil Monro on his medical history, [1881] LMA ACC/1063/2817.
19 Journal, SF MS 85.
20 James Whiteside, *Italy in the Nineteenth Century, Contrasted with Its Past Condition* (London: Richard Bentley, 1848), vol. 1, 5.
21 Bullar, *Letters from Abroad*, 171.
22 Bennet, *Treatment of Pulmonary Consumption*, 20.
23 Shore, *Journal*, 300.
24 Register of the British cemetery, Funchal ABM HTC/13. The register provides enough detail to make identification of British visitors among the generality of burials relatively straightforward.
25 Transcripts of burials at various places in France, incl. Pau, 1822–80 LMA DL/E/E/066/MS11222.
26 Letter to her husband, 29 January 1853 GA D873/C10.

27 Letter to his brother, 2 December 1861 LMA ACC/1063/1401.
28 Letter dated 5 November 1861 LMA ACC/1063/1400.
29 Letter to his father, 13 January [1864] LMA Acc. 1063/1418. This letter was mistakenly dated 1863 by Cecil and has consequently been misfiled.
30 Letter to his father, 1 April 1862 LMA ACC/1063/1408.
31 Bennet, *Mentone, the Riviera, Corsica and Biarritz*, 145.
32 Jacques-François Farina, *Le Climat de Menton* (Paris: Baillière, 1879), 118–20.
33 Hassall, *San Remo and the Western Riviera*, 18.
34 Report of the trustees, 16 January 1854 TNA FO72/850.
35 Young papers, NA YO/710.
36 Despatch from HM consul Mark to the Foreign Office, 6 January 1861 TNA FO72/1015.
37 Minutes of the agm of subscribers to the British church and burial ground, Funchal, 11 January 1862 TNA FO 63/891.
38 *ODNB*.
39 Letter from John Bidwell to HM consul Stoddart, 15 November 1842 TNA FO 63/553.
40 'A short account of Miss Macready's last illness and death, written by her nurse', n. d. LMA ACC/810/94.
41 Letter from HM consul Elmore to the Foreign Office, 3 May 1872 TNA FO 27/1961.
42 Letter to Arthur Otway, 18 January 1869, TNA FO 45/150.
43 Brown, *Wintering at Menton*, 166.
44 Miller, *Wintering in the Riviera*, 230–1.
45 Ibid., 230.
46 TNA FO 27/2454.
47 Clark, *The Sanative Influence of Climate*, viii.
48 Ibid., 276.
49 J. A. Mason, *A Treatise on the Climate and Meteorology of Madeira*, ed. James S. Knowles (London: Churchill, 1850).
50 Janković, *Confronting the Climate*, 142–6; Thomas Burgess, 'Comments on the Inutility of Resorting to the Italian Climate for the Cure of Pulmonary Consumption', *Lancet* (1850), i: 591–4.
51 Costello, *Béarn and the Pyrenees*, vol. 2, 11, 38–9.
52 *Lancet* (1842–3), i: 511–15.
53 Madden, *On Change of Climate*, 249.
54 Letter to the *Times* by X.Y.Z., 19 October 1866.
55 Letter to his brother, 22 February 1868 LMA ACC/1063/1523.
56 Janković, 'The Last Resort', 284–5.
57 Burgess, 'Comments on the Inutility of Resorting to the Italian Climate', 591.

58 Cotton, *The Nature, Symptoms, and Treatment of Consumption*, 241, 247–55.
59 Atkinson, *Change of Air*, 37, 44.
60 Ibid., 60–1.
61 Thorowgood, *The Climatic Treatment of Consumption*, 68–70.
62 Ireland, *The Climate of Madeira*, 18, 21.
63 Parkin, *Climate and Phthisis*, 79.
64 Ibid., 87.
65 Williams, *The Influence of Climate*, 15–18.
66 William Thomson, *On Phthisis and the Supposed Influence of Climate* (Melbourne: Stillwell & Knight, 1877), 9.
67 Williams, *The Influence of Climate*, 88–92, 113.
68 Bennet, *Mentone, the Riviera, Corsica and Biarritz*, 83.
69 Janković, *Confronting the Climate*, 135.
70 Thorowgood, *The Climatic Treatment of Consumption*, 9–11.
71 Hermann Weber, 'On the Treatment of Phthisis by Prolonged Residence in Elevated Regions', *Medico-Chirurgical Transactions* 52 (1869): 230.
72 Ibid., 258–60.
73 Hermann Weber, 'The High Alpine Valleys as Winter Health-Resorts for the Consumptive', *BMJ* 471 (1870), i: 43–4.
74 Susan Barton, *Healthy Living in the Alps: The Origins of Winter Tourism in Switzerland, 1860–1914* (Manchester: Manchester University Press, 2008), 20–1.
75 Weber, 'On the Treatment of Phthisis', *Medico-Chirurgical Transactions* 52 (1869): 251–2.
76 Barton, *Healthy Living in the Alps*, 180.
77 Weber, 'The High Alpine Valleys', *BMJ* 471 (1870), i: 43–4.
78 Frank B. Rogers, 'The Rise and Decline of the Altitude Theory of Tuberculosis', *Bulletin of the History of Medicine* 41, no. 1 (1969): 5.
79 *ODNB*.
80 Clifford Allbutt, 'On Davos as a Health Resort', *Lancet* (1877), ii: 555–7, 614–16; 'On the Treatment of Phthisis at Davos am Platz', *Lancet* (1878), i: 824–5; 'The Past Winter in Davos, *Lancet* (1879), ii: 76–8, 118–19.
81 Hermann Weber, 'The Hygienic and Climatic Treatment of Chronic Pulmonary Phthisis', Croonian Lecture III, *BMJ* 1266 (1885), i: 688–90.
82 Alfred T. Tucker Wise, *Davos Platz and the Effects of High Altitude on Phthisis* (London: Churchill, 1881), 49.
83 Isaac Burney Yeo, *Health Resorts and Their Uses: Being Vacation Studies in Various Health Resorts* (London: Chapman & Hall, 1882), 114.
84 Allbutt, 'On Davos as a Health Resort', *Lancet* (1877), ii: 575–7; (1879), ii: 76–8.
85 Barton, *Healthy Living in the Alps*, 43.

86 R. H. Otter, *Winters Abroad: Some Information Respecting Places Visited by the Author on Account of His Health, Intended for the Use of Invalids* (London: John Murray, 1882), 184.

87 [Mrs Macmorland], *Davos-Platz* (London: Edward Stanford, 1878), 13; Allbutt, 'On Davos as a Health Resort', *Lancet* (1877), ii: 575–7.

88 Otter, *Winters Abroad*, 187.

89 J. A. Symonds. 'Davos in winter', *Fortnightly Review* 30, no. 139 (1878): 79.

90 Pemble, *The Mediterranean Passion*, 255.

91 Quoted in Burney Yeo, *Health Resorts and Their Uses*, 122.

92 Marc Arnold, *Disease, Class and Social Change: Tuberculosis in Folkestone and Sandgate, 1880–1930* (Newcastle upon Tyne: Cambridge Scholars, 2012), 17.

93 Pemble, *The Mediterranean Passion*, 246.

94 'Phthisis', a pseudonymous British physician writing from Pisa, speculated that 'in some instances the ennui occasioned by protracted attendance upon a ruthless and immedicable disorder' persuaded practitioners to direct their patients south, 'On the Comparative Advantages of Southern Climates in Cases of Pulmonary Consumption, *Lancet* (1828–9), ii: 517.

95 *Liste der in Jahre 1844 Angekommenen und Abgereisten Kur-und Badegueste von Kissingen & Bocklet* [Kissingen, 1844] and subsequent editions; the editions for 1858, 1869 and 1878 show proportions of 10, 12 and 11 per cent, respectively.

96 Letters from Dr Frederick Rose of San Remo, *Times*, 24, 26 September 1872.

97 Alfred T. Tucker Wise, *The Alpine Winter Cure, with Notes on Davos Platz, Wiesen, St Moritz and the Maloja* (London: Baillière, Tindall, & Cox, 1884), 43.

98 Letter from J. A. Symonds to Sir Edward Sieveking, n. d. [*c*. 1882] WL MS 7029/16.

99 Wise, *The Alpine Winter Cure*, i–ii.

100 James Alexander Lindsay, *The Climatic Treatment of Consumption: A Contribution to Medical Climatology* (London: Macmillan, 1887), ix.

101 *BMJ* (1880), ii: 552–3.

102 For discussion of the diseases of 'Civilisation' see *Progress and Pathology: Medicine and Culture in the Nineteenth Century*, ed. Melissa Dickson, Emilie Taylor-Brown and Sally Shuttleworth (Manchester: Manchester University Press, 2020), especially, for present purposes, the editors' introduction.

103 Benjamin Ward Richardson, *Diseases of Modern Life* (London: Macmillan, 1876), 123.

104 Ibid., 497.

105 Morris, 'The Victorian Change of Air', 59.

106 Michael Worboys, 'The Sanatorium Treatment for Consumption in Britain, 1890–1914', in *Medical Innovations in Historical Perspective*, ed. John V. Pickstone (Basingstoke, Hampshire: Macmillan, in association with the Centre for History of Science, Technology and Medicine, University of Manchester, 1992), 49–52.

107 Travel journal of Revd Laughton Alison, LPL MS 4655, 25–6.

# Select Bibliography

## Archival sources


### The National Archives, Kew (TNA)

#### *Foreign Office records*

FO27 General correspondence, France (1781–1905).

FO45 General correspondence, Italy (1861–1905).

FO63 General correspondence, Portugal (1781–1905).

FO67 General correspondence, Sardinia (1781–1860).

FO72 General correspondence, Spain (1781–1905).

### Bedfordshire Archives (BA)

Letters to Sir William Edward Rouse-Boughton, incl. from his daughters at Pau, 1854–6 Richard Orlebar papers OR2298.

### Gloucestershire Archives (GA)

Blathwayt family papers D1799.

Marling family papers D873.

### Hampshire Archives and Local Studies (HA)

Journal of Walter Francis Wrottesley, 1862 Wrottesley papers 109M94/FW4/2.

Letters from Rev Thomas Baring to his brother from Nice, 1839–40 Baring papers 92M95/P7/1/41–46.

Letters of Joanna Bonham-Carter and other family members, 1843–50 Bonham-Carter papers 94M72/F532.

Letters from E. H. Bradby, travelling on the Continent, to his mother, 1847–59 Bradby of Hamble papers 46A06/A4/6/1–13.

Letters from 4th Earl of Carnarvon to his mother, 1869–72 Carnarvon of Highclere papers 75M91/L21.

Travel diaries of Helen Mason, 1857–9 Wickham papers 38M49/15–17.

## Lambeth Palace Library, London (LPL)

Tait papers, Official Letters, London, 1856–69; esp. overseas series, vols 409–24.

## Lancashire Archives (LA)

Garnett of Quernmore papers DDQ.

## London Metropolitan Archives (LMA)

'A short account of Miss Macready's last illness and death, written by her nurse', n.d. ACC/0810/094.

Letters and papers of Cecil James Monro (1833–1882), Monro family papers ACC/1063/580-2833.

Transcripts of baptisms, marriages and burials at various places in France, 1822–80, incl. burials at Pau, 1865–78 Diocese of London records DL/E/E/066/MS11222.

## Northamptonshire Archives (NA)

Letters from the Young family, travelling on the Continent, 1838–39 Young (Orlingbury) papers Y(O)/710.

## Royal College of Physicians Library, London (RCP)

Return by the British consul at Nice on local health conditions, 1829 MS 3082.

## Society of Friends Library, London (SF)

Memoranda of an excursion in the Mediterranean, Italy, Switzerland, France and Belgium, by Saunderson Walker, 1837 MSS 84–5.

### Stoke-on-Trent City Archives (STA)

'Daily journal of Mrs Louisa Wilmot Campbell', 1865–6. Ts copy SD 1705/MS 38.

### Surrey History Centre (SHC)

Letters from Elizabeth Wynter to her brother from Madeira, 1838–40 2185/79/49–55.

### Wellcome Library, London (WL)

Diary of Dr Robert James Lee as personal physician to Lord Harrington at Cannes, 1865–6 Western MS 3222.

Travel diary of Dr Charles Brodie Sewell, 1882 Western MS 4507.

### Wiltshire and Swindon History Centre (WS)

Letters from Lady Naesmyth to Richard Long, 1854–7 Lord Long papers 947/1904.

Letters from William Money-Kyrle to his parents, 1843–6 Money-Kyrle family papers 1720/843.

Talbot of Lacock archives 2664.

## Primary sources – online

*dilibri Rheinland Pfalz* (the digitization portal of Rhineland-Palatinate) has facsimiles of published *Kurlisten* for Ems (1818–1933, with gaps and some editions incomplete), Schwalbach (1840–5), Schlangenbad (1840–5) and Weilbach (1840–5) https://www.dilibri.de/.

Holy Trinity Church online archives, 1808–2018 Archivo e Biblioteca da Madeira (ABM), PT/ABM/HTC https://arquivo-abm.madeira.gov.pt/.

*Homburger Kur-und Bad-Listen,* 1834–1918 https://www.lagis-hessen.de/de/klhg/.

Lists of spa guests for Franzenbad, Karlovy Vary (Carlsbad) and Marienbad, 1686–1941 https://portafontium.eu/contents/kurliste/.

## Primary sources – newspapers and periodicals

*Association Medical Journal*

*Blackwood's Magazine*
*British Medical Journal*
*Edinburgh Medical Journal*
*Fortnightly Review*
*Illustrated London News*
*Lancet*
*London Medical Gazette*
*Medical Times and Gazette*
*Medico-Chirurgical Transactions*
*Times*

## Primary sources – published guidebooks

Baedeker, Karl, *Southern Germany and the Austrian Empire: Handbook for Travellers*, 1st edn (Coblenz: Karl Baedeker, 1868).

Baedeker, Karl, *Southern Germany and Austria, Handbook for Travellers*, 4th edn (Liepzig: Karl Baedeker, 1880).

Black, C. B., *Guide to the South of France and to the North of Italy* (London: Sampson Low, Marston, Low & Searle, 1873).

Cook, Thomas, *Cook's Handbook to the Health Resorts of the South of France and the Riviera* (London: Thomas Cook, 1878).

Cook, Thomas, *Cook's Handbook to the Health Resorts of the South of France and the Northern Coast of the Mediterranean*, new and revised edn (London: Thomas Cook, 1881–2).

Murray, John, *A Handbook for Travellers on the Continent: Being a Guide through Holland, Belgium, Prussia, and Northern Germany, and Along the Rhine, from Holland to Switzerland*, various editions, with minor alterations in title (London: John Murray, 1836–68).

Murray, John, *A Handbook for Travellers in Southern Germany: Being a Guide to Bavaria, Austria, Tyrol, Salzburg, Styria, etc.*, 3rd edn (London: John Murray, 1843).

Murray, John, *Handbook for Travellers in Southern Germany: Being a Guide to Würtemberg, Bavaria, Austria, Tyrol, Salzburg, Styria, etc.*, 10th edn (London: John Murray, 1867).

Murray, John, *Hand-book for Travellers in Northern Italy*, various editions (London: John Murray, 1842–58).

Murray, John, *Hand-book for Travellers in France*, various editions (London: John Murray, 1843–78).

## Primary sources – *Kurlisten*

### Carlsbad

see https://portafontium.eu/contents/kurliste/.

### Ems

see https://www.dilibri.de/.

### Homburg

see https://www.lagis-hessen.de/de/klhg/.

### Kissingen

*Liste der in Jahre 1844 angekommenen und abgereisten Kur-und Badegueste von Kissingen & Bocklet* (n.p., n.d.).
*Liste der im Jahre 1858 angekommenen und abgereisten Kur-und Badgäste von Bad Kissingen und Bocklet* (n.p., n.d.).
*Liste der im Jahre 1869 angekommenen und abgereisten Kur-und Bad-Gäste in Bad Kissingen, Bocklet und Brückenau* (n.p., n.d.).
*Liste der im Jahre 1878 angekommenen und abgereisten Kur-und Bad-Gäste in Bad Kissingen, Bocklet und Brückenau* (n.p., n.d.).

### Schlangenbad

see https://www.dilibri.de/.

### Schwalbach

see https://www.dilibri.de/.

## Primary sources – published books and pamphlets

Anon., *A Hot-Water Cure, Sought Out in Germany in the Summer of 1844. The Journal of a Patient* (London: Saunders and Otley, 1845).

Anon., *Madeira. A Brief Letter of Advice to an Invalid, in Reply to a Request for Information about Madeira as a Winter Residence. By an Ex-Invalid* (London: Bell and Daldy, 1859).

Aspinall, W. B., *San Remo as a Winter Residence by an Invalid, 1863–65*, 3rd edn, edited by his widow (London: William Hunt, 1869).

Atkinson, J. C., *Change of Air: Fallacies Regarding It* (London: John Ollivier, 1848).

Bennet, J. Henry, *Mentone and the Riviera as a Winter Climate* (London: Churchill, 1861).

Bennet, J. Henry, *Mentone, the Riviera, Corsica and Biarritz as Winter Climates* (London: Churchill, 1862).

Bennet, J. Henry, *Winter in the South of Europe: Or, Mentone, the Riviera, Corsica, Sicily, and Biarritz, as Winter Climates* (London: Churchill, 1865).

Bennet, J. Henry, *Treatment of Pulmonary Consumption by Hygiene, Climate, and Medicine* (London: Churchill, 1866).

Bennet, J. Henry, *Winter and Spring on the Shores of the Mediterranean: Or, the Riviera, Mentone, Italy, Corsica, Sicily, Algeria, Spain, and Biarritz, as Winter Climates* (New York: D. Appleton, 1870).

Bertall, C. A. d'Arnoux, *La Vie hors de Chez Soi (Comédie de Notre Temps … par Bertall)* (Paris: E. Plon et Cie, 1876).

Blackburn, Henry, *The Pyrenees: A Description of Summer Life at French Watering Places* (London: Sampson Low, Son, and Marston, 1867).

Bloxam, James Mackenzie, *The Climate of the Island of Madeira: And the Errors and Misrepresentations of Some Recent Authors on This Subject* (London: T. Richards, 1854).

Bodington, George, *An Essay on the Treatment and Cure of Pulmonary Consumption. By George Bodington, of Sutton Coldfield, A.D. 1840. Reprinted with a Preface by Dr Arthur E. Bodington* (Lichfield: Lomax's successors, 1906).

Brewster, Margaret Maria, *Letters from Cannes and Nice* (Edinburgh: Thomas Constable, 1857).

Brown, Alexander M., *Wintering at Menton on the Riviera, a Compagnon de Voyage with Hints to Invalids* (London: Churchill, 1872).

Brunton, Thomas Lauder, *Winter Health Resorts*, reprinted from *The Practitioner*, November 1884 (London: Adlard, 1884).

Bullar, William, *Letters from Abroad, from a Physician in Search of Health* (London: John Van Voorst, 1861).

Bunbury, Selina, *Rides in the Pyrenees*, 2 vols (London: Newby, 1844).

Burgess, Thomas H., *Climate of Italy in Relation to Pulmonary Consumption: With Remarks on the Influence of Foreign Climates upon Invalids* (London: Longman, Brown, Green and Longmans, 1852).

Carleton, Mrs, *Brief Advice to Travellers in Italy, Addressed to Persons Who Travel for Health, Economy, or Education* (Paris: Galignani, 1847).

Chambers, Thomas King, *Some Effects of the Climate of Italy* (London: Churchill, 1865).

Chambers, William, *Wintering at Mentone* (London: W. and R. Chambers, 1870).

Chapman-Huston, Desmond, *Sir James Reckitt, a Memoir* (London: Faber & Gwyer, 1927).

Chatterton, Lady Georgiana, *The Pyrenees with Excursions into Spain*, 2 vols (London: Saunders & Otley, 1843).

Clark, James, *Medical Notes on Climate, Disease, Hospitals, and Medical Schools in France, Italy and Switzerland: Comprising an Inquiry into the Effects of a Residence in the South of Europe, in Cases of Pulmonary Consumption* (London: printed for T. and G. Underwood, 1820).

Clark, James, *The Influence of Climate in the Prevention and Cure of Chronic Diseases, More Particularly of the Chest and Digestive Organs: Comprising an Account of the Principal Places Resorted to by Invalids in England, the South of Europe, etc …; and Directions for Invalids While Travelling and Residing Abroad* (London: John Murray, 1830).

Clark, James, *The Sanative Influence of Climate: With an Account of the Best Places of Resort for Invalids in England, the South of Europe, etc.* (London: John Murray, 1841).

Clark, James, *The Sanative Influence of Climate: With an Account of the Best Places for Resort for Invalids in England, the South of Europe, etc.* (London: J. Murray & J. Churchill, 1846).

Collins, Wilkie, *The Letters of Wilkie Collins*, ed. W. Baker and W. M. Clarke, 2 vols (London: Palgrave Macmillan, 1999).

Cooper, William White, *The Invalid's Guide to Madeira* (London: Smith, Elder, 1840).

Cotton, Richard Payne, *The Nature, Symptoms, and Treatment of Consumption* (London: Churchill, 1852).

*Correspondence between Dr Gillham and Other Medical Men in Madeira* (Funchal: at A.L. da Cunha's P. Office, 1847).

Costello, Louisa Stuart, *Béarn and the Pyrenees: A Legendary Tour to the Country of Henri Quatre*, 2 vols (London: Richard Bentley, 1844).

Cox, Joseph C., *Hints for Invalids About to Visit Naples; Being a Sketch of the Medical Topography of that City. Also an Account of the Mineral Waters of the Bay of Naples* (London: Longman, 1841).

Cumming, William Fullarton, *Notes of a Wanderer in Search of Health through Italy, Egypt, Greece, Turkey, up the Danube and down the Rhine*, 2 vols (London: Saunders & Otley, 1839).

Cunningham, Alison, *Cummy's Diary: A Diary Kept by R. L. Stevenson's Nurse, Alison Cunningham, while Travelling with Him on the Continent during 1863* (London: Chatto & Windus, 1926).

Davies, Revd E. W. L., *Algiers in 1857. Its Accessibility, Climate, and Resources Described with Especial Reference to English Invalids* (London: Longman, Brown, Green, Longmans and Roberts, 1858).

Denison, Albert [Lord Londesborough], *Wanderings in Search of Health* (London: printed for private circulation, 1849).

Downie, Sir Alexander MacKenzie, *A Practical Treatise on the Efficacy of Mineral Waters in the Cure of Chronic Disease, Illustrated by Cases; With an Appendix Containing, an Analysis of the Most Reputed Spas in Germany* (Frankfurt: Charles Jugel, 1841).

Downie, Sir Alexander MacKenzie, *The Spas of Homburg, Considered with Reference to Their Efficacy in the Treatment of Chronic Disease* (London: Churchill, 1842).

Drysdale, Alfred, *Wintering Abroad: Mentone and the Riviera* (London: printed by J. S. Virtue, 1884).

Dunbar, Lady Sophia, *A Family Tour Round the Coasts of Spain and Portugal during the Winter of 1860–1861* (Edinburgh: William Blackwood, 1862).

Eliot, George, *The George Eliot Letters*, ed. G. H. Haight, 9 vols (New Haven: Yale University Press, 1954–78).

Ellis, Sarah Stickney, *Summer and Winter in the Pyrenees* (London: Fisher, 1841).

Eyre, Mary, *A Lady's Walks in the South of France in 1863* (London: Richard Bentley, 1865).

Faber, C. B., *On the Influence of Sea-Voyages on the Human Body, and Their Value in the Treatment of Consumption* (reprints from *The Practitioner*, 1876–7).

Farina, Jacques-François, *Le Climat de Menton* (Paris: Baillière, 1879).

Farr, William, *A Medical Guide to Nice; Containing Every Information Necessary to the Invalid and Resident Stranger* (London: Churchill, 1841).

Francis, D. J. T., *Change of Climate Considered as a Remedy in Dyspeptic, Pulmonary, and Other Chronic Affections; With an Account of the Most Eligible Places of Residence for Invalids in Spain, Portugal, Algeria, etc.* (London: Churchill, 1853).

Galton, Douglas, *Report on the Works of Sewerage and Drainage Proposed for the Town of Cannes* (London: Wyman, 1883).

Grabham, Michael C., *The Climate and Resources of Madeira, as regarding Chiefly the Necessities of Consumption and the Welfare of Invalids* (London: Churchill, 1870).

Grant, Elizabeth, *A Highland Lady in France 1843–1845*, ed. Patricia Pelly and Andrew Tod (East Linton: Tuckwell Press, 1996).

Granville, Augustus Bozzi, *The Spas of Germany*, 2nd edn with a supplement (London: Henry Colburn, 1843).

Granville, Augustus Bozzi, *Kissingen, Its Sources and Resources. With Observations on Their Use and Efficacy in the Treatment of Disease* (London: G.W. Nickisson, 1846).

Granville, Augustus Bozzi, *Autobiography of A.B. Granville*, ed. Paulina B. Granville, 2 vols (London: Henry S. King, 1874).

Green, John Richard, *Stray Studies from England and Italy*, 2 vols (London: Macmillan, 1876).

Gregory, Desmond, *The Beneficent Usurpers: a History of the British in Madeira* (Rutherford, NJ, Farleigh Dickinson University Press; London: Associated University Presses, c. 1988).

Hare, Augustus J. C., *A Winter at Mentone* (London: Wertheim, MacIntosh, and Hunt, 1861).

Hassall, Arthur Hill, *San Remo and the Western Riviera* (London: Longman, Green, 1879).

Head, Francis Bond, *Bubbles from the Brunnens of Nassau by an Old Man* (London: John Murray, 1834).

Hoeber, Dr, *Bad Homburg and Its Resources for the Use of English Visitors Especially* (Bad Homburg: Louis Schick, 1875).

Hood, Thomas, *Up the Rhine*, 2nd edn (London: A.H. Baily, 1840).

Ireland, W. W., *The Climate of Madeira* (Edinburgh: Oliver and Boyd, 1869).

Jackson, Robert Edmund Scoresby, *Medical Climatology: Or, a Topographical and Meteorological Description of the Localities Resorted to in Winter and Summer by Invalids of Various Classes, at Home and Abroad* (London: Churchill, 1862).

James, M. Prosser, *A Visit to Vichy, Comprising a Sketch of Its Mineral Springs and Thermal Establishment, with a Notice on the Medicinal Uses of the Vichy Waters, Salts, and Lozenges* (London: William Williams, 1866).

Jeffreys, Julius, *A Few Remarks on Climate and the Rational Treatment of Affections of the Throat and Lungs by Means of Atmospheres of Soothing Properties* (London: Longmans, Brown, Green, and Longmans, 1849).

Johnson, Frederick H., *A Winter's Sketches in the South of France and the Pyrenees, with Remarks upon the Use of the Climate and Mineral Waters in the Cure of Disease* (London: Chapman & Hall, 1857).

Johnson, James, *Change of Air, or the Pursuit of Health and Recreation*, 3rd edn (London: S. Highley, 1832).

Johnson, James, *Pilgrimages to the Spas in Pursuit of Health and Recreation; With an Inquiry into the Comparative Merits of Different Mineral Waters* (London: S. Highley, 1841)

Kittoe, William Hamilton, *The Pocket Book of Practical Medicine; Or, Manual for Emergencies*, 3rd edn (London: Sherwood, Gilbert and Piper, 1844).

Lee, Edwin, *Notes on Italy and Rhenish Germany: With Professional Notices of the Climates of Nice, Pisa, Florence, Rome, and Naples, and of the Mineral Springs of Baden Baden, Wisbaden [sic], Schwalbach, Ems, and Aix la Chapelle* (Edinburgh: Laing and Forbes, 1835).

Lee, Edwin, *An Account of the Most Frequented Watering Places on the Continent: And of the Medicinal Applications of Their Mineral Springs* (London: Longman, Rees, Orme, Brown, Green and Longman, 1836).

Lee, Edwin, *A Treatise on Some Nervous Disorders; Being Chiefly Intended to Illustrate Those Varieties Which Simulate Structural Disease*, 2nd edn (London: Churchill, 1838).

Lee, Edwin, *Memoranda on France, Italy and Germany, with Remarks on Climates, Medical Practice, Mineral Waters, etc.* (London: Saunders & Otley, 1841).

Lee, Edwin, *The Baths of Germany, Considered with Reference to Their Remedial Efficacy in Chronic Diseases*, 2nd edn (London: Whittaker, 1843).

Lee, Edwin, *Practical Observations on Mineral Waters and Baths; With Notices of Some Continental Climates* (London: Churchill, 1846).

Lee, Edwin, *Continental Travel; With an Appendix on the Influence of Climate, the Remedial Advantages of Travelling, etc.* (London: W.J. Adams, 1848).

Lee, Edwin, *Bradshaw's Companion to the Continent; A Descriptive Hand-Book to the Chief Places of Resort: Their Characteristic Features, Climates, Scenery, and Remedial Resources, with Observations on the Influence of Climate and Travelling* (London: W.J. Adams, 1851).

Lee, Edwin, *Homburg and Its Mineral Waters, with a Notice of Nauheim* (London: Churchill, 1853).

Lee, Edwin, *Notes on Spain: With a Special Account of Malaga and Its Climate* (London: Hope, 1854).

Lee, Edwin, *The Effects of Climate on Tuberculous Disease: Being, with Additions, the Essay for Which the Fiske Fund Prize Was Awarded to Edwin Lee with an Appendix of Corroborative Observations and Notices of Several Places of Winter Resort* (London: Churchill, 1858).

Lee, Edwin, *Bradshaw's Invalid's Companion to the Continent: Comprising General and Medical Notices of the Principal Places of Resort* (London: W.J. Adams, 1861).

Lee, Edwin, *The Principal Baths of Germany, France, and Switzerland, Considered with Reference to Their Remedial Efficacy in Chronic Disease*, 4th edn, with alterations and additions. First volume Baths of Germany (London: Churchill, 1863).

Lee, Edwin, *Vichy and Its Mineral Springs. Extracted from the Fourth Edition of the Baths of France* (London: Churchill, 1866).

Lefevre, George William, *The Life of a Travelling Physician, from His First Introduction to Practice; Including Twenty Years' Wanderings through the Greater Part of Europe*, 3 vols (London: Longman, Brown, Green and Longmans, 1843).

Lloyd Evans, Mrs H., *Last Winter in Algeria* (London: Chapman & Hall, 1868).

Lyall, Alfred, *Rambles in Madeira and in Portugal in the Early Part of 1826* (London: C. and J. Rivington, 1827).

M'Cormac, Henry, *On the Nature, Treatment, and Prevention of Pulmonary Consumption, and Incidentally of Scrofula* (London: Longman, Brown, Green and Longmans, 1855).

Macmorland, Mrs, *Davos-Platz; A New Alpine Resort for Sick and Sound in Summer and Winter. By One Who Knows It Well* (London: Edward Stanford, 1878).

Macpherson, John, *The Baths and Wells of Europe: Their Action and Uses with Hints on Change of Air and Diet Cures* (London: Macmillan, 1869).

Macpherson, John, *The Baths and Wells of Europe: Their Action and Uses with Notices of Climatic Resorts and Diet Cures*, 2nd edn, revised and enlarged (London: Macmillan, 1873).

Madden, Thomas More, *On Change of Climate. A Guide for Travellers in Pursuit of Health* (London: T. C. Newby, 1864).

Madden, Thomas More, *The Spas of Belgium, Germany, Switzerland, France and Italy, a Hand-book of the Principal Watering Places on the Continent* (London: T.C. Newby, 1867).

Madden, Thomas More, *The Principal Health-Resorts of Europe and Africa for the Treatment of Chronic Diseases* (London: Churchill, 1876).

Marcet, William, *The Principal Southern and Swiss Health Resorts* (London: Churchill, 1883).

Mason, J. A., *A Treatise on the Climate and Meteorology of Madeira by the Late J.A. Mason, M.D.*, ed. James Sheridan Knowles (London: Churchill, 1850).

Matthews, Henry, *Diary of an Invalid Being the Journal of a Tour in Pursuit of Health in Portugal, Italy, Switzerland, and France in the Years 1817, 1818 and 1819*, 2nd edn (London: John Murray, 1820).

Miller, William, *Wintering in the Riviera with Notes of Travel in Italy and France and Practical Hints to Travellers* (London: Longmans, Green, 1879).

North, Marianne, *Recollections of a Happy Life, Being an Autobiography of Marianne North*, ed. Janet Catherine Symonds (New York: Macmillan, 1894).

Otter, R. H., *Winters Abroad. Some Information Respecting Places Visited by the Author on Account of His Health. Intended for the Use of Invalids* (London: John Murray, 1882).

Paris, T. Clifton, *Letters from the Pyrenees during Three Months' Pedestrian Wanderings amidst the Wildest Scenes of the French and Spanish Mountains in the Summer of 1842* (London: John Murray, 1843).

Parkin, John, *Climate and Phthisis: Or, the Influence of Climate in the Production and Prevention of Phthisis* (London: Longmans, Green, 1875).

Phelps, Revd W., *A Mirror of the Duchy of Nassau or an Historical Guide to the Brunnens of Wiesbaden, Ems, Schwalbach, Schlangenbad, Selters, Soden, and Weilbach* (Wiesbaden: printed for the author by A. Scholz, 1842).

Prytherch, F. H., *The Mineral Waters of Homburg and Kissingen Compared with a Medical Topography of Their Environs etc.* (Frankfurt: Charles Jugel, 1844).

Prytherch, F.H., *On the Mineral Waters of Homburg*, 3rd edn revised (London: Churchill, 1853).

Ramsay, Mrs, *A Summer in Spain* (London: Tinsley Brothers, 1874).

Richardson, Benjamin Ward, *Diseases of Modern Life* (London: Macmillan, 1876).

Shelley, Mary Wollstonecraft, *Rambles in Germany and Italy, in 1840, 1842, and 1843*, 2 vols (London: Edward Moxon, 1844).

Shore, Emily, *Journal of Emily Shore*, ed. and with an introduction by Barbara Timm Gates (Charlottesville: University Press of Virginia, 1991).

Siordet, James Lewis, *Mentone in Its Medical Aspect* (London: Churchill, 1863).

Smith, Adolphe, *The Garden of Hyères. A Description of the Most Southern Point on the French Riviera* (London: J. Evans, 1880).

Sparks, Edward I., *The Riviera: Sketches of the Health Resorts of the North Mediterranean Coast of France and Italy from Hyères to Spezia* (London: Churchill, 1879).

Starke, Mariana, *Letters from Italy, between the Years 1792 and 1798 … with Instructions for the Use of Invalids and Families Who May Not Choose to Incur the Expence of Travelling with a Courier*, 2 vols (London: R. Phillips: 1800).

Starke, Mariana, *Travels on the Continent: Written for the Use and Particular Information of Travellers* (London: John Murray, 1820).

Starke, Mariana, *Travels in Europe, for the Use of Travellers on the Continent*, 9th edn (Paris: Galignani, 1839).

Taylor, Alexander, *On the Curative Influence of the Climate of Pau, and the Mineral Waters of the Pyrenees, on Disease … and Their Principal Watering Places* (London: John W. Parker, 1842).

Taylor, Alexander, *A Comparative Enquiry as to the Preventive and Curative Influence of the Climate of Pau … with a Description of the Watering Places of the Pyrenees and of the Virtues of Their Respective Mineral Sources* (London: J. W. Parker, 1856).

Taylor, Sir Herbert, *The Taylor Papers, Being a Record of Certain Reminiscences, Letters and Journals in the Life of Lieut.-Gen. Sir Herbert Taylor*, arranged by Ernest Taylor (London: Longmans, Green, 1913).

Thomson, William, *On Phthisis and the Supposed Influence of Climate* (Melbourne: Stillwell & Knight, 1877).

Thorowgood, John C., *The Climatic Treatment of Consumption and Chronic Lung Diseases*, 3rd and enlarged edn (London: H. K. Lewis, 1868).

Travis, Nathaniel Allen, *Kissingen* (Frankfurt: Charles Jugel, 1846).

Trench, Revd Francis, *Diary of Travels in France and Spain, Chiefly in the Year 1844*, 2 vols (London: Richard Bentley, 1845).

Vavasour, Ann Lady, *My Last Lour and First work; Or, a Visit to the Baths of Wildbad and Rippoldsau* (London: Hugh Cunningham, 1842).

Viator Verax, *Cautions for the First Tour on the Annoyances, Short Comings, Indecencies and Impositions Incidental to Foreign Travel*, 4th edn (London: W. Ridgway, 1863).

Weld, Charles Richard, *The Pyrenees, East and West* (London: Longmans, Brown, Green, Longmans & Roberts, 1859).

White, Robert, *Madeira, Its Climate and Scenery: Containing Medical and General Information for Invalids and Visitors* (London: Cradock, 1851).

White, Robert, and James Y. Johnson, *Madeira Its Climate and Scenery a Handbook for Visitors* (Edinburgh: Adam and Charles Black, 1860).

Wilde, William Robert, *Narrative of a Voyage to Madeira, Tenerrife and along the Shores of the Mediterranean* (Dublin: W Curry, Jun., 1840).

Williams, Charles J. B., *Memoirs of Life and Work* (London: Smith, Elder, 1884).

Williams, Charles Theodore, *The Climate of the South of France, and Its Varieties Most Suitable for Invalids; With Remarks on Italian and Other Winter Stations* (London: Churchill, 1867).

Williams, Charles Theodore, *The Climate of the South of France as Suited to Invalids: With Notices of Mediterranean and Other Winter Stations* (London: Longmans, Green, 1869).

Williams, Charles Theodore, *The Influence of Climate in the Prevention and Treatment of Pulmonary Consumption, Lettsomian Lectures for 1876* (London: Smith, Elder, 1877).

Wilson, Erasmus, *A Three Weeks' Scamper through the Spas of Germany and Belgium, with an Appendix on the Nature and Uses of Mineral Waters* (London: Churchill, 1858).

Wilson, William S., *The Ocean as a Health-Resort: A Handbook of Practical Information as to Sea Voyages for the Use of Tourists and Invalids* (London: Churchill, 1880).

Wise, Alfred T. Tucker, *Davos Platz and the Effects of High Altitude on Phthisis* (London: Churchill, 1881).

Wise, Alfred T. Tucker, *The Alpine Winter Cure, with Notes on Davos Platz, Wiesen, St Moritz and the Maloja* (London: Baillière, Tindall, & Cox, 1884).

Wittitterly, John Altrayd [alias Elizabeth Carne], *Three Months' Rest at Pau, in the Winter and Spring of 1859* (London: Bell and Daldy, 1860).

Wortley, Lady Emmeline Stuart-, *A Visit to Portugal and Madeira* (London: Chapman and Hall, 1854).

Wortley, Lady Emmeline Stuart-, *The Sweet South*, 2 vols (London: printed for private circulation, 1856).

Yeo, I. Burney, *Health Resorts and Their Uses: Being Vacation Studies in Various Health Resorts* (London: Chapman & Hall, 1882).

## Secondary sources

Adams, Jane M., *Healing with Water: English Spas and the Water Cure, 1840–1960* (Manchester: Manchester University Press, 2015).

Andrews, Jonathon, 'Letting Madness Range: Travel and Mental Disorder, c.1700–1900', in *Pathologies of Travel*, ed. Richard Wrigley and George Revill (Amsterdam: Rodopi, 2000), 25–88.

Arcara, Stefania, 'Constructing the South: Southern Italy and the Mediterranean in British Culture, 1773–1926', PhD diss., University of Warwick, 1998.

Bailey, Peter, *Leisure and Class in Victorian England: Rational Recreation and the Contest for Control, 1830–1885* (London: Routledge, 1978).

Barton, Susan, *Healthy Living in the Alps: The Origins of Winter Tourism in Switzerland, 1860–1914* (Manchester: Manchester University Press, 2008).

Brown, G. H., *Lives of the Fellows of the Royal College of Physicians of London, 1826–1925* (London: Published by the College, 1955).

Buzard, James, *The Beaten Track: European Tourism, Literature and the Ways to Culture, 1800–1918* (Oxford: Clarendon Press, 1993).

Bynum, Helen, *Spitting Blood: The History of Tuberculosis* (Oxford: Oxford University Press, 2012).

Byrne, Katherine, *Tuberculosis and the Victorian Literary Imagination* (Cambridge: Cambridge University Press, 2011).

Corbin, Alain, *The Lure of the Sea: The Discovery of the Seaside in the Western World, 1750–1840*, trans. Jocelyn Phelps (Cambridge: Polity, 1994).

Dickson, Melissa, EmilieTaylor-Brown, SallyShuttleworth, eds, *Progress and Pathology: Medicine and Culture in the Nineteenth-Century* (Manchester: Manchester University Press, 2020).

Dormandy, Thomas, *The White Death: A History of Tuberculosis* (London: Hambledon Press, 1999).

Forsyth, William B., *The Wolf from Scotland; The Story of Robert Reid Kalley – Pioneer Missionary* (Darlington: Evangelical Press, 1988).

Foxhall, Katherine, *Health, Medicine, and the Sea: Australian Voyages, c. 1815–1860* (Manchester: Manchester University Press, 2012).

Frawley, Maria H., *Invalidism and Identity in Nineteenth-Century Britain* (Chicago: University of Chicago Press, 2004).

Gordon, Bertram M., 'Reinvention of a Spa Town: The Unique Case of Vichy', *Journal of Tourism History* 4, no. 1 (2012): 35–55.

Hamlin, Christopher, 'Chemistry, Medicine, and the Legitimization of English Spas, 1740–1840', in *The Medical History of Waters and Spas*, ed. Roy Porter, *Medical History* Supplement no. 10 (London: Wellcome Institute for the History of Medicine, 1990), 67–81.

Hembry, Phyllis, *The English Spa 1560–1815, a Social History* (London: Athlone Press, 1990).

Hembry, Phyllis, *British Spas from 1815 to the Present*, ed. and completed by W. Cowie and Evelyn E. Cowie (London: Athlone Press, 1997).

Holland, Robert, *The Warm South. How the Mediterranean Shaped the British Imagination* (New Haven: Yale University Press, 2018).

Hoolihan, Christopher, 'Health and Travel in Nineteenth-Century Rome', *Journal of the History of Medicine* 44, no. 4 (1989), 462–85.

Hoppen, K. Theodore, *The Mid-Victorian Generation* (Oxford: Oxford University Press, 1998).

Howarth, Patrick, *When the Riviera Was Ours* (London: Routledge, 1977).

Janković, Vladimir, 'The Last Resort: A British Perspective on the Medical South, 1815–1870', *Journal of Intercultural Studies* 27, no. 3 (2006), 271–8.

Janković, Vladimir, *Confronting the Climate: British Airs and the Making of Environmental Medicine* (New York: Palgrave Macmillan, 2010).

Lafagne, Pierre, *Spa and the English, or, English Influence in the History of Spa (Belgium Ardennes)* (Spa: Association for the Promotion and Encouragement of Tourism in Spa, 1948).

Langum, Virginia, '"A Paradise for Invalids": Medical Tourism and the Climate of Prejudice in Nineteenth-Century Madeira', *Nordic Journal of English Studies* 21, no. 2 (2022): 52–72.

Lawlor, Clark, and AkihitoSuzuki, 'The Disease of the Self: Representing Consumption, 1700–1830', *Bulletin of the History of Medicine* 74, no. 3 (2000), 458–94.

Lawlor, Clark, *Consumption and Literature; The Making of the Romantic Disease* (London: Palgrave Macmillan, 2006).

Lister, W. B. C., *A Bibliography of Murray's Handbooks for Travellers* (Dereham: Dereham Books, 1993).

Lyons, Martyn, *The Pyrenees in the Modern Era: Reinventions of a Landscape, 1775–2012* (London: Bloomsbury, 2018).

Mackaman, Douglas Peter, *Leisure Settings: Bourgeois Culture, Medicine, and the Spa in Modern France* (Chicago: University of Chicago Press, 1998).

McMurry, Nan Marie, '"Am I? I am in a Consumption": The Tuberculosis Patient, 1780–1930', PhD diss., Duke University, 1985.

Mitman, Gregg, *Breathing Space: How Allergies Shape Our Lives and Landscapes* (New Haven, London: Yale University Press, 2007).

Morgan, Marjorie, *National Identities and Travel in Victorian Britain* (Basingstoke: Palgrave, 2001).

Morris, Richard E., 'The Victorian Change of Air as Medical and Social Construction', *Journal of Tourism History* 10, no. 1 (2018), 49–65.

Mowl, Graham, and Michael Barke, 'Changing Visitor Perceptions of Malaga (Spain) and Its Development as a Winter Health Resort in the Nineteenth Century', *Studies in Travel Writing* 18, no. 3 (2014), 233–48.

Mullen, Richard, and James Munson, '*The Smell of the Continent*': *The British Discover Europe 1814–1914* (London: Macmillan, 2009).

Nicholls, Philip, 'Class, Status and Gender: Toward a Sociology of the Homeopathic Patient in Nineteenth-Century Britain', in *Patients in the History of Homeopathy*, ed. Martin Dinges (Sheffield: European Association for the History of Medicine and Health Publications, 2002), 142–51.

Oppenheim, Janet, '*Shattered Nerves*': *Doctors, Patients and Depression in Victorian England* (New York: Oxford University Press, 1991).

*Oxford Dictionary of National Biography*, ed. H. C. G. Matthew and Brain Harrison, 61 vols (Oxford: Oxford University Press, 2004).

Pemble, John, *The Mediterranean Passion: Victorians and Edwardians in the South* (Oxford: Clarendon, 1987).

Penez, Jérôme, *Histoire du Thermalisme en France au XIXe Siècle: Eau, Médicine et Loisirs* (Paris: Econimica, 2005).

Porter, Roy, 'The Patient in England, c. 1660–c. 1800', in *Medicine in Society: Historical Essays*, ed. Andrew Wear (Cambridge: Cambridge University Press, 1992), 91–118.

Porter, Roy, 'Consumption: Disease of the Consumer Society?', in *Consumption and the World of Goods* ed. John Brewer and Roy Porter (London: Routledge, 1993), 58–81.

Rogers, Frank B., 'The Rise and Decline of the Altitude Theory of Tuberculosis', *Bulletin of the History of Medicine* 44, no. 1 (1969), 1–16.

Rothman, Sheila M., *Living in the Shadow of Death: Tuberculosis and the Social Experience of Illness in America* (New York: Basic Books, 1994).

Scull, Andrew, Charlotte MacKenzie and Nicholas Hervey, *Masters of Bedlam: The Transformation of the Mad-Doctoring Trade* (Princeton, NJ: Princeton University Press, 1996).

Smith, F. B., *The Retreat of Tuberculosis, 1850–1950* (London: Croom Helm, 1988).

Sommer, Hermann, *Zur Kur nach Ems: ein Beitrag zur Geschichte der Badereise von 1830 bis 1914* (Stuttgart: Franz Steiner, 1999).

Steward, Jill R., ' "On the Continong": Britons Abroad and the "Business of Travel", 1820–1914', in *The British Abroad since the Eighteenth Century*, ed. Martin Farr and Xavier Guégan, 2 vols (Basingstoke: Palgrave Macmillan, 2013), vol. 1, 77–100.

Steward, Jill R., 'Moral Economies and Commercial Imperatives: Food, Diet and Spas in Central Europe, 1800–1914', in *Mineral Springs Resorts in Global Perspective*, ed. John K. Walton (London: Routledge, 2014), 109–31.

Steward, Jill R., 'The Role of Inland Spas as Sites of Transnational Cultural Exchange in the Production of European Leisure Culture (1750–1870)', in *Leisure Cultures in Urban Europe, c. 1700–1870*, ed. Peter Borsay and Jan Hein Fumée (Manchester: Manchester University Press, 2016), 234–59.

Tucoo-Chala, Pierre, *Pau, Ville Anglaise: Promenades Historiques* (Pau: Société Nouvelle d'Editions Régionales et de Diffusion, 1979).

Turner, E. S., *Taking the Cure* (London: Michael Joseph, 1967).

Walton, John K., ed., *Mineral Springs Resorts in Global Perspective: Spa Histories* (London: Routledge, 2014).

Walton, John K., 'Coastal Resorts and Cultural Exchange in Europe, 1780–1870', in *Leisure Cultures in Urban Europe, c. 1700–1870*, ed. Peter Borsay and Jan Hein Fumée (Manchester: Manchester University Press, 2016), 260–77.

Withey, Lynne, *Grand Tours and Cook's Tours, a History of Leisure Travel, 1750 to 1915* (New York: William Morrow, 1997).

Warboys, Michael, 'The Sanatorium Treatment for Consumption in Britain, 1890–1914', in *Medical Innovations in Historical Perspective*, ed. John V. Pickstone (Basingstoke, Hampshire: Macmillan, in association with the Centre for History of Science, Technology and Medicine, University of Manchester, 1992), 47–71.

Warboys, Michael, *Spreading Germs: Disease Theories and Medical Practice in Britain, 1865–1900* (Cambridge: Cambridge University Press, 2000).

Wrigley, Richard, 'Pathological Topography and Cultural Itineraries: Mapping "Mal'aria" in 18th and 19th-Century Rome', in *Pathologies of Travel*, ed. Richard Wrigley and George Revill (Amsterdam: Rodopi, 2000), 207–28.

# Index

www.ingramcontent.com/pod-product-compliance
Lightning Source LLC
LaVergne TN
LVHW020202140225
803739LV00003B/118